Hypoxia, Polycythemia, and Chronic Mountain Sickness

**The Johns Hopkins Series in Contemporary Medicine
and Public Health**

Consulting Editors

Hypoxia, Polycythemia, and Chronic Mountain Sickness

Robert M. Winslow, M.D.

Chief, Division of Blood Research
Letterman Army Institute of Research
Presidio of San Francisco, California

and

Carlos Monge C., M.D.

Professor of Physiology,
Cayetano Heredia University,
Lima, Peru

The Johns Hopkins University Press
Baltimore and London

The Johns Hopkins University Press
701 West 40th Street
Baltimore, Maryland 21211
The Johns Hopkins Press Ltd., London

The paper used in this publication meets the minimum requirements of American
National Standard for Information Sciences—Permanence of Paper for Printed
Library Materials, ANSI Z39.48-1984.

Library of Congress Cataloging-in-Publication Data

Winslow, Robert M., 1941–
Hypoxia, polychythemia, and chronic mountain
sickness.

(The Johns Hopkins series in contemporary medicine
and public health)
Bibliography: p.
Includes index.
1. Mountain sickness. 2. Polycythemia. 3. Anoxemia.
I. Monge Cassinelli, Carlos. II. Title. III. Series.
[DNLM: 1. Anoxia. 2. Polycythemia. WD 715 W78lh]
RC103.A4W56 1987   616.9′893   87-3805
ISBN 0-8018-3448-1 (alk. paper)

Contents

List of Figures   *ix*

List of Tables   *xiii*

Foreword, by Steven Muller   *xv*

Acknowledgments   *xvii*

Introduction   *1*

1   *The History of Chronic Mountain Sickness*   *5*
   1.1   The First Descriptions of Mountain Sickness   5
   1.2   Paul Bert and the French Physiologists   6
   1.3   Joseph Barcroft's Expedition to Cerro de Pasco   8
   1.4   Carlos Monge M.   9
   1.5   North American Contributions to the Knowledge of Mountain Sickness   12
   1.6   Alberto Hurtado and Co-workers   13
   1.7   Recent Expeditions and the Consolidation of Information   14
   1.8   Leadville, Colorado   15
   1.9   Chile   16
   1.10   Geographic Differences between Asia and South America   17

2   *High-Altitude Natives and Chronic Mountain Sickness*   *19*
   2.1   High-Altitude Natives   20
   2.2   Clinical Features of Chronic Mountain Sickness   21
   2.3   The First Recorded Case of Chronic Mountain Sickness   23
   2.4   Pathologic Findings   27
   2.5   The Carotid Bodies   30

3   *Red Cells, Red Cell and Plasma Volumes, and Their Regulation*   *31*
   3.1   The Hemoglobin and Hematocrit Values   31
   3.2   The Morphology of Red Cells at High Altitudes   39
   3.3   Nutrition and the Production of Red Cells   41
   3.4   Erythropoietin   42
   3.5   Erythropoiesis at High Altitudes   44

3.6   Renal Hemodynamics and Erythrocytosis   46
3.7   The Measurement of Red Cell and Plasma
        Volumes   48
3.8   The Regulation of Red Cell and Plasma Volumes   54

4   *The Structure and Function of Hemoglobin at High Altitudes*   *55*
4.1   The Blood Oxygen Equilibrium Curve   55
4.2   The Structure and Function of Hemoglobin   57
4.3   Older Studies of Blood Oxygen Affinity   59
4.4   The Role of 2,3-DPG   64
4.5   The Blood Oxygen Affinity in vivo   66
4.6   The Bohr Effect   70
4.7   The Blood Oxygen Affinity and Chronic Mountain
        Sickness   74

5   *Circulation*   *75*
5.1   Physiologic Considerations   75
5.2   Systemic Circulation   78
5.3   Cor Pulmonale and Chronic Mountain Sickness   79
5.4   Electrocardiographic Findings   81
5.5   Cardiac Output   84
5.6   Pulmonary Circulation   89
5.7   Cerebral Circulation   92
5.8   Circulation in Skeletal Muscles   94

6   *Ventilation*   *97*
6.1   Morphometry   98
6.2   Lung Capacities   99
6.3   Pulmonary Diffusing Capacity   102
6.4   Normal Control of Ventilation   104
6.5   Ventilation in High-Altitude Natives   108
6.6   The Effect of Age on Ventilation   109
6.7   The Control of Ventilation during Sleep   111
6.8   Ventilation and Chronic Mountain Sickness   114
6.9   Excessive Polycythemia in Lowlander Sojourners   116
6.10 Pregnancy   117

7   *Renal Function in High-Altitude Polycythemia*   *119*
7.1   Renal Functions   119
7.2   Renal Hemodynamics in High-Altitude Natives   124
7.3   Renal Excretion of Bicarbonate   133
7.4   Renal Excretion of Acid   133
7.5   Renal Excretion of Sodium in Response to
        Angiotensin   135

7.6   Maximal Urinary Concentrating Capacity   136
7.7   Maximal Tubular Free-Water Reabsorption
       Capacity   136
7.8   Renal Oxygenation   138
7.9   Renal Abnormalities in High-Altitude Natives   138
7.10   The Polycythemic Kidney as a Model   141

8   *Exercise Capacity*   *142*
8.1   Andean High-Altitude Natives   143
8.2   North American Natives   156
8.3   Himalayan Natives   157
8.4   The Effect of Polycythemia on Exercise   158
8.5   The Economy of Oxygen Uptake during Exercise   159

9   *The Comparative Physiology of Hypoxemic Polycythemia*   *162*
9.1   Polycythemia and Hemoglobin Oxygen Affinity   162
9.2   Tissue PO_2 and Adaptation to High Altitudes   168
9.3   Properties of Red Cells   170
9.4   Chronic Mountain Sickness in Animals   172
9.5   Animal Models   173
9.6   Comparisons of Animals with Humans   175

10   *Bloodletting*   *177*
10.1   The Effect of Polycythemia on Gas Exchange   177
10.2   Bloodletting in High-Altitude Natives   179
10.3   Studies of Bloodletting in Cerro de Pasco   179
10.4   Exercise Performance after Hematocrit Reduction   182
10.5   Invasive Gas Transport Measurements   186
10.6   Conclusions from Hematocrit-Reduction Studies   201

11   *Summary and Conclusions*   *203*
11.1   The History of Chronic Mountain Sickness   203
11.2   High-Altitude Natives and Chronic Mountain
       Sickness   204
11.3   Red Cells, Red Cell and Plasma Volumes, and Their
       Regulation   205
11.4   The Structure and Function of Hemoglobin at High
       Altitudes   207
11.5   Circulation   208
11.6   Ventilation   209
11.7   Renal Function in High-Altitude Polycythemia   210
11.8   Exercise Capacity   211

11.9   The Comparative Physiology of Hypoxemic
         Polycythemia   211
11.10   Bloodletting   212
11.11   The Integration of Physiologic Variables   213
11.12   A Public Health Note   215

Notes   *217*

Glossary   *223*

References   *227*

Index   *251*

Figures

2.1   A typical subject with chronic mountain sickness   22

3.1   Normal hematocrit values at sea level as a function of age for 7,426 normal males and 7,704 normal females in the United States   32

3.2   The hematocrit as a function of age in subjects in Cerro de Pasco (4,300 m) and Morococha (4,500 m)   34

3.3   Hemoglobin variation with altitude   35

3.4   A comparison of two Peruvian communities at the same altitude   37

3.5   The distribution of hematocrit values at sea level, Cerro de Pasco, and Morococha   38

3.6   The mean corpuscular hemoglobin concentration at sea level, Cerro de Pasco, and Morococha   40

3.7   Serum ferritin and free erythrocyte protoporphyrin in Morococha   41

3.8   Reticulocytosis after injection of plasma from high-altitude natives or controls into normal sea-level volunteers   45

3.9   The dependence of hematocrit on red-cell volume   51

4.1   The normal whole-blood-oxygen equilibrium curve   56

4.2   The advantages of the sigmoid shape of the oxygen equilibrium curve   56

4.3   Barcroft's data on oxygen equilibrium   61

4.4   The metabolism of glucose by erythrocytes   65

4.5   The distributions of 2,3-DPG concentrations at sea level and at high altitude   66

4.6   The distributions of P50 at sea level and at high altitude   68

4.7   The suspension effect of red cells on apparent blood pH   70

4.8   The in vivo oxygen equilibrium curve at Morococha   72

4.9   The relationship between P50 and hematocrit in natives of Morococha   73

5.1   The dependence of blood viscosity on hematocrit in natives of Cerro de Pasco   76

5.2   The relationships of pressure, venous return, and cardiac output   77

5.3   The mean pulmonary-artery pressure in three cases of chronic mountain sickness, as a function of time of residence at sea level   80

5.4   Mean QRS vectors for a sample of native residents of Cerro de Pasco   82

5.5   The heart-rate response to imposition of a square-wave work
      load   88
5.6   Sea-level and high-altitude curves for the appearance of dye
      in the femoral artery after injection into the antecubital vein   89
5.7   The mean circulation time and cardiac index as a function of
      hematocrit   91
5.8   The relationship between the hematocrit and measured
      arteriovenous oxygen difference across the brain in high-
      altitude residents breathing either ambient air or oxygen   94
6.1   An O_2-CO_2 diagram, showing the composition of alveolar
      gas in acclimatized subjects at high altitude   98
6.2   The age dependence of chest morphometry   100
6.3   The relationship between vital capacity and height in
      Sherpas, western trekkers, and Quechua Indians in
      Morococha and Cerro de Pasco   102
6.4   The ventilatory response to hypoxia   106
6.5   Cardiac conduction in a high-altitude native   107
6.6   Hypoxic ventilatory sensitivity in acclimatized lowlanders
      and Quechua Indians with and without chronic mountain
      sickness   110
6.7   The normal decrease of PaO_2 with age   111
6.8   The hematocrit and the resting ventilatory rate   112
6.9   The relationship between hypoxic ventilatory response and
      frequency of sleep apnea in Caucasian lowlanders and
      Sherpas at 5,400 m   113
6.10 The ventilatory response to isocapnic hypoxia in normal
      high-altitude residents and in those with chronic mountain
      sickness   115
6.11 The relationship between the hematocrit and SaO_2 while
      subjects are awake and during various stages of sleep   115
7.1   The renal circulation   120
7.2   The hormonal control of renal function   123
7.3   Renal hemodynamics in sea-level controls, high-altitude
      natives, and natives with chronic mountain sickness   125
7.4   The dependence of the filtration fraction on the hematocrit   126
7.5   The relationship between the logarithm of blood viscosity
      and the hematocrit at two shear rates   127
7.6   The relationship between the parameters of renal function
      and blood viscosity at two shear rates   128
7.7   The dependence of an effective flow of renal plasma (ERPF)
      on the hematocrit   129
7.8   The relationship between the GFR and the ERPF in residents
      of Morococha   130

7.9   The relationship between the filtration fraction and blood
      viscosity in Peruvian sea-level residents and high-altitude
      natives   131
7.10 The relationship of pH, bicarbonate, and PCO_2 in the blood
      plasma   132
7.11 A semilogarithmic plot of ten parameters of the acid-base
      equilibrium studied before and after a constant intravenous
      infusion of ammonium chloride   134
7.12 The renal physiologic changes induced by angiotensin   135
7.13 The maximal urinary concentration after water deprivation
      and administration of pitressin in sea-level residents and
      high-altitude natives   136
7.14 The maximal tubular reabsorption capacity studied in
      hydropenic conditions by mannitol infusion   137
7.15 An example of the relationship between C_{osm} and urine
      volume (V) during osmotic diuresis   137
7.16 Renal PvO_2 as a function of PaO_2, calculated from a
      theoretical model that includes the polycythemic response to
      changes in PaO_2 in Peruvian natives   139
8.1   A comparison of the ventilatory response to exercise in a
      resident of Cerro de Pasco with that in an acclimatized
      lowlander   148
8.2   A comparison of the ventilatory response to exercise in
      sedentary and athletic acclimatized lowlanders with that in
      natives of Morococha at submaximal and maximal exercise   149
8.3   The lack of correlation between the ventilatory response to
      exercise and the hematocrit, age, or maximal exercise   150
8.4   Changes in the arterial blood gases during exercise in a
      native of Cerro de Pasco   154
8.5   The accumulation of lactic acid in three natives of Cerro de
      Pasco   155
8.6   The theoretical relationship between "available" O_2 and
      hematocrit   159
8.7   The relationship between the hematocrit and maximal
      exercise capacity in natives of Cerro de Pasco   160
9.1   The logarithm of P50 as a function of the logarithm of the
      body weight of a group of mammals   163
9.2   The logarithm of 2,3-DPG concentration as a function of the
      logarithm of body weight   164
9.3   P50 values in mammals and birds   165
9.4   The oxygen affinity and oxygen capacity of toad blood   166
9.5   Mixed venous PO_2 for various animals at sea level and at
      high altitude   169

9.6   The velocity constant of red-cell oxygenation as a function
      of the reciprocal of the red-cell radius   171
9.7   A comparison of the body-weight, brain-weight, and blood-
      volume fractions in mice at sea level and at high altitude   174
9.8   The brain hematocrit as a function of the body hematocrit in
      mice at sea level and at high altitude   175
10.1 The time course of the change in hematologic parameters
      during phlebotomy in a polycythemic subject   181
10.2 An analysis of arterial blood during exercise in three
      subjects in Cerro de Pasco   187
10.3 QRS complexes recorded during exercise cycling   190
10.4 The effect of hemodilution on pulmonary circulation   191
10.5 Incremental exercise tests before and after hemodilution   192
10.6 The ventilatory threshold, determined by plotting $\dot{V}_E$ against
      $\dot{V}O_2$ 193
10.7 Steady-state exercise tests before and after hemodilution   194
10.8 Parameters of oxygen transport during exercise   195
10.9 A comparison of the cardiac index (CI) and (a-$\bar{v}$) O_2 with
      previous studies   199
11.1 Physiologic variables in the etiology of chronic mountain
      sickness   214

Tables

1.1   Red-cell counts made by Viault in 1889   7

2.1   A comparison of the heights and weights of subjects at low and high altitudes   21

3.1   The hemoglobin and hematocrit values in high-altitude populations   35

3.2   Red-cell indexes in subjects at low and high altitudes   39

3.3   Kidney oxygenation in subjects at low and high altitudes   48

3.4   Red-cell and plasma volumes at sea level and high altitudes   49

3.5   Hemodilution of selected subjects at Cerro de Pasco   50

3.6   A comparison of the means for HB, HV, PLV, RCV, and HB/HV measurements   52

3.7   Correlation coefficients for VH, PLV, and RCV measurements   53

4.1   Arterial measurements, Cerro de Pasco, 1921–22   60

4.2   Barcroft's in vitro experiment, Cerro de Pasco, 1921–22   61

4.3   Blood oxygenation data of Aste-Salazar and Hurtado   63

4.4   Blood-gas and pH values in high-altitude natives   71

5.1   Cardiovascular findings in high-altitude natives   80

5.2   Electrocardiographic findings in natives of Cerro de Pasco   81

5.3   Maximal work and heart rate in natives of Cerro de Pasco   87

5.4   Pulmonary circulatory measurements of subjects at low and high altitudes   90

6.1   Anthropometric data in high-altitude natives   99

6.2   Respiratory adaptation to high altitudes   101

6.3   Vital capacity of high-altitude populations   102

6.4   Isocapnic hypoxic responses in natives of Morococha   114

6.5   Ventilatory measurements, Tibetans at 3,890 meters   116

7.1   Renal oxygen-transport values in subjects at low and high altitudes   124

7.2   Renal hemodynamics in high-altitude natives   131

7.3   Tubular reabsorption of sea-level and high-altitude subjects   133

7.4   Urinary protein excretion rates and creatinine clearances in residents of low and high altitudes   140

7.5   Urinary protein excretion rates and creatinine clearances in high-altitude natives with a nephropathy of unknown origin   140

8.1   Maximal O_2 uptake in high-altitude natives   143

8.2   Exercise capacity in natives of Lima and Morococha   145

8.3   Maximal work in high-altitude natives and acclimatized lowlanders   146

8.4   Exercise capacities in high-altitude Indians and in athletic
      and sedentary lowlanders   147
8.5   Ventilation with various inspired PO_2 149
8.6   Hemodynamic measurements in natives of Lima and
      Morococha   152
8.7   Oxygen transport in a Sherpa and in acclimatized lowlanders 157
10.1 Pulmonary functions in polycythemia vera   178
10.2 Effects of familiarity on exercise test results   180
10.3 Exercise results in subjects chosen for phlebotomy or
      hemodilution   182
10.4 The ventilatory response to exercise   183
10.5 The effect of hematocrit reduction on exercise performance 185
10.6 Changes with hemodilution in subject 3680   188
10.7 Blood-gas measurements during constant work-rate exercise
      in subject 3680   194
10.8 Pulmonary gas exchange during constant work-rate exercise
      in subject 3680   196
10.9 Hemodynamics during constant work-rate exercise in subject
      3680   197

Foreword

With *Hypoxia, Polycythemia, and Chronic Mountain Sickness,* the Johns Hopkins University Press continues a tradition of publishing works that reflect the interests and strengths of two of the academic divisions of the university with which the name Johns Hopkins is perhaps most closely associated worldwide: the School of Medicine and the School of Hygiene and Public Health. It seems fitting that the press that bears the name of Johns Hopkins should present works that address significant issues in the allied areas of medicine and public health and, in the case of this particular work, it also seems fitting that its foreword should be written by the incumbent president of the Johns Hopkins University. Almost forty years ago, Dr. Isaiah Bowman, one of my predecessors as president, contributed the foreword to *Acclimatization in the Andes,* a landmark book by the father of one of the coauthors of this volume.

As a distinguished geographer with first-hand knowledge of Peru, Dr. Bowman was eminently qualified to comment on the 1948 volume by Dr. Carlos Monge M. As a political scientist, I cannot assess the scientific merits of this comprehensive text on chronic mountain sickness by Dr. Robert M. Winslow and Dr. Carlos Monge C.; that judgment has already been made through the press's peer review procedures. I can, however, comment on some of the cultural and sociological implications of the conclusions drawn by the authors.

The view of Winslow and Monge C. that humans who exist in high altitudes do *not* necessarily represent a genetically different breed of human being challenges the ideas set forth in the work by the senior Dr. Monge and invites further investigation by geneticists. The comparative genetic studies that the authors advocate are now possible to conduct more definitely than ever before, thanks to the sophisticated equipment and techniques increasingly available to researchers. Results from this kind of study could validate or disprove the hypothesis that Himalayan populations are not as susceptible to chronic mountain sickness as Andean and North American populations because of the genetic adaptation of Tibetans to high altitudes over a much longer period of time.

Comparative studies will undoubtedly lead to important findings about possible genetic differences, but they will not deal directly with the health problems of individuals who, by happenstance of birth, will live at high altitudes in the late twentieth century and into the twenty-first century. The same advanced telecommunications technology and rapid forms of transportation that enable scientists to conduct in vivo studies with relative ease of access to populations in the Andes and the Himalayas also expose the inhabitants of these areas to a Western way of life with all its advantages and disadvantages.

Winslow and Monge C. point out that, in the case of the Andean populations, obesity, smoking, and a more sedentary way of life—in spite of the cult of physical fitness which pervades many Western societies—are characteristics of a Western life-style that can contribute to the incidence of chronic mountain sickness and that can be exacerbated by the environmental pollution to which workers in the mines are subjected. As Dr. Bowman noted in 1948, the mines in Peru are, for the most part, at high altitudes, and that still holds true in the 1980s for the most important mines in Peru as well as in Bolivia and Chile. In spite of the fact that the economies of these three nations continue to depend heavily on mining, and in spite of more enlightened occupational and environmental health and safety practices developed in the Western world over the last forty years, the health problems—of which chronic mountain sickness is but one—of the high-altitude people who almost exclusively make up the work force in the mines have not been addressed adequately. Several factors seem to contribute to this situation: the relative inaccessibility of these populations; the minority status of the Andean peoples, particularly in Chile and Peru; the language differences between these peoples and those governing them; and the lack of formal education. It is difficult if not impossible to change any of these factors except for improved education.

The authors quite properly insist that the research efforts that have led to a better understanding of chronic mountain sickness must be directed vigorously to the improvement of the health of high-altitude residents. The governments have a responsibility to implement and enforce proper environmental controls in the workplace. The fields of medicine and public health also have a responsibility to train the next generation of medical and public health practitioners to serve these populations more effectively and to prepare them for a healthy life in the decades to come.

We have come a long way in forty years in the study of chronic mountain sickness, and the work of Dr. Winslow and Dr. Monge C. significantly advances our knowledge of this condition. Their text builds on the fund of data that has accumulated since the pioneering work of Viault, Barcroft, and Monge M. and summarizes an important body of research. Winslow and Monge C. focus attention on the special health needs of high-altitude humans and remind us that human beings have an extraordinary ability to adapt to their environment but also have limits that must be recognized in order to preserve and enhance the quality of their existence.

Steven Muller, Ph.D.
President, The Johns Hopkins University

Acknowledgments

This book presents our views on some of the problems of high-altitude adaptation, particularly in long-term residents of the mountains who develop chronic mountain sickness. The topics we emphasize reflect our own beliefs on the etiology of this fascinating "loss of adaptation." Many of our colleagues do not share all of our opinions, and some of them would very likely have stressed other aspects of adaptation to high altitudes. Therefore, a large debt of gratitude is due the Johns Hopkins University Press, whose support and encouragement throughout the project was essential. At times, our families and co-workers in our respective institutions did not appreciate our interest in the problems of high-altitude man. To them we express our thanks for their patience and indulgence.

Our work in the mountains of Peru would not have been possible without the financial support of the National Science Foundation, and the guidance of Ms. Christine French, Latin American Cooperative Science Program. In addition, we are grateful to the National Heart, Lung, and Blood Institute, the Centers for Disease Control, and the Cayetano Heredia University, for allowing us the flexibility to be away from our primary duties for the prolonged periods needed for expedition work. We are also grateful to Corning Instruments and to Advanced Products for allowing us to use important items of equipment in the field.

Many individuals helped directly in the expeditions. Nancy Winslow organized the supplies and equipment in exacting detail and obtained most of our blood data in the field. Carter Gibson, Biomedical Engineering and Instrumentation Branch, NIH, fabricated, repaired, and helped operate our computerized exercise gas analysis equipment. Other North American collaborators included Sam Charache, Johns Hopkins University School of Medicine; Ed Brown, Rick Krouskop, and Ned McDonald, Mt. Sinai School of Medicine; Harvey Klein, National Institutes of Health; and Earl Dixon, Tuskegee Institute.

In Peru, collaboration with José Whittembury, Juan D'Brot, Oscar Moran, and Ernesto Gonzales was indispensable. In addition, special thanks must be given to Mr. G. Fitsmaurice in Morococha and to Mr. Atencio in Cerro de Pasco, who maintained the laboratories in excellent condition and looked after our personal needs while working in the mountains. Centromín, the Peruvian national mining company, provided medical records of our subjects and permitted them to participate in our studies. They too provided indispensable help.

Many informal discussions were held over the course of this work with colleagues who generously shared their experience, expertise, and opinions with us. Some of those who were especially helpful were Robert Berger, Ed DeLand, Bruce Dill, Robert Grover, Bernard Holland, Sukhamay Lahiri, John Reeves, and John West. While we acknowledge the contributions of these friends and colleagues, the views presented in the following pages do not necessarily reflect their opinions; the authors take full responsibility for the content, and for any errors, in this book.

Finally, we wish to acknowledge the cooperation and participation in our studies of the Indian natives of Morococha and Cerro de Pasco. In the course of our work, we developed tremendous respect and admiration for these gentle, humble people. So far, they have contributed more to science than we have contributed to their health. This book is dedicated to them, in the hope that an increased understanding of their patterns of adaptation to hypoxia may eventually lead to improved health for them.

Hypoxia, Polycythemia, and Chronic Mountain Sickness

Introduction

Chronic mountain sickness (Monge's disease) is the occurrence of symptomatic, excessive polycythemia in long-term residents of high altitudes. Hypoxia is the stimulus to erythropoiesis; symptoms result from a severe expansion of the blood volume and a consequent burden on the circulatory system. The cure for this syndrome is descent to sea level or phlebotomy.

For many years, chronic mountain sickness was thought to be a disease, in the sense that pathologic causes were sought. However, none has been found, in spite of a wide variety of studies and theories. Our hypothesis is that the symptoms are caused, in this case, by an over-response of normal physiologic mechanisms. The cure, whether descent or phlebotomy, is entirely straightforward. Why, then, should a book be devoted to this entity? The answer is that normal physiologic mechanisms are not usually thought to cause disease, and to understand chronic mountain sickness we must therefore consider the definition of normality in an environment that is hostile to humans. One major goal of this book is to examine systematically the evidence for pathologic processes in subjects with chronic mountain sickness in order to support our conclusions regarding its etiology.

Only a small fraction of permanent residents manifest chronic mountain sickness. The majority of persons who take up residence in the high mountains develop a tolerance to the conditions there. This process is called "acclimatization" and is a testament to the profound flexibility of the human body. The limit of this flexibility is at issue here, not a precise focus on chronic mountain sickness as a clinical entity. In this sense, hypoxia, polycythemia, and chronic mountain sickness represent a model for understanding normality and, in particular, variations of normal that, under some stressful circumstances, may lead to symptomatic illness.

A second goal for the book is to explore the concept of acclimatization. The term is used in many ways by physiologists to mean tolerance to an extreme environment. But there is no strict definition of what acclimatization really is. For some, it is the disappearance of the symptoms of acute exposure to altitude experienced, for example, by skiers or mountain climbers after a few days. For others it is a complex of adjustments in long-term residents of high altitude. Carlos Monge Medrano (1884–1964), considered chronic mountain sickness to be a loss of acclimatization by such long-term residents, implying that those who did not have chronic mountain sickness were, by definition, acclimatized.

People have taken up permanent residence in the Andes of South America, at altitudes of 14,000–15,000 feet, for many reasons, including the presence there of rich deposits of ores and precious metals. This population, made up mainly of Quechua Indians, is isolated and very stable, making it a unique group for the study of the chronic effects of hypoxia in human physiology and medicine. There is a popular and romantic view that these people represent a "superhuman" subset of the human race; their feats of strength and stamina are legendary. Many observers hold the belief that these people are genetically "adapted" to this environment, and a third goal of this book is to consider the evidence for and against this belief.

After many years of experience studying high-altitude natives, we have come to the view that life in the high mountains, particularly in the Andes, is harsh, difficult, and demanding. The living conditions on the high plateaus are not well appreciated except by firsthand observation because there is no written record from the Inca civilization. Instead, there is an oral history, and the daily conditions of life are described eloquently in the following translation of a Quechua song, "To Be Wandering."[1]

> Oh perhaps my mother was the vicuña of the pampas
> or my father was the mountain stag
> to be wandering,
> to walk without rest
> through the mountains and the pampas
> hardly wrapped by wind,
> in the creeks and on the hills
> clothed by wind and cold.
>
> Oh I was born in the nest of the pukupuku
> to cry out in the day,
> to cry out in the night
> like the pukupuku chick
> hardly wrapped by wind.

These verses illustrate vividly that, in addition to a thin atmosphere, the high plateaus of the Andes are cold, windy, desolate, and sparsely populated. High-altitude natives most commonly remain in the mountains for economic or family reasons. Some of them are so isolated that they have no idea of the severe limitations under which they live. The Indians of the Inca empire were astonishingly well organized and sophisticated, and there were practical reasons for their living in the mountains. One that is too little appreciated is that the western coastal regions of the South American continent constitute the dryest desert on earth. The valleys at moderate altitude were much more conducive to an agrarian economy. The introduction of commercial mining after the Spanish conquest was an additional stimulus to permanent residence in the mountains.

Although there is less known about natives of the high Asian plateaus, information is rapidly becoming available. In recent years, a dogma has arisen that natives of the Himalayas do not develop chronic mountain sickness because of a longer period for genetic adaptation of the populations there. In spite of a paucity of supporting evidence, this hypothesis has gained wide acceptance.

The study of the physiologic mechanisms of acclimatization may also provide a model to understand related sea-level problems. For example, there is great interest in the effects of blood viscosity in the etiology of stroke and heart disease. Recent evidence suggests that reducing the hematocrit to normal or even subnormal levels can increase cerebral blood flow in sea-level residents. Polycythemia is known to be a risk factor in the genesis of coronary artery disease. A controversy has arisen over the question of "blood doping," a means of increasing the hematocrit by autologous blood transfusion to improve athletic performance. Physicians do not agree on whether the hematocrit in subjects with chronic lung disease should be therapeutically reduced to a normal level. In addition, because high viscosity could increase the risk of stroke or frostbite in mountain climbers, phlebotomy or hemodilution (replacement of red cells by plasma or a substitute) is advocated by some, even though the oxygen content of the blood would be reduced.

Carlos Monge M., a pioneer in the study of high-altitude natives, laid the foundation for the Peruvian Institute of Andean Biology at San Marcos University and provided the first clinical description of chronic mountain sickness. Monge's early work on the syndrome that bears his name was directed at a definition of the pathologic basis of what he considered the "disease of the Andes." In his later work he appreciated the multifaceted nature of this disorder, and his integration of biology, medicine, anthropology, and sociology stimulated new approaches to high-altitude problems. In this book, we have tried to carry on in this tradition in considering chronic mountain sickness from several different aspects.

In 1977 the authors met for the first time and found that we shared many common opinions on approaches to high-altitude problems, particularly polycythemia and chronic mountain sickness. For example, we believe that careful study of the physiologic changes that accompany exposure to high altitude must not be influenced by the belief that natives are, by definition, completely acclimatized. Over the years, we have been impressed at the physiologic variability in high-altitude natives with regard to acclimatization. Furthermore, some of the responses to hypoxia do not appear to be entirely beneficial.

In our attempt to build our case that chronic mountain sickness is caused by normal physiologic mechanisms, we have selected for review what we judge to be the pivotal experimental work on this entity accumulated over more than sixty years. In doing so, we present some information that either has not been previously published or has been published in hard-to-obtain medical sources. We also review the pertinent results of our own collaboration during several scientific expeditions to the Peruvian Andes, beginning in 1978.

We have made no attempt to prepare a high-altitude encyclopedia or a travelogue; these have been developed by other authors. Rather, we focus on high-altitude polycythemia, classically considered to be a condition of the loss of acclimatization, as a model to understand the acclimatization process. Our studies and review of a number of related subjects have led us to the view that polycythemia, whether physiologic or excessive, may be maladaptive. In addition to the fascination this subject holds for understanding adaptive mechanisms, it is of practical importance to a large number of people who live and work in the mountains. We hope that this book will contribute to a better understanding of the health of these people.

CHAPTER ONE
The History of Chronic Mountain Sickness

While the great majority of persons residing permanently at altitudes between 10,000 feet and 14,000 feet have apparently "adapted" to the thin air there, others develop a sickness called "chronic mountain sickness." They are usually older, and they suffer with a variety of symptoms including headache, bone pain, confusion, sleeplessness, and a subjective feeling of congestion of the head. Because they are usually persons who were previously well, and because descent to a lower altitude is curative, this syndrome has been considered to represent a loss of the body's ability to acclimatize to high altitude. The number of sufferers with chronic mountain sickness is not known, but it is not a large number, compared to other causes of morbidity and mortality. Rather, its fascination is with the idea of acclimatization, and its loss. Therefore, the study of this clinical entity is intimately bound to the understanding of the acclimatization process.

Permanent life in the high mountains is a subject that has interested physiologists and other scientists since Paul Bert. Perhaps chronic mountain sickness represents the ultimate test of whether people can truly adjust to life in a rarefied atmosphere. As such, it provides the opportunity to investigate many different physiologic concepts and mechanisms. In addition, the story of the evolution of thinking about chronic mountain sickness is a rich fabric woven from the development of scientific methods, nationalism, the establishment of individual scientific careers, and the economics of mountain industry. The story is sometimes scientific and always human; it is a story of the explosion of scientific methods in the twentieth century and of the individuals who have used those methods to understand high-altitude natives.

1.1 The First Descriptions of Mountain Sickness

Father Acosta was the first to record his sufferings while crossing the Andean divide on the Peruvian Cordillera (Acosta 1608). Since that description, Peru has been a focus for high-altitude studies. Acosta's original publication in 1573 (Bonavía et al. 1984, 1985) is usually considered to be typical of writings on acute mountain sickness, a condition known to the native population as "Soroche" (Monge M. 1948; Gilbert 1983a). Although careful reading of Acosta's writings suggests his ailments may not have been entirely due to Soroche, Acosta was certainly the first to point out that the condition of the air in the mountains was inappropriate for human respiration: "I am persuaded that the element of air there is so thin and delicate that

5

it doesn't provide for human respiration which needs it to be thicker and more tempered" (Monge M. 1948, 3).

1.2 Paul Bert and the French Physiologists

Modern investigations into the physiologic response to the high-altitude environment began with the great French physiologist Paul Bert. His widely ranging interests included engineering, law, politics, and medicine, and he was trained in physiology by Claude Bernard (Olmsted 1952). His book *La Pression Barométrique* was a pioneer work on barometric pressure at high altitude (Bert 1878, 1943). In a variety of experiments on animals in low-pressure chambers and in man during balloon ascents in the Alps, he proved that oxygen was essential for survival.

Bert was also the first to suggest that changes in the blood might allow the possibility of tolerance to high-altitude exposure. In his 1878 book he wrote, "We might ask first whether, by a harmonious compensation of which general nature history gives us many examples, either by a modification in the nature of quantity of hemoglobin, or by an increase in the number of red blood corpuscles, his blood had become qualified to absorb more oxygen under the same volume, and thus to return to the usual standard of the seashore" (Bert 1943, 1000). Bert even suggested that the way to test this hypothesis would be to collect the blood of a person or animal who was a resident of high altitude and to measure its O_2 capacity. The opportunity arose a few years later, when a colleague sent him some samples of blood from La Paz, Bolivia, collected from native domestic animals. Bert showed that the O_2 capacity of these samples was 16–20 milliliters/deciliter, compared to 10–12 milliliters/deciliter in domestic French animals (Dill 1938).

Bert's friend and colleague Dennis Jourdanet also had a strong interest in adaptation to high altitude. As a surgeon in Mexico, Jourdanet observed that some of his patients' blood was very thick, but that they occasionally had symptoms that were identical to those of anemic lowlanders. In his book, *Anemia of Altitudes*, he suggested that "anoxemia" could occur, either at sea level or at high altitude (Jourdanet 1863). Jourdanet and Bert both believed that acclimatization to high altitude would take generations, but this view was politically unpopular because the French government, under Napoleon III, was eager to establish an empire in Mexico (Erslev 1981). In an effort to bolster the government's position in this controversy, a French Army physician, L. Coindet, published a short pamphlet (Coindet 1863) that attempted to demonstrate that lowlanders could acclimatize in a rather short period (Erslev 1981).

The dispute between Bert and Jourdanet on the one hand and Coindet on the other was finally settled by the French physician François Viault, who at Bert's suggestion traveled from Lima to Morococha (altitude 4,500 m) by train in 1889 (Viault 1890). He was accompanied by a Peruvian, Dr. J. Mayorga, and the two studied themselves, a dog, a cock, and a male llama, in addition to residents and Indian natives (table 1.1). Their findings seemed to support Bert's theory of an increased O_2 carrying capacity at high altitude. However, Viault also used a mercury pump to measure O_2 capacity in a variety of animals.[1] These first blood gas measurements to be made in the field on fresh samples led Viault to conclude that anoxemia does not exist in animals living at high altitude. However, Bert had already demonstrated the useful concept of PaO_2 in the interpretation of anoxemia, and Viault's findings were never generally acknowledged.

Viault wrote, "One may suppose a priori that the physiological reason that allows man and animals to endure the very rarefied atmosphere of high places must be a result of either: an increase in frequency of respiratory movements; or an acceleration of the heart beat that would return more blood to the lung; or an increase in the respiratory element of the blood, that is to say, the red blood cells; or a greater respiratory capacity of the hemoglobin; or finally, and this is difficult to evaluate, a reduction in the oxygen needs of the tissues, that is to say, a decrease in the amount of tissue oxidation, or even a higher work efficiency for the oxidation that has occurred" (West 1981, 333). This enumeration of the possible physiologic adaptive mechanisms in hypoxia is as relevant today as it was in 1890. Viault's chief contribution, however, was that he measured his own red blood cell count, which increased from five million to eight million after twenty-three days at Morococha.

Viault interpreted polycythemia as a mechanism for adaptation to low

Table 1.1.   Red-cell counts made by Viault in 1889

Subject	Corpuscles
In Lima, October 4, 1889 (eve of my departure to the Cordillera) my blood contained per cubic millimeter	5,000,000
In Morococha, October 19 (after 15 days in the Cordillera)	7,100,000
Dr. Mayorga (ditto)	7,300,000
Mayorga, same (living 3 years at mine)	7,840,000
R. Prieto, kitchen boy, half-breed	6,770,000
Dittman, German mine administrator	7,920,000
Atchachay, Indian	7,960,000
Margarita, Ind	7,080,000
Charpentier, son of French parents, butler	6,000,000
Rossi, Italian, at Oroya	6,320,000
My blood, October 27	8,000,000
Dr. Mayorga (ditto)	7,440,000
Strong young bitch	9,000,000
Strong one-year-old cock	6,000,000
Male llama	16,000,000

Source: Viault 1890.

barometric pressure. No doubt a red blood cell count of sixteen million per cubic millimeter found in the llama must have convinced him of the importance of polycythemia as a compensatory mechanism. His early interpretation must have been the starting point for the widespread acceptance for many years of the belief that polycythemia was one of the fundamental physiologic responses to a hypoxic environment.

1.3   Joseph Barcroft's Expedition to Cerro de Pasco

The year 1921 marked the first of a series of Andean expeditions in which physiologic experiments were carried out in the field. This is significant, because it was the beginning of the collection of data from native human subjects. The expedition was led by Joseph Barcroft, the prominent Cambridge physiologist, during the winter of 1921–22 to Cerro de Pasco, Peru (4,300 m). Although mainly devoted to the respiratory physiology of the members of the party, it also included a few measurements in natives (Barcroft et al. 1923). Barcroft was very impressed by the physical capacities of the natives of the Peruvian Andes. In his 1923 report, he included photographs of a woman carrying a heavy load uphill, and of miners carrying 80 pounds of ore up from the mine shafts. Pertinent results of this expedition will be discussed in later chapters, but Barcroft believed that acclimatization, be it short- or long-term, was influenced primarily by three factors: an increase in ventilation, providing an alveolar pO_2 10–12 torr higher than it would be otherwise, a rise (left-shift) of the hemoglobin-oxygen dissociation curve, providing augmented oxygen uptake in the lung, and an increase in the number of red cells in the circulation.

Barcroft, however, seems to have been ambivalent on the issue of acclimatization, because in a later publication he concluded that acclimatization to high altitude does not exist (Barcroft 1925). He generalized this concept even to permanent residents or natives of high altitude. In the last chapter of his book, he concluded: "And this redistribution of disadvantages appears to be the real essence of acclimatization. The acclimatized man is not the man who has attained to bodily and mental powers as great in Cerro de Pasco as he would have in Cambridge (whether that town be situated in Massachusetts or in England). Such a man does not exist. All dwellers at high altitude are persons of impaired physical and mental powers. The acclimatized man is he who is least impaired, or, in other words, he who has made least demand upon his reserve. At rest he will appear like the dweller of the plain, but exercise will always bring him to a standstill sooner at the higher altitude" (Barcroft 1925, 176).

1.4 Carlos Monge M.

In the same year that Barcroft's report appeared, Carlos Monge Medrano, a private physician in Lima, encountered in his clinical practice a man with a syndrome closely resembling polycythemia vera. This man would later become the first reported case of chronic mountain sickness (see chap. 2). Monge's experience with high-altitude matters dated from his examination for his entrance into the medical school of San Marcos University. At that time, he was asked a question about the hematologic response to high altitude, and he was prepared with the correct answer, since, even as an undergraduate, he was familiar with the writings of Viault.

After receiving the M.D. degree from San Marcos, Monge went on to earn a degree in tropical medicine in London in 1912, then spent another year in Paris, where polycythemia vera was known as "Váquez's disease." He noted that his patient was a native of Cerro de Pasco and that while he remained at sea level, his symptoms of polycythemia disappeared. He presented a communication to the National Academy of Medicine of Lima, entitled "Sobre un caso de Enfermedad de Váquez (Sindrome eritrémico de altura)," on a case of Váquez's disease (erythremic syndrome of altitude) (Monge M. 1925). Although he used the term *Váquez's disease* because the patient had marked polycythemia, he believed that the condition was caused by the patient's residence at high altitude and was cured by descent to sea level. The symptoms recurred when the patient returned to high altitude. In fact, this clinical record was one discussed later by Monge M. in his 1928 book. The subtitle of the 1925 paper, "Erythremic Syndrome of Altitude," leaves no doubt that he related the disease to the high-altitude environment.

Monge M. believed that it was unfair to regard a high-altitude native as a transplanted sea-level person, and that either person, living at high altitude or sea level, suffered when forced to live in the other environment. Monge later became professor of medical Nosology at the Faculty of Medicine of the University of San Marcos of Lima. His contributions to the study of the Andean dweller went beyond the field of clinical medicine into public health, anthropology and sociology; they are described in a biographical note by David Bruce Dill in *The Physiologist* (Dill 1973).

Barcroft and Monge apparently were unaware of each other at the time of Barcroft's 1921–22 expedition. Barcroft dealt directly with the authorities at the Cerro de Pasco Mining Company, which operated with considerable independence in Peru at the time. The cooperating physicians were North Americans working at Chulec Hospital in la Oroya. Monge, who was by now professor of medicine at San Marcos University, was not yet interested in high-altitude problems.

In 1925, Monge M. did not seem to be aware of Barcroft's description of the 1921–22 Cerro de Pasco expedition in the *Transactions of the Royal*

Society (London) (Barcroft et al. 1923), since he made no mention of it in his report. But he must have read Barcroft's book of 1925, *The Respiratory Function of the Blood: Lessons from High Altitude* (Barcroft 1925), soon after its publication, because in 1927 he had already made his own expedition to Cerro de Pasco as a reaction to Barcroft's interpretations.

Monge and Barcroft did not meet until 1928 and, while they were friends, they developed divergent points of view on the completeness of acclimatization of high-altitude natives. Barcroft seems to have thought of them as sea-level persons struggling against a hostile environment, while Monge felt that they were adapted to their environment and should be considered in a completely different context from sea-level residents.

In response to Barcroft's opinions Monge (1948, xiii) later wrote:

> Andean man being different from sea-level man, his biological personality must be measured with a scale distinct from that applied to the men of the lower valleys and plains. Logically the high-altitude Indian and Indo-Spanish peoples of America must be considered in the light of the deterministic forces of an oxygen-deficient environment. The climatic imperatives determine and sustain an adaptive equilibrium. Ignorance of these postulates has led eminent men of science to make shocking errors of interpretation. Hence the incredible statement of Professor Barcroft, the Cambridge physiologist, who [stayed] . . . three months at Cerro de Pasco (4300 meters), while emphasizing the enormous physical resistance of Andean man.
>
> For our part, as early as 1928 we proved in the Paris Medical School that Professor Barcroft was himself suffering from a subacute case of mountain sickness without realizing it. His substantial error is easy to explain as resulting from an improper generalization on his part of what he himself felt and applying his reactions to Andean man in general. He did not realize that in Cambridge (Massachusetts or England) man lives at practically 0 meters of altitude, 760 mm of atmospheric pressure and 150 mm of oxygen tension; in Cerro de Pasco he lives at 4,300 meters of altitude, 430 mm of atmospheric pressure and at 86 mm of oxygen tension. And that consequently Andean man must be physically distinct from sea-level man and requiring much further research before one may define, let alone apply, the terms inferior and superior.

Monge's expedition to Cerro de Pasco in 1927 culminated in his classic book *La Enfermedad de los Andes,* which contains the first widely quoted description of chronic mountain sickness, or Monge's disease (Monge M. 1928). In this book, Monge M. claimed the existence of fully acclimatized high-altitude natives but called attention to the fact that some people may never acclimatize. He considered chronic mountain sickness as an instance in which acclimatization is lost.

Monge M. believed that Barcroft's expedition was concerned with what he called "adaptive disease," which may or may not eventually culminate in acclimatization. (This same concept would be used years later by Hans Selye in his consideration of adaptive disease in the presence of chronic stress.) This historical episode is important because Monge M. believed in the existence of full acclimatization in most high-altitude natives, but loss of acclimatization was to be the condition that would bear his name. Both of these concepts are difficult to support with clear scientific documentation, and, as subsequent chapters indicate, heated disagreements on acclimatization and its possible reversal in chronic mountain sickness have marked the literature in this fascinating field.

What moved Monge M. so strongly to demonstrate the capacity for acclimatization in high-altitude natives or long-term residents when he had described the loss of acclimatization as his first contribution to the field? More than this, why did he entitle his book *The Disease of the Andes* if his intention was to emphasize normality rather than failure to acclimatize? Was he intent on showing Barcroft to be wrong? Perhaps part of the answer is that in addition to his desire to show that the great majority of high-altitude people were well acclimatized, he was also intensely nationalistic. In his later years, he devoted all of his attention to social research aimed at understanding and helping Andean natives. In any case, Monge M. was an astute clinician, and his finding of a new clinical entity must have given him great academic satisfaction. His selection of the title of his 1928 book implies that he was more interested in the pathology than in the normality of his people. These ambiguous feelings are still present in many investigators of high-altitude peoples.

In 1929 Professor G. H. Roger, dean of the Faculty of Medicine of Paris University, invited Monge M. to publish a new edition of his book in French (Monge M. 1929). In the preface, Roger proposed for the first time that "l'Erytremie des altitudes" be named "la maladie de Carlos Monge" (Monge's disease). This book contributed to the widespread interest in high-altitude investigations, and a long series of scientific studies of Andean natives followed.

Curiously, Monge himself was never particularly interested in the specificity of this clinical entity. In his paper of 1942 on chronic mountain sickness, invited by the editors of *Science,* he stated, "From our point of view, chronic mountain sickness means non-acclimatization, that is, impaired adaptation, and loss of acclimatization. It may pass through a severe stage, so-called acute mountain sickness. To be borne at high altitude does not confer immunity" (Monge M. 1942, 82). He reinforced this point in a later paragraph: "From this condensed description it is seen that the fundamental characteristic of high altitude disease which has made us group it as a nosologic entity, is the fact that all the symptoms subside or disappear as soon as the patient is brought down to sea level. This feature is undoubtedly due to a common cause, anoxemia" (84). He always used the general term *high-altitude disease* for all the forms of mountain sickness and was some-what intrigued and amused at the efforts made by his scientist friends to clearly identify chronic mountain sickness as Monge's disease. Nevertheless, in his later years he agreed with his son, Carlos Monge Cassinelli, on the modern definition of Monge's disease as a loss of acclimatization due to hypoventilation in the absence of pulmonary disease (Monge M. and Monge C. 1966, Monge C. and Whittembury 1976b).

The last twenty-five years of Monge's scientific career were devoted to his leadership as dean of San Marcos University, and establishment of the Institute of Andean Biology. This involved a constant negotiation with a governmental structure not oriented to scientific research, an activity at which he must have been a master. With his support and encouragement, a cadre of well-trained, capable young Peruvian scientists and physicians followed him. As the work of these men incorporated the latest in technical advances, learned in leading universities of the world, Monge's academic attention turned more and more to sociological and historical considerations. This work culminated in publication, in 1948, of his book *Acclimatization in the Andes,* a rich compilation of early Spanish and Indian writings about the high Andes and the people who lived there. He mustered strong evidence for the physical capabilities of the high-altitude natives but wrote of "climatic aggression" as an etiologic factor in high-altitude diseases.

1.5   North American Contributions to the Knowledge of Mountain Sickness

In 1935 an ambitious expedition organized by Ancel Keys, who was assistant professor of biochemistry at the Mayo Foundation for Medical Research, studied high-altitude physiology in the Andes of northern Chile (Keys 1936). E. S. G. Barron, who had been a medical intern under Monge M. at San Marcos University, was a member of the expedition team. In the report of this expedition, which appeared in the October 1936 issue of *The Scientific Monthly,* Keys stated: "At Ollagüe, Drs. Talbott and Barron discovered two cases of Monge's disease, a chronic form of mountain sickness recently described by Dr. Carlos Monge of Lima" (300). In the November 1936 issue of *American Journal of the Medical Sciences,* two members of the expedition, J. H. Talbott and D. B. Dill, reported one case of chronic mountain sickness but made no mention of Barron's description of another case during the same expedition. Nevertheless, they attributed to Barron the proposal for the eponym Monge's disease (Talbott and Dill 1936).

Since Barron never mentioned his own finding, it is fair to say that the first report of a case of Monge's disease in the North American literature was that of Talbott and Dill. Monge's first paper on the subject of high-altitude disease in the North American literature appeared in 1937 in *Archives of Internal Medicine;* a brief introduction by Barron again used the eponym Monge's disease (Monge M. 1937). It is intriguing to notice that these scientists, all of them friends of Monge M., did not seem to be aware of Roger's proposal in the preface of Monge's 1929 book.

1.6 Alberto Hurtado and Co-workers

Alberto Hurtado was perhaps the most prolific and influential of the young Peruvians who followed Monge M. in studies of high-altitude dwellers. Hurtado received his medical degree from Harvard University, where his M.D. thesis was on pulmonary physiology. When Hurtado returned to Peru, Monge was organizing his 1927 Cerro de Pasco expedition, and he invited the younger man to join him. After the expedition, Hurtado worked for the Cerro de Pasco Mining Company at La Oroya as a physician and studied blood gases in silicotics. He later returned to North America for further training in respiratory physiology at the University of Rochester, New York, then returned to Peru to join the San Marcos Institute of Andean Biology, where Monge was director. He remained in Peru until his death in 1984.

Hurtado and Monge worked almost independently at San Marcos University, and frequently they disagreed on many aspects of high-altitude physiology. However, it was Hurtado who was mainly responsible for assuring that the eponym Monge's disease be restricted to a clinical picture related to the loss of adaptation in a person previously acclimatized to high altitude. In 1942 Hurtado showed that chronic mountain sickness cases had accentuated polycythemia and desaturated blood beyond the physiologic limits for the corresponding altitude. He related the cause of the exaggerated polycythemia to the increased degree of desaturation. Hurtado summarized his work in the *Handbook of Physiology* (Hurtado 1964), which became the classic description of the physiology of the high-altitude native.

In his paper in the *Journal of the American Medical Association* (Hurtado 1942), Hurtado suggested the possibility that fibrosclerotic changes in the lungs may be the organic cause of chronic mountain sickness, but he later argued against the possibility of an organic cause with Professor Donald Heath in the 1971 Ciba Foundation symposium held in Hurtado's honor (Heath 1971). This is an important point for the concept of loss of acclimatization in the absence of pulmonary disease. Monge himself, in his 1928 book, intentionally studied cases of mountain sickness specifically selected among the agricultural population around Lake Titicaca, Peru, in order to avoid any possibility of ambient pollution, which may have caused organic lung disease in the mining areas of Cerro de Pasco, where his original patients lived.

Hurtado (1960) and Velásquez (1972) described hypoventilation in cases of chronic mountain sickness in Morococha. In addition, they observed that patients with the disease hyperventilated less in response to CO_2 administration than did the healthy high-altitude controls. They concluded that this was due to a loss of sensitivity of the respiratory center. In 1964, Carlos Monge C. and co-workers confirmed the relative hypoventilation of chronic mountain sickness by direct arterial puncture and gas analysis (Monge C., Lozano, and Carcelén 1964).

They showed an average $PaCO_2$ of 40 torr at Cerro de Pasco, indicating a total loss of the hypoxic ventilatory drive to hypoxemia in their patients.

1.7   Recent Expeditions and the Consolidation of Information

Earlier concepts have been refined by advances in technology and improvement in travel. By the 1960s it was possible to perform nearly any experiment in Morococha that was possible in a modern sea-level laboratory. In 1966, Severinghaus and co-workers, following initial observations in Argentina by Chiodi, postulated that alveolar hypoventilation resulted from irreversible insensitivity of the peripheral chemoreceptors to the hypoxic stimulus as a consequence of chronic exposure to hypoxia (Severinghaus, Bainton, and Carcelén 1966). In 1975 a Peruvian, Francisco Sime, correlated age with total ventilatory rate and hematocrit, and concluded that at this altitude age can be a cause of chronic mountain sickness and that humans may show a limited capacity to acclimatize (Sime, Monge C., and Whittembury 1975).

The pathologists Arias-Stella and Saldaña gained international recognition from their classical description of the pathologic anatomy of the bronchopulmonary tree in high-altitude natives (Arias-Stella and Saldaña 1963). Later, Arias-Stella provided a histologic description of the enlarged carotid bodies of high-altitude natives (Arias-Stella 1969), and Saldaña observed that most of the chemodectomas[2] found in Lima were in patients who had previously lived in the mountains (Saldaña, Salem, and Travezán 1973).

Curiously, chronic mountain sickness has never been considered to be primarily a hematologic disease, even though excessive polycythemia is its main manifestation and the cause of its symptoms. Moreover, since the work of Paul Bert, polycythemia has been considered to be an adaptive (beneficial) mechanism, and few observers have considered chronic mountain sickness to be an instance of a normal control mechanism gone awry. Merino (1950) continued the systematic study of hematologic aspects of life at high altitude, later extended by C. Reynafarje (Reynafarje et al. 1964) to studies of iron turnover, and by Sánchez (Sánchez, Merino, and Figallo 1970) to sophisticated measurements of red cell and plasma volumes. These workers established that high-altitude polycythemia is mediated by the hormone erythropoietin, whose elaboration is due to hypoxia.

Peñaloza and Sime (1971), using modern techniques of electrocardiography, vectorcardiography, and catheterization, provided an extremely valuable set of data describing the pulmonary and systemic circulations in high-altitude natives. Their work included careful descriptions of the circulatory changes in chronic mountain sickness, and the separate effects of hypoxia and polycythemia in the etiology of cor pulmonale.

In 1976, Monge C. and his co-worker José Whittembury, on the basis of numerous studies in comparative physiology, concluded that humans have a sea-level design, whether they are sea-level or high-altitude natives, and that their adaptation is mainly phenotypic and reversible (Monge C. and Whittembury 1976a). Although they did not share Barcroft's extreme view of the lack of acclimatization, neither did they agree with Monge M., who believed that Andean dwellers belong to a special variety of the human race.

In the light of the known clinical benefit of phlebotomy in polycythemic high-altitude natives and recent evidence for compromised cerebral blood flow with even marginal elevations of hematocrit, it was of interest to us to question the value of the extreme red cell response demonstrated by some high-altitude natives. In a series of three expeditions, one to Morococha and two to Cerro de Pasco, Winslow and co-workers demonstrated improved work capacity in some high-altitude natives after removal of blood, either by simple phlebotomy or by hemodilution[3] (Winslow et al. 1979). These studies showed, from clear physiologic measurements, that high-altitude natives at 4,300 meters are compromised in their exercise capacity and that polycythemia does not serve to compensate. The results support the opinions of Barcroft, Monge C., and Whittembury that humans are essentially cut from a sea-level mold. Acclimatization to high altitudes occurs only in the sense of "tolerance" to extreme environmental exposure. There is a wide range of abilities for this adaptation, however, just as there is a wide range of abilities for athletic performance at sea level. In this sense, Monge M. was also correct in his belief in acclimatization. The key seems to be in biological variability, and its manifestation under the stress of hypoxia.

1.8   Leadville, Colorado

In the late 1940s, Carlos Monge M. visited the Colorado mining town of Leadville, Colorado (altitude 3,100 m), where he observed cases of chronic mountain sickness similar to those at higher altitudes in the Andes. Since that time, a number of Peruvian scientists have worked in the laboratories of the cardiovascular division of the Department of Medicine, University of Colorado, in collaboration with North American scientists. Dr. Robert

Grover, now professor emeritus, began his work in Leadville in 1960, primarily on pulmonary hypertension. Grover and his colleagues initially surveyed the population of Leadville and found that polycythemia was a very common problem. They were struck with the finding of normal hematocrit values as well, hence they became intrigued with the problem of individual variation.

Also intrigued by this variation, Dr. John Weil, of the University of Colorado, initiated a series of important studies on the control of ventilation. Weil found that the hypoxic ventilatory response was reduced in Leadville natives, in agreement with the results of Chiodi, Severinghaus, and Sørensen, but with the additional important observation that this "blunting" is acquired, not inherited. Weil and co-workers found a correlation between arterial desaturation and hematocrit, but they could not establish that the blunted ventilatory response to hypoxia was the causative factor in the development of polycythemia. This led to the important studies of Kryger and co-workers on arterial saturation during sleep. They found that in subjects which excessive polycythemia, saturation fell to very low levels in sleep, but that desaturation was not correlated with hypoxic ventilatory response when awake. Although much remains to be learned about the control of blood oxygenation during sleep, the current feeling of the Colorado group is that loss of the hypoxic ventilatory response per se does not cause problems, but that it permits desaturation from other causes to persist, as in obesity, chronic obstructive lung disease, and upper airway obstruction. As will be seen in subsequent chapters, the symptom complex of chronic mountain sickness may be a vicious cycle composed of sleep hypoxia, depressed ventilation, polycythemia, pulmonary engorgement, lung stiffness, further hypoxia, and so forth.

1.9   Chile

Although the Chilean Andes was the location of the important 1935 expedition, high-altitude research in Chile was limited until 1977, when a research center was created at Chuquicamata mining company (Centro de Investigaciones Ecobiológicas y Médicas de Altura, de Codelco-Chile. Roy H. Glover Hospital, Chuquicamata; director, Dr. Raimundo Santolaya). This center is situated at 2,800 meters and has an environment similar to that of Leadville, Colorado. It has the great advantage of being located near the Chilean altiplano, where populations of isolated Andean natives can be studied at altitudes of about 3,800 meters. Santolaya (Santolaya et al. 1981) compared hematocrits in a large number of nonminers from the Chuquicamata with two populations of Andean natives, finding significant differences between communities at similar altitudes. He concluded that residents of the altiplano have lower hematocrits than residents of the westernized Chuquicamata, despite living close to 1,000 meters higher. He suggested that factors other than altitude are important. These include obesity, sedentarism, smoking, and environmental contamination, conditions that are nearly absent on the altiplano. Santolaya considers the definition of physiologic levels of polycythemia and excessive polycythemia to be a relative matter.

The Argentinian Andes were also the location of pioneer studies by the physiologist Hugo Chiodi in the Instituto de Biología de la Altura, Universidad Nacional de Tucumán, S. S. de Jujuy, Argentina. Chiodi (1957) performed important studies with newcomers and long-term residents, and he was also interested in chronic mountain sickness. He personally became sensitive to high altitude and developed hemiparesis whenever he went to high places. His insistence on calling these episodes chronic mountain sickness was an irritation to Hurtado, but it amused the younger investigators who worked with him.

1.10   Geographic Differences between Asia and South America

One remarkable aspect of Monge's disease is its apparent rarity in the Himalayas: no case has been described in the Western literature. There has been much speculation about this, including the hypothesis that South American Indians have lived at high altitudes for only twenty thousand to thirty thousand years, whereas the high Tibetan plateau has been populated for at least five hundred thousand years (Monge C. and Whittembury 1982). Thus, perhaps insufficient time has passed for evolutionary adaptation in Andean natives. Beall has even suggested a fundamental physiologic difference between these two groups in regard to erythropoiesis (Beall 1983). It is also possible, however, that the two regions differ in other environmental factors or that the populations have different diets or migratory habits. Moreover, Himalayan natives have not been studied in as much detail as their Andean counterparts.

One of the authors observed a young high-altitude Sherpa porter on the 1981 American Medical Expedition to Everest who had a hematocrit of 72 percent and typical symptoms of chronic mountain sickness, which he had suffered for several years. However, a diagnosis of chronic mountain sickness requires the exclusion of pulmonary disease or other causes of secondary polycythemia, which would require a more extensive clinical evaluation. This was not possible in that remote place.

Geographic differences between the Andes and the Himalayas could be important in the apparent difference in the incidence of chronic mountain sickness. The Andean range is situated on a continental divide; the Himalayan range is not. Therefore, the rivers of the Himalayas have cut deep gorges between the mountains, so most of the passes are at lower altitudes than those of the Andes (Gilbert 1983b). This means that permanent settlements can be established at lower altitudes in the Himalayas, even though the mountains are much higher. Further careful comparative studies of these two areas may lead to more information of great interest.

CHAPTER TWO

High-Altitude Natives and Chronic Mountain Sickness

The Quechua-speaking peoples in South America probably date from a downward migration of Asian people from the Bering Strait forty thousand to one hundred thousand years ago (MacNeish 1971). This population reached its maximum during the Inca empire, suffered a catastrophic decline after the Spanish conquest, and has now regained its earlier number. Quechua-speaking people can be found throughout modern Peru, much of Ecuador, and in northern Argentina and Chile.

Because the Incas had no written history, details about their early civilization are sparse, but they were probably strictly mountain dwellers until ten thousand to fifteen thousand years ago, when communication began between the highland and coastal communities. At that time, more efficient economies were developed that exploited both the agricultural potential of the altiplano and the abundance of fish in the coastal waters.

The Inca rulers exerted considerable control over population movements. They were careful to limit vertical migration because of the known difficulties of highlanders to adapt to the coastal desert environment, as well as the reverse (Monge M. 1948, 1–25). They also relocated many communities after conquest, probably to facilitate domination. But this practice also had the effect of preventing extreme genetic isolation (Garruto and Hoff 1976). The Spaniards further relocated many natives to exploit them as labor for the mines. At present, modern railroads and highways link many of even the most remote communities in the Andean altiplano with sea-level population centers, so the genetic homogeneity cannot be easily characterized. Nevertheless, in a careful study of genetic traits in Nuñoa, Peru, Garruto estimated that, for this community, the rate of immigration into the population, thus the gene flow, is only 10 percent to 15 percent per generation, but the immigration is mainly from neighboring communities (Garruto and Hoff 1976). He estimated the rate of emigration from the community to be about 2.5 percent and did not regard the combined figures as affecting the overall gene pool significantly.

The Inca rulers were careful not to allow prolonged interchange of high- and low-altitude residents. It was the practice of the Inca to renew the armies of the coastal regions often so that no highland native would have to remain there for a prolonged period (Monge M. and Monge C. 1966, 73). This practice derived from the known fact that after such relocation many diseases were more common.

The birth of the first Spaniard in South America did not take place until fifty years after the founding of Potosí, Peru (4,500 m) Monge M. and Monge C. 1966, 74). This birth, called the miracle of Saint Nicholas of Tolentino, illustrates that acclimatization has a long-term dimension. In fact, this problem of Spanish infertility was one of the reasons the capital of Peru was transferred from Jauja (3,300 m) to Lima (sea level) by Pizarro. As described by Father Cobo in 1897, (Monge M. and Monge C. 1966, 73–74).

> The Indians are healthiest and where they multiply the most prolifically is in the same cold air-tempers, which is quite the reverse of what happens to children of the Spaniards, most of whom when born in such regions do not survive. But where it is most noticeable is in those who have half, a quarter, or any admixture of Indian blood; better they survive and grow; so that it is now a common saying based on everyday experience that babies having some Indian in them run less risk in the cold regions than those not having the admixture.

These brief historical reflections are the only indications available for the genetic adaptation of high-altitude Andean natives. In the future it should be possible to exploit the new technology of cell culture and restriction endonuclease mapping to obtain further information about the genetic makeup of high-altitude populations and whether they may be genetically adapted to the environmental conditions of the mountains. The well-documented infertility of the early Spaniards is an intriguing indication that some type of long-term acclimatization, whether it is genotypic or phenotypic, takes place.

2.1   High-Altitude Natives

High-altitude natives are subject to many stresses; cold, ionizing radiation, dry air, and hypoxia are just a few of them. In addition, their diet is different from that of populations living at lower altitudes (see, for example, Frisancho, Borkan, and Klayman 1976). Nevertheless, it seems that the general body habitus of these natives is not different from that of their lowland counterparts. To compare, however, it is necessary to select groups at different altitudes who share as many characteristics of race, diet, occupation, and age as possible.

High-altitude natives are not necessarily different from lowlanders of the same race in regard to height and weight (table 2.1). However, Indian and Sherpa natives of both high and low altitudes are significantly taller than Quechua Indians, while their weights are about the same. Furthermore, the Aymara Indians of the Bolivian and Chilean altiplano (altitude 3,900 m) are taller and heavier than the Quechua Indians.

One might expect the body composition values of high-altitude natives to differ from sea-level values, but data are fragmentary. In one study of Ladakhis (Bharadwaj et al. 1977), the high-altitude natives were found to have significantly more bone mineral than did related sea-level subjects.

Table 2.1. A comparison of the heights and weights of subjects at low and high altitudes

Race	Location	N	Height (cm)	Weight (kg)	Source
Quechua	Nuñoa (3,900 m)	95	159.2 ± 5.7	55.5 ± 5.4	(1)
	Morococha (4,500 m)	478	159.0	55.4	(2)
	Chiclayo (sl)	44	156.6 ± 6.2	—	(3)
Aymara	Isluga (3,900 m)	43	165.0	60.4	(4)
Indian	Ladakh (3,920 m)	45	163.0 ± 4.8	55.5 ± 4.8	(5)
	Madras (sl)	30	166.9 ± 6.8	55.9 ± 5.7	(5)
Sherpa	Khumbu (3,800 m)	68	162.3 ± 7.6	55.7 ± 5.6	(6)
	Kalimpong (sl)	166	158.5 ± 5.6	50.4 ± 5.4	(6)

Sources: (1) Frisancho 1976; (2) Hurtado 1932a; (3) Lasker 1962; (4) Santolaya 1983; (5) Bharadwaj, Verma, Zachariah et al. 1977; and (6) Gupta and Basu 1981.

This difference was felt to be a result of the stimulation of lifelong accelerated erythropoiesis. Body water, fat, and lean body mass were, however, not distinguishable.

A very important difference in body configuration appears to be in the dimensions of the chest. The South American Indian typically has a "barrel" configuration, while Himalayan natives do not. Careful comparative studies have been carried out (Beall 1982) to support this subjective impression. The relationship between vital capacities, anthropometric dimensions, and ventilation will be discussed in detail in chapter 6.

2.2 Clinical Features of Chronic Mountain Sickness

Some high-altitude subjects, particularly in the Andes, develop excessive symptomatic polycythemia (chronic mountain sickness), a clinical entity that lacks clear definition (see chap. 1). The subjects, usually adult males, generally suffer from symptoms of an expanded blood volume. They are likely to complain of decreased exercise tolerance and bone pain and are easily fatigued by the lightest work. They characteristically complain of dyspnea, insomnia, dizziness, headache, and confusion, and occasionally they report a history of hemoptysis. The impairment of mental function was strikingly apparent in the first description of the syndrome (Monge M. 1925) and is typified by a middle-aged man the authors studied in Cerro de Pasco, whose hematocrit was 72 percent (fig. 2.1). Asked to pedal a cycle ergometer to measure his exercise capacity, he was unable to coordinate the movements of his legs to turn the pedals. He complained that he understood the instructions but was unable to comply. After his hematocrit was reduced to 45 percent by phlebotomy, he was able to perform the test without difficulty.

On physical examination, the subjects appear strikingly cyanotic (fig.

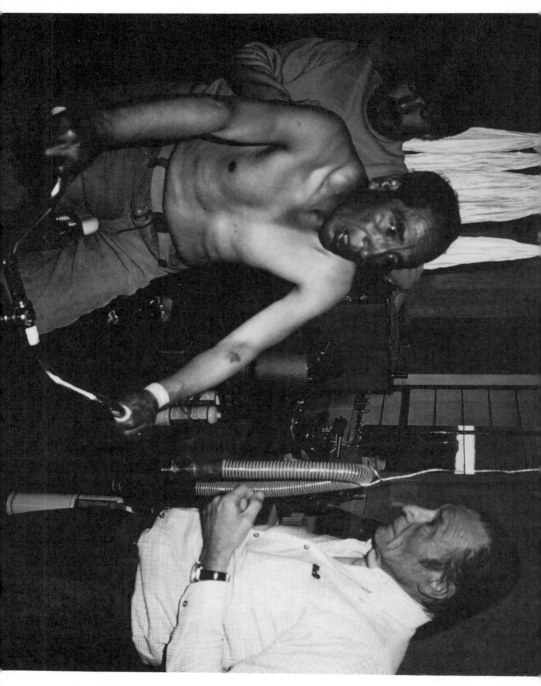

Figure 2.1. A typical subject with chronic mountain sickness. This man's hematocrit was 72 percent.

2.1). This appearance is due to a combination of polycythemia, hemoglobin desaturation, and deep pigmentation of areas of the skin exposed to the sun. The face and hands, in particular, may seem almost black. The mucous membranes of the mouth and the throat are deeply cyanotic. Many subjects do not appear to be alert and sometimes have a fixed gaze. The eyes are watery; the conjunctivae are markedly hyperemic, with prominent capillary patterns; and the retinal vessels are dilated and engorged. The chest has a characteristic "barrel" configuration and appears to be in fixed hyperexpansion. Indeed, anthropomorphic studies (Hurtado 1932a) have shown this configuration to be characteristic of Andean natives in general and not restricted to subjects with chronic mountain sickness. The cardiac pulmonic second sound is frequently accentuated, and systolic murmurs are common (Peñaloza and Sime 1971). Occasional subjects may have moderate symptomatic diastolic, and sometimes systolic, hypertension as well.

Radiographic examination of the chest reveals increased cardiac size, mainly due to right ventricular hypertrophy. However, the right atrium and pulmonary artery often appear to be enlarged also. The pulmonary vasculature is engorged, and left ventricular hypertrophy occurs in many advanced cases. The electrocardiogram often shows a p-pulmonale pattern, right QRS axis deviation, increased R wave in the left chest leads, and a biphasic T wave in the right chest leads.

As the age of the subject increases, more evidence of congestive heart failure is likely to be found. This includes marked dyspnea, both at rest and after even mild exertion, prominent distension of surface veins, peripheral edema, and progressive cardiac dilation.

2.3 The First Recorded Case of Chronic Mountain Sickness

Many of the clinical findings in cases of chronic mountain sickness are those of polycythemia and an expanded blood volume. Polycythemia vera is a syndrome recognized since 1892 to occur at sea level (Váquez 1892; Osler 1903), and it was not initially clear that the high-altitude cases of polycythemia were due to hypoxia. In 1925, Carlos Monge M. reported to the Peruvian Academy of Medicine what he believed was the first case of polycythemia ever to be described in Peru (Monge M. 1925). His patient, a resident of Cerro de Pasco (4,300 m), had a red cell count of 8.86 million, considerably higher than those of other residents of that altitude. The case report is unique because of the remarkable acuity of the subject's own description of his symptoms, particularly the characteristic impaired mental function. For this reason, and because heretofore it has been unavailable in English translation, the report is quoted in detail here.

Clinical history: Mr. N. N., age 38. Occupation engineer, status married. Weight 156 pounds.

Chief complaint: Patient called attention to the change of color of the skin and of the face.

Past history: No syphilis or gonorrhea. Normal birth, some childhood disease: measles, mumps, bronchitis, typhoid at the age of 8, jaundice at 11.

History of present illness: In September he took a trip to Huarochirí;[1] when he arrived in this place he felt acute pain in the lower extremities, which was diagnosed as rheumatism. He was forced to return to the capital, where it took two months for him to recover completely. In June 1909 he went to Cerro de Pasco, where he settled and lived in good health. The following data are taken from a written report administered by him.

"During 1910 I slept very little, or rather I spent sleepless nights. In the first month of the year 1911 I reached a point where I lay down only one night of the week, sometimes two, and slept for about two hours in the daytime. I worked every day from 7 to 10 am. I noticed that by 10 my work was completely wrong; when I recovered my lucidity I confirmed the mistakes that I had committed. I was unaware of what I was doing when I worked. After that time, life became normal. Seven months after being installed at the smelter, I suffered once again from a bout of acute rheumatism and remained in bed for three days, without being able to move my neck. (It should be mentioned once again that in this attack there was no disturbance at all in the joints, while the disease was reduced to acute pain.) I returned to Cerro to live the life of a clubman until October 1912, when I suffered from strong pain around the waist, which did not allow me to stand up. I had to stay in bed for five days without any relief; after five days I suddenly felt better and returned to my occupation as if nothing had happened. One month later I got married and returned to my ordinary life. In February 1913 I started feeling pain once again in my bones, especially in the lower extremities. The doctor treated me, but there was no improvement, and he recommended that I come to the coast. I was practically crippled, or rather I had to use sticks to walk because my feet could not support my body (my weight had dropped from 163 to 131 pounds). In this state I left Cerro. When I reached Matucana I left one stick in Chosica and the other in Desamparados and I was able to walk perfectly, although pain remained in all the bones of the body. I stayed for a month in Lima without the pains disappearing. I went to Huacachina, took cod liver oil, and after 65 baths returned to Cerro, cured.[2] I no longer felt any of those symptoms except occasionally pains in the bones of the lower extremities, as though I had been tied, and I attributed no greater importance to it.

"During the last three years, I have noticed a purple color of my face persisting even in Lima for fifteen days; probably from 1917 this color returned but did not persist in Lima. Five years ago a dentist showed me the presence at the bottom of the palate of a wine-colored strip. In recent years congested lips, eyes, and throat were most noticeable. In September 1923 I started to feel nausea lasting for a short time and occasionally repeatedly, alternating with a cloudiness of vision that prevented me from seeing in one eye and sometimes in both, and in one case I went blind for five minutes. The doctor recommended that I come to Lima to consult an ophthalmologist, which I did. He gave me glasses and recommended that I see a physician. After fifteen days in the capital without feeling any symptoms I returned to Cerro, and once again the same phenomenon occurred; it disappeared when I returned to Lima (December 1923)."

Up to now it had been impossible to obtain a description by a talented patient who described his case with the certainty of a clinician. It should be added, moreover, that by going deeply into the interrogation it was possible to observe that the patient had suffered from discrete epistaxes, that he had a sensation of losing his consciousness in cases of sudden effort, that the osteocopic pains, in indefinite location for him, did not leave him, and that occasionally he suffered from generalized acute pains that forced him to take absolute rest, after which they disappeared and he returned to normal life, agitated by these disturbances.

Physical examination: The patient is a man of good constitution, who has a deeply marked aspect typical of those coming from the Sierra although he may be in Lima for fifteen days. Attention is called to the purple color that he described, the wine red color of his face, more accentuated at the cheeks, chin, and particularly the ears. The visible mucosae also have the same characteristics, while the nasal openings and the edges of the lips show a more marked wine color and the eyes are enormously congested with palpebral lines that seem to shed blood. An identical color is observed in the skin of the extremities, particularly that of the upper limbs, and, although the contrast between the skin of these regions and of the body is visible, it may be estimated that the teguments as a whole offer a reddish tonality that the patient asserts does not correspond to the former color of his normal skin. The ramifications of the veins are easily noticeable and are easily drawn over all the extremities and the veins of the forehead.

Respiratory system: The nasal mucosae have a violaceous appearance. The same color is seen on the laryngeal membranes. Apart from it, nothing abnormal is noticed. The Traube space has a slight compactness in its external portion.

Digestive system: the mouth offers a color similar to that of the mucosae of the nose. Attention is drawn particularly to a wide red strip that covers all the posterior part of the mucosa of the palate, ending in a perfectly outlined edge. The pharyngeal mucosa shows a similar aspect. The rest of the examination did not indicate anything important.

Circulatory system: Easily noticeable venous network over the entire body surface, particularly at the extremities. The examination of the capillaries at the level of the ungueal edge makes it possible to see them tortuous, dilated, and enlarged. The maximum tension is 15, the minimum tension 8.

Lymphatic system: Discrete lymph node enlargement. Spleen increased in volume by percussion.

Genitourinary system: Normal
Nervous system: Normal
Locomotor system: Normal
Organs of senses: Examination of the retina. Dr. Dammert found no abnormalities other than the very congested venous vessels of the retina. Moreover, the patient is astigmatic and somewhat hypermetropic in the left eye. Dr. Dammert provided the information that he has noted in his records identical lesions in the patient, whom we had examined previously in 1922.

Analysis of the blood (Dr. Monteverde)

Red cells	8,860,000
Leucocytes	10,000
Polymorphonuclear leucocytes	62%
Lymphocytes	30%
Mononuclear cells	8%
Anisocytosis	slight
Coagulation time	11 minutes
Viscosity of the blood	8 (Hess)
Hemoglobin	21.10 (Sahli)
Azotemia	0.03%
Wasserman reaction	negative
Granulocytes	normal

Analysis of the urine

Volume	1500 cc
Specific gravity	1.019
Reaction	acid
Color	4 Vogel
Odor	Sui generis
Appearance	clear
Sediment	none
Urea	15.13%
Chlorides	14.63%
Phosphates	1.80%
Uric acid	0.46%
Abnormal elements	none
Spectroscopic examination	normal
Examination of the sediment:	Rare leukocytes, vesical cells and amorphous earthlike phosphates.

This sickness and other related ones that altitude can create can cause temporary or transient work invalidism. The need for us to have a better knowledge of the national pathology incites us to propose the following conclusion for the consideration of the Academy of Medicine: In view of the health disturbances that may be caused by a stay in high altitudes, the academy presents to the medical body of these regions, the scientific institutions, and the study of the poly-cythemic syndrome so as to evaluate the seriousness of the damage that may be caused and to recommend therefore provisions as required.

It is not clear whether at the time of this report Monge believed this to be a case of Váquez's disease (polycythemia vera) or of a new syndrome charac-teristic of life in the high mountains. In his introduction to the report, he stated, "The fact of the prolongation of hyperglobulia[3] for a certain time in people coming from Cerro de Pasco and in general from regions located on the high plateaus of the Sierra is very well known. It is for the least a syndrome which occurs often when reaching these altitudes and which is designated by the name of Macolca." However, he apparently did not be-lieve it was a normal reaction to the altitude:

> It is important to mention that there are persons predisposed to this type of manifestation and that very often each time they go up to those places the painful symptoms become more marked. . . . On the other hand, the existence of cases of the Váquez's disease could be suspected in regions located at 5,000 meters altitude above sea level, seeing that there is no other pathogenic cause more obvious than altitude to excite abnormally the bone marrow. And actually the reports which I have been able to collect on various occasions have revealed to me a syndrome characterized by osteocopic[4] pains, called rheumatic, of such inten-sity that they cause the patient to stay in bed and that they only improved when they came down to Lima; the preservation of a reddish and congested appearance of the face in spite of a long stay on the coast and many subjective manifestations as signs of it; all this is sufficient to suspect the possibility of a case of Váquez's disease.

Monge was also impressed with the bony pain, which he believed to be evidence for marrow involvement: "There is no doubt at all about the role which the marrow of the bones must be playing in its determination and certainly there must be work arising through the spirit of scientific research of the doctors in these regions giving a conclusive demonstration about the real cause."

2.4 Pathologic Findings

The lack of distinctive gross pathologic findings in cases of chronic moun-tain sickness sparked a controversy among observers of the disorder. The problem is that very few data are available and, because no clear single etiol-ogy has been established, some authors have advocated their own different points of view to the exclusion of others.

Fernán-Zegarra and Lazo-Toboada (1961) provided the first autopsy description of a person who had been diagnosed as suffering from chronic mountain sickness. The subject was a thirty-five-year-old man, a native of 4,300 meters altitude, who suffered from progressive dyspnea and congestive heart failure and who died in Aerequipa (altitude 2,400 m). An autopsy showed a heart that weighed 750 grams, with biventricular hypertrophy. In the lungs, marked peripheral arterial hypertrophy with medial thickening was noted. The subject, who also suffered from lordoscoliosis, died of intractable cardiac insufficiency.

Two additional cases were reported in 1969 (Reátegui-López 1969). These patients also had right ventricular hypertrophy and pulmonary peripheral arterial thickening. Both obese, they, too, died with severe cardiac insufficiency.

Perhaps the best studied and final case was described by Arias-Stella (Arias-Stella, Kruger, and Recavarren 1973). This patient was a forty-eight-year-old woman who had lived her entire life at Cerro de Pasco. She had a clinical picture typical of chronic mountain sickness, with cyanosis, peripheral edema, hemoptysis, and pulmonary edema. Her hemoglobin concentration was 21.6 grams/deciliter, and she also had pronounced kyphoscoliosis. An autopsy revealed a heart that weighed 320 grams, with right ventricular hypertrophy. The liver, kidneys, brain, and lungs were all congested, and bilateral pleural effusions were found. Histologic examination of the lungs showed intense muscularization of the peripheral arterial vessels and intimal sclerosis. This subject also had a nodular goiter and adrenal hyperplasia, both presumed to be incidental findings. In 1967, Monge M. commented on the case, "Evidently this is a case of chronic mountain sickness, primary because of loss of acclimatization, or secondary due to other causes. I have seen similar cases but have not dared to report them because of insufficient clinical data. I remember one patient who developed extreme anasarca and eliminated her edema simply by coming down to the coast" (quoted in Arias-Stella and Topilsky 1971).

This opinion seems to have stimulated Arias-Stella to classify cases of excessive polycythemia according to presumed etiology:

Type I. Failure to acclimatize. These subjects are born at sea level and fail to acclimatize. Monge M. alluded in general terms to subjects of this type (Monge M. 1942), but gave no details of specific cases. Arias-Stella drew a parallel between these cases and Brisket disease of cattle, described by Hecht (Hecht et al. 1962).

Type II. "Monge's syndrome." These subjects, born either at sea level or at high altitude, appear to acclimatize for a time, then lose acclimatization because of superimposition of some underlying disease upon chronic hypoxia. These underlying processes, illustrated by the cases whose autopsy material is available, include obesity, kyphoscoliosis, neuromuscular disease of the chest, or emphysema. Arias-Stella drew the analogy between Type II chronic mountain sickness and "primary hypoventilation syndrome" occurring at sea level (Rodman and Chase 1959; Richter, West, and Fishman 1957; Bergofsky and Holtzman 1967).

Type III. "Monge's disease." This is the type believed to have been described by Monge M. (1928), and further studied by Hurtado (1942) and Peñaloza (Peñaloza, Sime, and Ruiz 1971). They proposed that the subjects, high-altitude natives, lost their peripheral chemoreceptor sensitivity and developed progressive hypoventilation. The studies by Severinghaus and Carcelén (1964) were felt to support this mechanism.

Arias-Stella reviewed the above cases and presented his classification at a symposium sponsored by the Ciba Foundation, "High Altitude Physiology: Cardiac and Respiratory Aspects," held in honor of Hurtado (Arias-Stella and Topilsky 1971). At that time, he believed that all cases in whom autopsies had been performed were examples of types I and II chronic mountain sickness. He apparently felt, however, that type III cases do exist but had never come to autopsy.

In the discussion of Arias-Stella's paper, the Liverpool pathologist Donald Heath challenged the existence of Monge's disease (type III). He cited the inadequacy of the methods used to prepare tissues for histologic examination and suggested that all chronic mountain sickness is due to impaired lung function at high altitudes. To this challenge Hurtado responded, "I don't agree with the view that we are not justified in speaking of Monge's disease until we know its pathological anatomy. On such a vein we would be forced to eliminate most mental diseases" (Peñaloza, Sime, and Ruiz 1971).

This discussion and the confrontation that followed seem to have arisen from the fact that for many years attention was focused on the role of the lung in O_2 transport. Most of these studies were carried out before much was known about the neural control of ventilation and the desaturation that can occur during sleep in some hypoxic subjects. Moreover, little was known about the control of erythropoiesis and the effects of erythropoietin, the effect of blood viscosity on cardiac output, or even of the control of O_2 transport by red cells and the role of hemoglobin O_2 affinity. Hurtado's comment was prophetic in that chronic mountain sickness is probably more complex than initially believed, and it would not be particularly helpful to ignore a clinical syndrome because a characteristic pathologic anatomy cannot be described. Subsequent chapters of this volume review current thinking about the involvement of various organs and control systems and attempt a synthesis of O_2 transport mechanisms based on information that has become available since the 1971 Ciba symposium.

2.5   The Carotid Bodies

One of the most provocative findings from pathologic studies of high-altitude natives is enlargement of the carotid bodies. When Arias-Stella compared forty-two subjects in Lima with forty-two in Cerro de Pasco who came to postmortem examination, he found that in the high-altitude natives the carotid bodies could be as large as 1.5 centimeters in diameter (Arias-Stella 1969). The increase was due to hyperplasia of type I glomic cells. He also noted vascular engorgement, as well as intense vacuolization of the chief cells. Atlhough it was observed that the carotid body size and weight generally increased with age, Arias-Stella concluded that chronic hypoxia probably stimulated the hyperplasia in the high-altitude residents (Arias-Stella and Recavarren 1973).

The carotid bodies constitute the peripheral chemoreceptor site for the regulation of respiration in hypoxia. However, in spite of intensive investigations, the mechanism by which the stimulus (hypoxia) is translated into a response (neural stimulation of ventilation) is not completely known (Biscoe 1971). It is clear that chronic exposure to high altitudes leads to hyperplasia of the glomic cells: the incidence of chemodectomas is ten times higher in high-altitude natives than in sea-level subjects (Saldaña, Salem, and Travezán 1973). These unusual tumors are also associated with chronic obstructive lung disease at sea level (Chedid and Jao 1974). In addition, animals native to high altitudes have larger carotid bodies, and pathologic examination of them has shown proliferation and vacuolization of the light variant of the glomic chief cells (Edwards, Heath, and Harris 1971).

Proof of a cause-and-effect relationship between hypoxia and enlarged carotid bodies has been elusive. In autopsy studies of subjects with chronic obstructive lung disease, Edwards and co-workers found a correlation between the size of the carotid bodies and the degree of right ventricular hypertrophy. However, in these subjects, the right and left ventricular hypertrophies were also correlated, so a direct cause-and-effect relationship was uncertain. More recently it has been found that rats develop right ventricular hypertrophy after removal of the carotid bodies and that removal abolishes the hypoxic ventilatory drive (Chiocchio et al. 1984).

These studies and others suggest that the carotid bodies may prove to be central in the etiology of chronic mountain sickness. A working hypothesis may be formulated that, because of chronic exposure, the response of these organs is blunted, resulting in the typical reduced hypoxic ventilatory response that characterizes high-altitude natives. It remains only to explore the relationship between blunted hypoxic ventilatory regulation and erythropoiesis.

CHAPTER THREE

Red Cells, Red Cell and Plasma Volumes, and Their Regulation

Since Viault noted for the first time that the number of red cells increases at high altitudes, descriptions of acclimatization to high altitudes have cited polycythemia as one of the principal reactions of normal humans. Thus, with regard to red cells, "More is better" is the accepted axiom. However, polycythemia is the cause of symptoms in high-altitude natives with chronic mountain sickness. These fascinating cases have now raised a doubt, shared by many physiologists and high-altitude physicians: excessive poly-cythemia may be maladaptive and an "optimal" hematocrit exists for a given altitude (Aggio et al. 1972). Sea-level studies have demonstrated that cerebral blood flow is reduced when the hematocrit exceeds 45 percent (Humphrey et al. 1979), perhaps explaining the cerebral symptoms in chronic mountain sickness. Moreover, there is growing concern that excessive polycythemia in sojourners at high altitudes also may be maladaptive (Messmer 1975).

Perhaps the traditional opinion of the value of a high hematocrit came from sea-level experience. Patients with anemia may be incapacitated by weakness, and some studies have suggested that athletic performance can be improved by autologous transfusions, or "blood doping" (Buick et al. 1980; Woodson 1984). This is obviously a very complex matter, requiring consideration of many physiologic variables, including cardiac, pulmonary, and vascular properties, in addition to the capacity of the blood to transport oxygen. This chapter reviews observations on the degree of erythroid activity in high-altitude natives, their red cell properties, the normal mechanism of erythropoiesis at high altitudes, and the relationships between red cell and plasma volume. Subsequent chapters consider interacting properties of other organ systems.

3.1 The Hemoglobin and Hematocrit Values

The traditional view is that erythropoiesis is one of the main adaptations to high altitudes. Nevertheless, the relationship between the stimulus, hypoxia, and the response, polycythemia, still is unclear. There is no doubt that extremely high hematocrits can be found in high-altitude native populations and that mean hematocrits and hemoglobins are higher in these subjects, but the value of polycythemia as a compensatory mechanism was questioned even in the pioneering observations of Viault, and objective evidence of its physiologic advantage is still lacking. Arguments in favor of the benefit of an increased red-cell volume have been mainly theoretical, not experimental.

3.1.1   Normal Values

A major problem in studying polycythemia at high altitudes is the lack of normal values for hemoglobin or hematocrit that can be compared with sea-level data.[1] In normal sea-level subjects, hematocrit and hemoglobin concentrations increase with age up to about twenty years, but the actual values depend on sex and nutritional status. Figure 3.1 shows the dependence of hematocrit on age in approximately eighteen thousand normal persons surveyed by the U.S. National Center for Health Statistics between 1976 and 1980 (Fulwood 1982). In males, after increasing to age twenty, the hematocrit tends to be level up to the maximum age of the survey, seventy-four years. In females, the values continue to increase, perhaps reflecting the cessation of menstrual blood loss in later life. Still, the mean postmenopausal hematocrit in women is lower than it is in men. Very little is known about whether or not this difference occurs in high-altitude natives, because most surveys report only data from males.

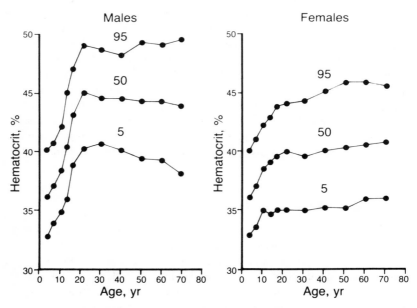

Figure 3.1.   Normal hematocrit values at sea level as a function of age for 7,426 normal males and 7,704 normal females in the United States. The 95th, 50th, and 5th percentile values are indicated. (Data from Fulwood 1982, with permission).

A most curious feature of the normal data in figure 3.1 is that there is a perceptible increase in hematocrit with age after twenty years within the top 5 percentile. In contrast, for the bottom 5 percentile, there is a distinct decrease with age. This observation raises the question of whether there is a normal range of marrow sensitivity, such that those with sensitive marrows respond more briskly with age than the average person to the normal decrease in PaO_2 (see chap. 6). If so, this would have important consequences for prediction of which individuals may be at risk for developing chronic mountain sickness at high altitude. Whatever the explanation, the data illustrate the fact that there is a wide variation in normal hematocrits, and it would be very important to understand what determines the hematocrit within this normal range.

An attractive hypothesis might be that there are different erythropoietic "set points" for different individuals. For example, a person's sea-level hematocrit could determine his erythropoietic response to acute hypoxia. That is, if the hematocrit is in the high-normal range at sea level, then the response to hypoxia might also be in the high-normal range. Perhaps if we understood why a person's "set point" for hematocrit is high, normal, or low, we would understand who would be susceptible to chronic mountain sickness.

3.1.2   High-Altitude Values

Data as extensive as the sea-level figures discussed above are not available for high-altitude populations, but limited surveys have been carried out. Normal hematocrit values were studied in Leadville, Colorado, in 355 boys and girls aged ten to eighteen years (Treger, Shaw, and Grover 1965). These investigators found that hematocrit increased as it does at sea level in this age range, but that all values were higher at all ages. No evidence was found for iron deficiency in either boys or girls, but no comparable data are available for older age groups. This study shows that the hypoxic stimulus affects persons of all ages.

Whittembury and Monge C. (1972) suggested that hematocrit increases with age in adult natives of the Peruvian Andes. On obtaining hematocrit values in a number of subjects studied sequentially at different ages, they observed that the hematocrit increased with time (fig. 3.2). They suggested that chronic mountain sickness is an accentuated tendency to polycythemia that occurs normally with age. They further suggested that age-dependent polycythemia is caused by an age-dependent loss of ventilation, and arterial hypoxemia. However, Chiodi (1978) pointed out that many of Whittembury and Monge's values that correlated with age were in subjects whose age was less than twenty, and in these subjects an increase is to be expected (cf. fig. 3.1). Examination of mass plots of hematocrit versus age is probably

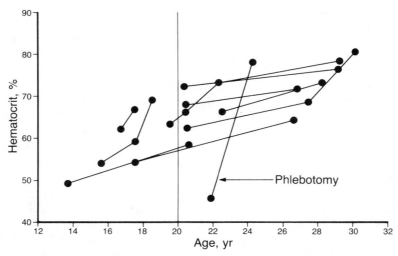

Figure 3.2.   The hematocrit as a function of age in subjects in Cerro de Pasco (4,300 m) and Morococha (4,500 m). The vertical line indicates the age at which adult values are expected (see fig. 3.1). The subject whose hematocrit changed the most had undergone phlebotomy at the younger age. (Whittembury and Monge C. 1972)

useless, since the variation in hematocrit is so great in high-altitude populations. The hypothesis that chronic mountain sickness results from the normal aging process, as suggested by Whittembury and Monge C., will require longitudinal data collected over many years.

3.1.3   Geographic Differences

High hematocrits and hemoglobins traditionally have been observed in northern Peru, Bolivia, Chile, the North American Rocky Mountains, and on the Tibetan plateau. Lower, almost sea-level, normal values have been observed in southern Peru and Nepal. Moreover, in some instances, the same authors have reported different values depending on the site of their studies, and significant differences seem to occur between Peruvian sites separated in altitude by only a few hundred meters. Some of the more complete sets of data for adult subjects are summarized in table 3.1 and figure 3.3.

Care must be exercised in interpreting comparisons between data obtained by different workers at different times. For example, in Hurtado's first study (Hurtado 1932b), he used a simple optical device to estimate hemoglobin concentration, and in the second sample (Hurtado, Merino, and Delgado 1945), he used a more sophisticated photoelectric instrument.[2] Note that the hemoglobin concentration (16.0 g/dl) he measured in 1932

Table 3.1. The hemoglobin and hematocrit values in high-altitude populations

N	Altitude (m)	Location	Hb (g/dl)	Hct (%)	Source
132	4,500	Morococha	16.0 ± 1.0	71.1 ± 7.6	(1)
175	0	Lima	16.0 ± 0.8	48.6 ± 2.3	(2)
40	3,700	Oroya	18.8 ± 1.5	54.1 ± 3.9	(2)
32	4,500	Morococha	20.8 ± 1.7	59.9 ± 5.6	(2)
46	4,500	Morococha	20.2 ± 2.3	61.0 ± 8.0	(3)
85	3,600	La Paz	18.2 ± 1.1		(4)
75	4,300	Cerro de Pasco		55.0	(3)
44	4,200	Nuñoa	17.3 ± 1.5	51.4 ± 3.9	(5)
370	10	Isla Chincha	13.8 ± 1.1		(6)
258	1,130	Chilete	13.8 ± 1.2		(6)
104	1,200	Ancos	14.8 ± 1.3		(6)
268	2,300	Arequipa	15.4 ± 1.4		(6)
408	3,475	Pasto Bueno	18.0 ± 1.5		(6)
271	3,720	Buldibuyo	17.8 ± 1.3		(6)
531	4,600	San Antonio	20.6 ± 1.7		(6)
126	3,400	Nepal	16.1 ± 1.2		(7)

Sources: (1) Hurtado 1932b; (2) Hurtado, Merino, and Delgado 1945; (3) Winslow and Monge, unpublished; (4) Arnoud et al. 1979; (5) Garruto and Dutt 1983; (6) Cosio and Yataco 1968; and (7) Beall and Reichsman 1984.

Note: All locations except Nepal are in South America.

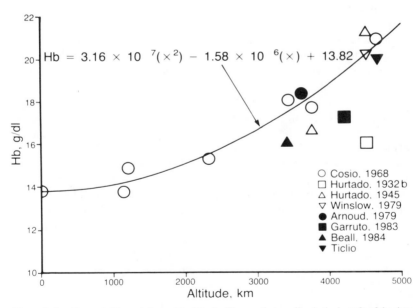

$$Hb = 3.16 \times 10^{-7}(x^2) - 1.58 \times 10^{-6}(x) + 13.82$$

○ Cosio, 1968
□ Hurtado, 1932b
△ Hurtado, 1945
▽ Winslow, 1979
● Arnoud, 1979
■ Garruto, 1983
▲ Beall, 1984
▼ Ticlio

Altitude, km

Hb, g/dl

Figure 3.3. Hemoglobin variation with altitude. The continuous line is the best fit of the data of Cosio and Yataco (1968), collected at different altitudes. While most other Peruvian observations generally agree with this line, the values from Nuñoa (*filled box*, Garruto and Dutt 1983), Morococha (*open box*, Hurtado 1932b; *open triangle*, Hurtado, Merino, and Delgado 1945), and Nepal (*filled triangle*, Beall and Reichsman 1984) are all below the line.

35

was normal by his own 1945 standard. The mean hematocrit he found at
Morococha, 61.1 percent, was much higher than his own value in 1945,
which compared well with the mean value the authors found at the same
location in 1978. Beall found apparently lower values for hemoglobin in
Nepal than those reported from Peru, but the blood was obtained by finger-
stick[3] and the measurements were made with a simple optical comparator
method (Beall and Reichsman 1984). Both Beall and Reichsman (1984) and
Garruto and Dutt (1983), also pointed out that great care in such studies must
be taken to compare the ages of the subjects, because hemoglobin concentration increases until late adolescence (cf. fig. 3.1).

Other technical considerations also must be mentioned in regard to comparative studies. First, the anticoagulant used for the blood is important.
Oxalate shrinks red cells, reducing the observed hematocrit and increasing
the apparent intracellular hemoglobin concentration. When heparin is used,
it must be provided in the proper amount or a degree of coagulation will
occur, also spuriously lowering the hematocrit. Most important, the speed
and the radius of centrifugation of the hematocrit centrifuge must be adequate for samples of blood in which the hematocrit is high (Hurtado, Merino, and Delgado 1945; Winslow, Samaja, and West 1984). Thus, definitive
comparison of different populations will probably await studies carried out
by the same team, using the same techniques and equipment.

A more serious but perhaps more interesting consideration in comparative studies is the problem of the environment. The inhabitants of Morococha and Cerro de Pasco are miners; many work underground, where
they are constantly exposed to dust in poorly ventilated mines. The authors
have toured the mine shafts in Morococha and observed that most miners
prefer not to wear the masks and breathing devices issued them by the
mining companies. Thus, silicosis is widespread, and, while we usually
claim to exclude subjects with lung disease, only sophisticated measurements of pulmonary diffusing capacity and lung mechanics would be likely
to reveal significant impairment of O_2 transfer. In contrast, the natives of
southern Peru (Nuñoa) are traditionally agrarian (Garruto and Dutt 1983)
and are not exposed to such contaminants. In northern Chile, the altiplano is
an extremely dry desert; natives there are subject to dehydration and intense
ultraviolet radiation. Nepalese natives, whose environment is relatively
unpolluted, live in homes without proper ventilation in which open fires are
used for cooking. Finally, natives of the Tibetan plateau are exposed to very
dusty air, and bronchitis (and chronic mountain sickness) are said to be
common.

An interesting example of the difficulties in comparing populations is
shown in figure 3.4. Cosio (1965) obtained blood samples from both surface
and underground workers in the neighboring towns of Ticlio and San Antonio, Peru, both primarily mining communities at 4,600 meters altitude.

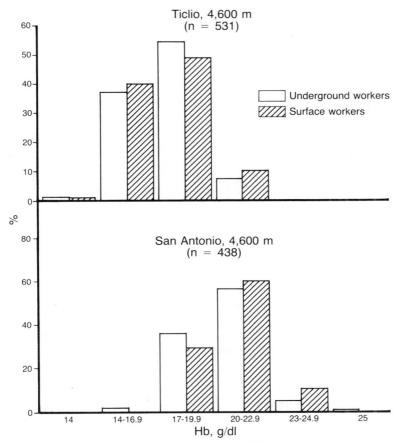

Figure 3.4. A comparison of two Peruvian communities at the same altitude. The hemo-globins at San Antonio are higher in both surface and underground workers than they are at Ticlio. (Data from Cosio 1965, with permission.)

Hematologic measurements were made using the same techniques at both sites. The number of samples was high—531 in Ticlio and 438 in San Antonio. Nevertheless, Cosio found a significantly higher mean hemo-globin concentration in the San Antonio residents, and the difference did not correlate with the place of work of the subjects, surface or underground. The subjects had the same racial background, so the difference must be due to factors that were not measured. Further studies, with a strong epidemiologic approach, will be needed to clarify these puzzling observations.

Few published studies provide data in sufficient detail to test whether the distribution of hematocrits is normal in high-altitude populations. This is not

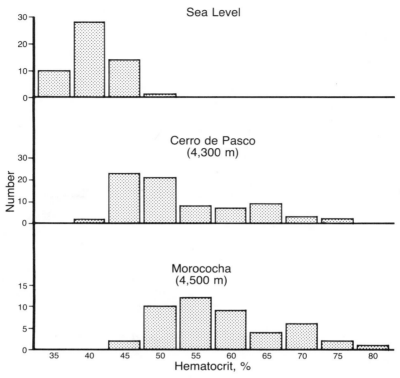

Figure 3.5. The distribution of hematocrit values at sea level, Cerro de Pasco, and Morococha. (Winslow and Monge, unpublished data.)

the fault of the authors, in most cases, but is dictated by the competition for precious journal pages. Figure 3.5 illustrates the importance of this consideration. In two high-altitude samples, Morococha and Cerro de Pasco, the distribution of subjects is skewed significantly to higher values. Thus, the median hematocrit is lower than the mean. In fact, if the median hematocrits from these two samples are compared with the low values from either Nuñoa (Garruto and Dutt 1983) or Nepal (Beall and Reichsman 1984), the putative difference between the two populations disappears! In other words, normal regulation of red cell production may be the same in natives of either location, but Morococha, in particular, seems to have a high incidence of pathologically elevated hematocrits (chronic mountain sickness). Only careful epidemiologic studies can determine whether, in fact, the incidence of chronic mountain sickness is different in various areas of the world; mass plots without analysis of the distributions are unlikely to resolve the question.

Table 3.2.   Red-cell indexes in subjects at low and high altitudes

	Sea-level Caucasian	Sea-level Indian	La Oroya Indian (3,700m)	Morococha Indian (4,500m)
	N = 175	*N = 25*	*N = 40*	*N = 32*
Rbc (10⁶/mm)	5.14 ± .34	5.00 ± .32	5.67 ± .39	6.15 ± .57
Retic (%)	.5 ± .3	—	.8 ± .5	1.5 ± .6
Hct (%)	46.8 ± 2.3	44.0 ± .3	54.1 ± 3.9	59.9 ± 5.6
Hb (g/dl)	16.0 ± .8	14.7 ± 1.0	18.8 ± 1.5	20.8 ± 1.7
MCV (fl)	91.3 ± 4.5	88.0 ± 4.6	95.2 ± 5.5	97.5 ± 6.3
MCH (pg/cell)	31.2 ± 1.9	29.6 ± 2.2	33.0 ± 2.4	33.9 ± 2.5
MCHC (g/dl)	34.1 ± 1.4	33.4 ± 1.2	34.8 ± .9	34.7 ± 1.0

Source: Hurtado, Merino, and Delgado 1945.
Note: rbc = red blood cells, Retic = reticulogytes, MVC = mean cell volume, MCH = mean cell hemoglobin, MCHC = mean cell hemoglobin concentration.

3.2   The Morphology of Red Cells at High Altitudes

Hurtado's study of men in Morococha (Hurtado 1932b) led to the conclusion that the typical red cell of high-altitude natives contains 15 percent less hemoglobin, is 16 percent larger, and, therefore, has a significantly lower mean corpuscular hemoglobin concentration (MCHC) than that of sea-level controls. He also found an increased resistance to osmotic lysis in Morococha. These results were explained by the hypothesis that the high-altitude natives had a younger population of red cells. The studies were repeated in 1945 with modern techniques (Hurtado and Delgado 1945); no significant differences between MCHC values for sea-level and two high-altitude populations were demonstrated (table 3.2).

In studies by the authors, mean corpuscular hemoglobin concentration values were compared for sea level, Cerro de Pasco, and Morococha (fig. 3.6). A larger variation occurs in the Cerro de Pasco data than in either of the other two. The mean value at Morococha (33.4 g/dl) is significantly lower (*p* = .0001) than the Cerro de Pasco value (36.0 g/dl), which is not distinguishable from the sea-level mean (Wintrobe 1981). Only in Morococha do we find a significant negative correlation between MCHC and hematocrit. These observations are in agreement with Hurtado's data of 1932 (but not 1945) and are consistent with a younger population of red cells in Morococha.

Why should the hematocrit and MCHC be so different in Morococha compared with Cerro de Pasco, when their altitudes are within 300 meters of each other? The difference is unlikely to have to do with technique because our studies were done by the same observers using the same instruments and methods. This is a question of great importance, because the similarity of

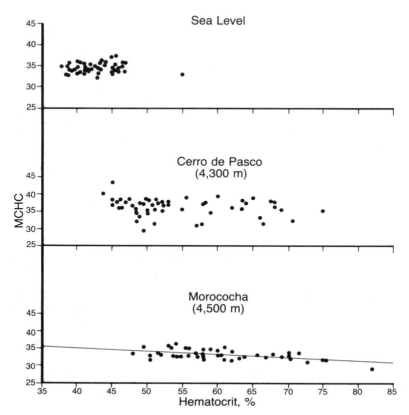

Figure 3.6.   The mean corpuscular hemoglobin concentration (*MCHC*) at sea level, Cerro de Pasco, and Morococha. The correlation is not significant at sea level ($r = .06$) but is weakly so at Cerro de Pasco ($r = .32$, $p = .02$). At Morococha, the relationship is highly significant ($r = .50$, $p = .001$). (Winslow and Monge, unpublished data.)

altitudes suggests that other factors in addition to hypoxia may regulate erythropoiesis, particularly in Morococha. However, the relationship of hemoglobin concentration with altitude is parabolic (fig. 3.3), so at higher altitudes a larger effect of small changes in altitude will be expected. This point, worth emphasizing, will reappear in later chapters: we believe that, because of the nonlinearity of some physiological responses with increased altitude, there exists a "critical altitude" above which humans do not acclimatize well. This altitude need not be the same for all individuals.

3.3   Nutrition and the Production of Red Cells

One possible explanation for the difference in apparent hematologic response to hypoxia in Morococha and Cerro de Pasco is that dietary or nutritional habits may differ. Figure 3.7 presents measurements of ferritin[4] and free erythrocyte protoporphyrin (FEP)[5] in the authors' Morococha subjects. Ferritin is apparently independent of hematocrit, and almost all the subjects have values in the normal range. That body iron stores do not limit erythropoiesis is shown by the fact that the low ferritin values are fairly evenly distributed over the entire hematocrit range. The FEP, which is a measure of inefficient heme synthesis, can be elevated in conditions of accelerated hemoglobin synthesis (Wintrobe 1981). Figure 3.7 also shows a

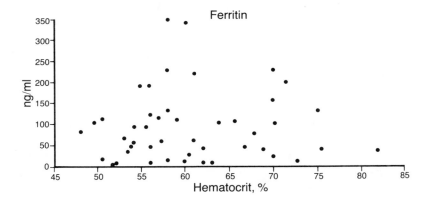

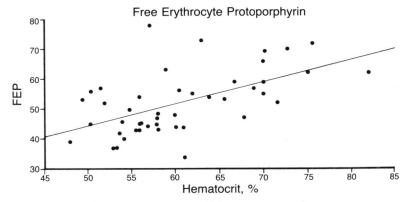

Figure 3.7.   Serum ferritin and free erythrocyte protoporphyrin in Morococha. Ferritin is not correlated with hematocrit. Although the correlation between FEP and hematocrit is significant ($r = .56, p = .001$), all values are within the normal sea-level range. (Winslow and Monge, unpublished data.)

significant correlation between FEP and hematocrit in Morococha, but all values were within the normal range, suggesting that limited hemoglobin synthesis does not explain the hematocrits in the lower ranges in figure 3.5.

Because hematocrit appears to be a parabolic function of altitude, and because viscosity is an exponential function of hematocrit, a very strong relationship exists between altitude and the resistive load on the circulation. This concept has strengthened our belief in a critical altitude, the altitude above which a person's ability to acclimatize may be exceeded. The exact altitude for an individual may be influenced by such factors as age, ventilation, physical activity, nutritional status, and so on. In any case, it appears that nutritional deficiencies do not play an important role in regulation of hematocrit, as first pointed out by Adams and Shresta (1974) for Himalayan natives.

3.4   Erythropoietin

If the variable response to altitude cannot be explained by iron metabolism or other nutritional factors, perhaps its basis is in the marrow control of erythropoiesis. Humoral regulation of the red cell volume, although suspected for many years, was not proven until Erslev (1953) found clear evidence of an erythropoietic factor in blood of anemic rabbits. The agent, a glycoprotein, was named erythropoietin (EPO). Erythropoietin was extensively purified, and Jacobson and co-workers showed that the kidney is responsible for the bulk of its production (Jacobson et al. 1957). Whether renal EPO is the sole regulator of red cell production has been a controversial issue. In adult rats, at least 10 percent of the total EPO may be produced in the liver (Erslev et al. 1981); EPO is produced also in the carotid bodies of cats (Tramezzani, Monita, and Chiocchio 1971). Recent studies show that EPO also can be released from alveolar and splenic macrophages that have been exposed to silica (Rich and Kubanek 1980). However, it is not known whether these cells actually produce the hormone or merely serve as storage sites.

Human studies of extrarenal EPO production are, of course, more difficult and rely mainly on clinical observation. Anephric subjects still maintain a level of erythropoiesis, albeit lower than that of normal humans (Erslev et al. 1968). However, such subjects can increase EPO production in response to hypoxia (Nathan et al. 1964) or hemorrhage (Naets and Wittek 1968). The site of this EPO production is not established, but human liver cells can produce it, as shown in patients with hepatocellular carcinoma (Mirand and Murphy 1971). Indeed, many cell types may have the potential to produce the hormone.

Although EPO probably is the principal controller of the rate of erythropoiesis, other factors can modulate its effects. Halvorsen (1966) argued that the central nervous system plays a role in erythropoiesis, because direct stimulation of the hypothalamus seems to increase the number of reticulocytes in peripheral blood. This observation, however, may be difficult to interpret, because the hypothalamic-pituitary axis can also be involved in plasma volume regulation, which in turn may affect oxygen delivery. Dietary protein intake (Alippi et al. 1979), environmental contamination (Koller, Exon, and Nixon 1979), and partial pressure of CO_2 (Zucali, Lee, and Mirand 1978) can also increase EPO production. The modulating effect of CO_2 may well be due to stimulation of respiration, however. The effect of thyroxine on protein synthesis may also play a role in regulation of the production of EPO (Erslev et al. 1981). Perhaps in view of the complex interactions of these variables, it should not be surprising that red cell production varies so much among individuals, even at sea level.

The kidney senses the lack of oxygen and responds by producing EPO. The mechanism of this sensing process is interesting, but not yet completely clear. It is tempting to imagine a physiologic analog of an oxygen electrode that can detect reduced concentration of oxygen. However, consider subjects with mutant hemoglobins with a high affinity for oxygen. In these rare cases, the plasma concentration of oxygen (PO_2) and the oxygen content of the blood are high, but the kidney still senses a lack of available oxygen. The hemoglobin molecule is altered genetically so as to increase its affinity for oxygen, in some cases dramatically. Thus, hypoxia is a result of a decreased *rate* of oxygen transfer to the sensing sites. Polycythemia is caused not by hypoxia, but by the molecule's inability to release its oxygen to the tissues. These subjects have an intact erythrypoietin mechanism, as demonstrated by EPO secretion in response to phlebotomy (Adamson et al. 1972). The only symptoms carriers of these proteins experience are those of polycythemia, not unlike those reported by patients with chronic mountain sickness. Thus, the sensing mechanism in the kidney is probably a composite function of available oxygen that includes blood flow, hemoglobin concentration, and oxygen affinity.

One major block in understanding the role of EPO at high altitude has been the lack of a widely available assay. For many years the standard method was a mouse bioassay (Popovic and Adamson 1979). Many animals were needed for each point, because their responses vary considerably and because standard curves must be prepared for each assay, requiring hundreds of mice for one set of measurements. Recently, radioimmunoassays have been developed (Sherwood and Goldwasser 1979), but still no satisfactory commercial assay is available. This situation should be rectified soon, however, and studies in high-altitude natives should contribute to our understanding of chronic mountain sickness and the control of erythropoiesis.

3.5   Erythropoiesis at High Altitudes

Although it is generally accepted that the polycythemia of high altitudes results from hypoxic stress, this relationship has not always been obvious. In 1925 the possibility was still entertained that chronic mountain sickness was simply polycythemia vera (Osler-Váquez's disease) in high-altitude natives. Later, Merino and Reynafarje (1952) reported an important series of bone marrow examinations in sixteen healthy natives of Morococha. They noted extreme hyperplasia of the erythroid cells but not of the leukocyte or platelet precursors. They concluded correctly that this finding, typical of hypoxic stress, was quite different from the picture of polycythemia vera and, combined with the absence of splenomegaly in their subjects, indicated a different etiology.

The mechanism of increased erythropoiesis noted by Viault (see chap. 1) appears to be a rapid rise in serum EPO after exposure to high altitudes. Faura and co-workers (Faura et al. 1969), using the mouse bioassay, measured urinary EPO in seven lowlanders who had been taken quickly to Morococha (4,500 m). After an initial latent period of six hours, they noted that EPO rapidly rose to reach a peak in twenty-four hours and then fell to a new plateau (about twice sea-level normal) in forty-eight hours. In a similar study of five lowlanders in Colorado, serum EPO reached a peak forty-eight hours after a two-hour ascent to 4,360 meters and remained significantly elevated for nine days (Abbrecht and Littel 1972). After that, however, the serum EPO was indistinguishable from sea-level normal. It is not known whether individual variation in EPO response can explain the variation in erythropoietic response, but based on a few subjects (Milledge and Cotes 1985), there seems to be no striking correlation.

The fall in serum EPO to sea-level control values in lowland sojourners at high altitudes is a troublesome observation because it occurs before the hemoglobin concentration changes significantly. This seems to argue against a simple feedback interaction between EPO and the red cell volume. Perhaps erythroid cells are sensitized to EPO after initial stimulation. Alternatively, the rate of EPO turnover could be increased after initial stimulation, precluding its accumulation in the blood. Perhaps, however, there are other unknown components of the control system. Finally, the bioassay is not well suited to measurements of near-normal values. Immunologic techniques that quantitate antigenic material (rather than biologic activity) may provide better data.

In contrast to sojourners, highland natives of Peru clearly have an elevated steady-state EPO concentration. Merino (1956), in an extraordinary experiment, injected pooled plasma from natives of Morococha into volunteers in Lima and showed a pronounced reticulocytosis compared with control recipients of normal plasma (fig. 3.8). Reynafarje and co-workers

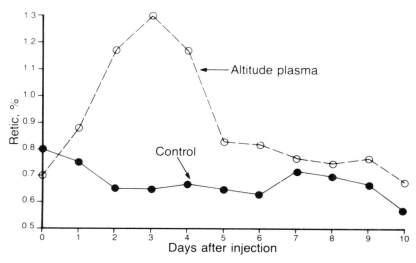

Figure 3.8. Reticulocytosis after injection of plasma from high-altitude natives or controls into normal sea-level volunteers. (With permission, from Merino 1956.)

(Reynafarje et al. 1964) showed that plasma from high-altitude natives accelerated the uptake of radioactive iron when injected into rats. When the EPO bioassay became available, Faura and co-workers (Faura et al. 1969) demonstrated its elevation in the urine of Morococha residents. However, whether EPO and hemoglobin concentration show a dose-response relationship remains to be determined. That is, it still is unknown whether variation in EPO explains the striking variation in hemoglobin concentration in high-altitude (or sea-level) natives.

The characterization of the erythropoietic mechanism at high altitudes is complicated somewhat by studies with natives taken suddenly to sea level. Plasma from such subjects depressed iron utilization when injected into rats (Reynafarje et al. 1964), and similar results were found using a different EPO assay system (Faura et al. 1969). These studies suggest an inhibitor of erythropoiesis, but similar effects have been observed in subjects with very low EPO concentrations (Birgegard et al. 1982) and may be due to unspecific properties of serum that are usually masked by EPO. The presence or absence of an EPO antagonist could be crucial for understanding the etiology of chronic mountain sickness. Perhaps the newer assay techniques for EPO will help clarify this important point.

3.6   Renal Hemodynamics and Erythrocytosis

Reduced blood flow resulting from the high viscosity, diminished red cell flow through the kidney, and renal hypoxia and stimulation of EPO production would lead to a vicious cycle of higher viscosity, lower flow, exaggerated hypoxia, and further erythrocytosis. Erslev proposed that this cycle does not occur because a reduction of renal blood flow produces a proportional reduction of glomerular filtration rate (see chap. 7 for a discussion of renal function at altitude), diminished reabsorption of sodium, and diminished O_2 consumption (Erslev, Caro, and Besarab 1985). This reduction in metabolic rate would, thus, prevent tissue hypoxia and avoid the excessive release of EPO.

Erslev draws upon three sources of support for the concept that polycythemia reduces renal blood flow. The first is an in vitro approach showing that O_2 flow,

$$(1/\text{viscosity}) \times (\text{hematocrit})$$

when plotted as a function of hematocrit, shows a sharp maximum at normal hematocrit values. The second is an experimental study of PO_2 in air and peritoneum air pockets in rats and mice with hematocrits varied by bleeding or by hypertransfusion (Thorling and Erslev 1968). In this case a broad optimum was obtained, but at very high hematocrits there was a tendency for PO_2 to decrease, providing the needed stimulus to initiate the vicious cycle of polycythemia. The third argument rests on experiments in dogs showing that O_2 transport to the kidney declines sharply above a hematocrit of about 60 percent (Fan et al. 1980). In the case of anemia, the authors assume that because of the low viscosity, the renal blood flow should be high but that the low hemoglobin concentration (low red cell concentration) will produce a low red cell flow and tissue hypoxia, with consequent release of erythropoietin. In this case a high renal O_2 demand will accentuate the production of erythropoietin.

In polycythemia vera, deWardener showed that kidney blood flow is above normal and diminishes after bloodletting (deWardener, McSwiney, and Miles 1951). Therefore, the inverse correlation between hematocrit and renal blood flow proposed by Erslev is not only absent, but reversed. In hypoxic polycythemia of high altitudes, Monge C. (unpublished) found no correlation between blood viscosity and renal blood flow (see fig. 7.6). In two subjects who were studied several years apart and who displayed an increase in hematocrit with age, the renal blood flow also increased, showing the reverse of the trend found in polycythemia vera. Also, in three cases of chronic mountain sickness involving very high hematocrits, renal blood flow was above the levels found in normal natives and in sea-level controls (Lozano and Monge C. 1965). Cases of congenital cyanotic heart disease with polycythemia also showed an increased renal blood flow (Scott and Elliott 1950). One may conclude that in humans polycythemia does not lead to a diminished renal blood flow, making unnecessary the mechanisms proposed by Erslev to explain the lack of excessive erythropoietin secretion.

Renal vein catheterization in Peruvian high-altitude natives (Rennie, Lozano, Monge, et al. 1971) allowed the measurement of renal blood flow by the Fick principle at an average hematocrit of 68 percent. The study confirmed the normality of renal blood flow found in the other studies by the clearance technique. It also demonstrated a normal O_2 consumption by the hypoxemic kidney, suggesting that a moderate drop in the filtration rate found in these cases did not reduce the metabolic rate.

Renal function in anemic humans was demonstrated in the early report of Bradley and Bradley (1945). In this condition the renal blood flow is significantly diminished. Here again the inverse correlation between hematocrit and renal blood flow suggested by Erslev is not only absent, but reversed.

Having reviewed the relevant renal function data in anemic and polycythemic humans, one may attempt to explain the erythropoietic response in these conditions in terms of conventional renal physiology. Anemia will markedly reduce renal O_2 transport by the double action of reduced renal blood flow and reduced hematocrit. This most probably will induce kidney tissue hypoxia and subsequent release of erythropoietin. Normoxic polycythemia would increase red cell transport by keeping renal blood flow normal or high and also would increase the hematocrit. No release of erythropoietin above the normal level is expected in this situation. In hypoxic polycythemia, because blood flow remains unchanged or slightly elevated, the tissue PO_2 will depend on how much the elevated hematocrit can compensate for the drop in PaO_2.

A mathematical model has been used to describe the balance between renal O_2 supply and demand (Monge C. 1983). In the calculations, PvO_2 was calculated from physiological parameters related to hypoxemia and polycythemia. The PvO_2 was taken as an approximation of tissue PO_2.

Table 3.3 shows the calculated values of PvO_2 when PaO_2 is 50 torr (altitude about 4,500 m) and 95 torr (sea level), when hemoglobin concentration is 23 grams/deciliter (4,500m) and 15 grams/deciliter (sea level). Values in parentheses are actual values found by renal vein catheterization in one of the experimental studies (Rennie, Lozano, Monge, et al. 1971). It may be seen that in hypoxic polycythemia (third row) the high hemoglobin concentration prevents a marked drop of $P\bar{v}O_2$ in the systemic circulation, but it does not do so in the kidney. The corresponding values in the systemic circulation are 42 torr for normoxia and 39 torr for hypoxia. In the kidney the values are 63 torr for normoxia and 48 torr for hypoxia. The second row indicates that the absence of polycythemia affects very little the kidney PvO_2 in the hypoxic condition. Since polycythemia has little effect in correcting

Table 3.3.   Kidney oxygenation in subjects at low and high altitudes

	Hb (g/dl)	PaO_2 (torr)	$P\bar{v}O_2$ (torr)	
			Systemic	Kidney
Sea level	15	95	42	63 (67)
High-altitude	15	50	35	46
High-altitude/polycythemic	23	50	39	48 (46)

Note: Calculated mixed venous PO_2 at stimulated sea level and at high altitude. Values in parentheses are from Rennie et al. (1971).

kidney hypoxia, an increase in erythropoietin is expected in this case. The increased release of erythropoietin in Peruvian high-altitude natives is in accord with the model and with actual measurements of renal vein PvO_2.

Therefore, there is no need to postulate a reduction of the kidney metabolic rate in polycythemia as a need to avoid the overproduction of erythropoietin secondary to an assumed reduction in renal blood flow and glomerular filtration rate. The release of erythropoietin in anemia, normoxic polycythemia, and hypoxic polycythemia can be explained in terms of conventional principles of renal physiology and experimental observations.

The tendency of certain individuals to develop excessive polycythemia with symptoms of chronic mountain sickness may well be due to the poor regulatory function of the kidney on erythropoietin production in hypoxemic polycythemia. This could explain not only the known fact that hypoxemia leads to polycythemia, but also why at the same level of hypoxemia some individuals develop chronic mountain sickness and others maintain moderate levels of polycythemia.

The different conclusion reached on this subject by Erslev may be, in part, due to his use of animal data. Many species differences are well-recognized with regard to the physiological adjustments to hypoxia.

3.7   The Measurements of Red Cell and Plasma Volumes

Symptoms of chronic mountain sickness result from expansion of the circulating blood volume and increased viscosity. The diagnosis is usually based on symptoms of plethora and a hematocrit that is in excess of that observed for the general population at the same altitude. At sea level, polycythemia may be due to a variety of causes, and careful measurement of the red cell volume is the cornerstone of the differential diagnosis. However, remarkably few direct measurements of red cell volume are available for high-altitude subjects, in spite of the well-documented problems in diagnosis of polycythemia at sea level (Valentine et al. 1968; van Assendelft 1984). The reason for this lack of information is, of course, that the modern measurement of red cell volume requires radioisotopic techniques, often impossible in remote areas.[6]

The classic data are those collected by Hurtado (Hurtado, Merino, and Delgado 1945) using Evans blue dye estimations of plasma volume[7] (table 3.4). In that study, red cell and total blood volumes were inferred from the venous hematocrit. A severely expanded red cell volume was noted, and the blood volumes in chronic mountain sickness subjects were enormous.

The authors' own studies illustrate some of the pitfalls that can be encountered in the estimation of red cell and plasma volume. In a study of the effects of hemodilution in high-altitude natives, the opportunity arose to compare estimates of red cell volume made with Hurtado's assumptions to those obtained by modern methods. In stages, whole blood was removed (approximately 500 to 1,000 ml at a time) from several subjects and replaced with an equal volume of saline containing 5 percent albumin. The amount of red cells to be removed was calculated from the estimated red cell volume, with the objective of achieving a final hematocrit of 50 percent or less.

Red cell volume was also measured with ^{51}Cr-labeled autologous red cells in four subjects before hemodilution. In three of these and in an additional three, red cell volume was estimated from the quantity of red cells removed and the change in venous hematocrit. It was expected that mixing labeled red cells would be very slow because of the sluggish circulation associated with polycythemia. Surprisingly, equilibration of the injected red cell label was complete within five minutes, regardless of the subject's hematocrit. In sea-level studies, equilibration of injected red cell label has

Table 3.4.   Red-cell and plasma volumes at sea level and high altitudes

Altitude (m)	Remark	N	Hct (%)	PLV (ml/kg)	RCV (ml/kg)	TBV (ml/kg)
			Sea Level			
0	Vital Red	10	45.7	46.2	39.0	85.4
0	Evans Blue	26	44.9	47.1	38.8	86.5
3,700	Vital Red	30	54.9	48.9	59.7	108.7
4,500	Vital Red	6	61.3	46.1	74.1	120.8
4,500	Evans Blue	11	63.9	36.2	64.1	100.3
			Silicosis			
3,700	Sat >84%	19	65.4	39.3	75.0	114.6
3,700	Sat 72–83%	17	70.5	37.3	94.1	133.5
3,700	Sat 60–71%	4	76.0	45.0	145.3	191.3
3,700	Sat <60%	3	65.9	52.5	103.2	156.6
			Chronic Mountain Sickness			
4,500	CMS	6	77.8	37.9	139.0	180.9

Source: Hurtado, Merino, ad Delgado 1945.
Note: PLV = plasma volume, RCV = red cell volume, TBV = total blood volume.

been shown to be complete in about two minutes (Bauer et al. 1975; Prankerd 1963; Root, Roughton, and Gregersen 1946), suggesting that our subjects did not have significant pools of stagnant red cells.

The observed red cell volumes (RCV) in our subjects are shown in table 3.5. In all cases, the measured red cell volume is about twice that predicted by the sea-level formulas

The various calculations were carried out as follows. The initial venous hematocrit (HV1) is

$$HV1 = RCV/TBV1 \times 1/(HB1/HV1) \qquad (3.1)$$

where TBV1 is the initial total blood volume and HB1/HV1 is the ratio of body hematocrit to venous hematocrit.[8] The final venous hematocrit (HV2) can be described similarly:

$$HV2 = (RCV - dRCV)/TBV2 \times 1/(HB2/HV2) \qquad (3.2)$$

where TBV2 is the final total blood volume, dRCV is the volume of red cells removed, and HB2/HV2 is the body-to-venous hematocrit ratio after hemodilution.

In analyzing the authors' data (Winslow, Monge C., and Klein 1987), it

Table 3.5.   Hemodilution of selected subjects at Cerro de Pasco

	Subject Identification Number					
	1680	3280	3680	3780	3880	3980
Age (yr)	46	59	54	73	57	41
Height (cm)	161	151	148	156	148	164
Weight (kg)	61.5	61.5	50.2	58.7	69.7	61.0
[51]Cr RCV (ml/kg)	46.7	51.3	47.9	—	—	49.7
Initial Hct (%)	69.0	66.0	62.0	69.0	69.9	67.0
#1 vol removed (ml)	1060	1000	1000	1075	1000	1000
Red cells (%)	60.8	57.0	51.0	55.3	61.0	58.0
RBC removed (ml)	644	570	510	595	610	580
#2 vol removed (ml)	1100	1080	1000	780	1000	1000
Red cells (%)	54.8	53.0	43.5	53.0	53.0	50.0
RBC removed (ml)	603	572	435	429	530	500
#3 Vol removed (ml)	1020	440	220	—	1000	640
Red cells (%)	41.7	42.0	27.7	—	46.0	41.0
RBC removed (ml)	425	185	61	—	460	262
#4 vol removed (ml)	—	—	—	—	320	—
Red cells (%)	23.0	—	—	—	—	—
RBC removed (ml)	—	—	—	—	73.6	—
RBC removed (ml/kg)	27.2	21.6	20.0	17.4	24.0	21.0
Final Hct (%)	50	53	42	53	47	46
Predicted final Hct (%)	45	46	36	—	—	39
Estimated RCV (ml/kg)	98.8	109.7	62.0	75.0	73.2	67.0

Source: Winslow and Monge, unpublished data.

was concluded that they could be explained only by significant variation in the HB/HV ratios. The ratios for subjects 1680, 3280, and 3680, respectively, are 1.51, 1.14, and 1.01 (table 3.5). These values are high, but very few measurements in high-altitude natives are available for comparison.

Figure 3.9 shows a comparison of the earlier studies, the authors, and more recent data both at high altitude and at sea level obtained with ^{51}Cr-labeled red cells. The line in figure 3.9 was calculated by starting with sea-level values for red cell volume and plasma volume and increasing the red cell volume, assuming a constant plasma volume. Note that most of the Hurtado data fall close to or below this line (high red cell volumes), while the more recent data are all in agreement with each other and are above the line. Figure 3.9 also shows that our ^{51}Cr results compare favorably with measurements in sea-level polycythemia vera subjects (Berlin, Lawrence, and Gartland 1950). Moreover, ^{51}Cr data collected by Sánchez (Sánchez, Merino, and Figallo 1970) agree with both the polycythemia vera group and our results.

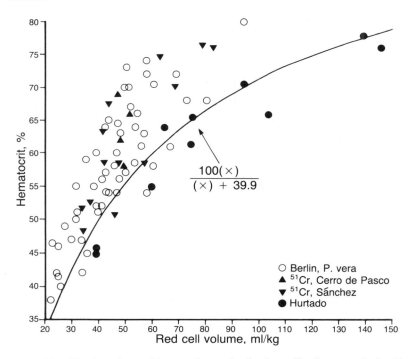

Figure 3.9. The dependence of hematocrit on red-cell volume. The line was calculated by assuming a body-to-venous hematocrit ratio of 1 and constant plasma volume at all hematocrits. The polycythemia vera data are from Berlin, Lawrence, and Gartland (1950). The ^{51}Cr data are from Klein (1983) and Sánchez, Merino, and Figallo (1970). Estimates based on plasma volume measurements are from Hurtado, Merino, and Delgado (1945).

These calculations strongly suggest the possibility that the differences in directly measured ^{51}Cr-labeled red cell volumes and those inferred from dye dilution measurements are due to a discrepancy between the body and capillary hematocrits. This has been shown to be a source of error in total blood volume measurements in sea-level subjects (Nusynowitz, Blumhardt, and Volpe 1974; Lawson 1964).

The values for HB/HV predicted in the authors' subjects are higher than the means reported for sea-level subjects (see table 3.6). The mean value for HB/HV in normal sea-level subjects is about 0.87 (Nusynowitz, Strader, and Waliszewski 1970; Lertzman et al. 1964; Retzlaff et al. 1969). However, the values for polycythemic subjects have been reported to be 0.913 ($N = 20$) in polycythemia vera (Lertzman et al. 1964), and 0.96 ($N = 13$) in high-altitude natives (Sánchez, Merino, and Figallo 1970). The variation in these measurements seems to be directly related to the absolute mean venous hematocrit. The range of values in the P. vera patients was from 0.69 to 1.18. Sánchez also found a higher range in HB/HV in high-altitude natives (0.96, $N = 13$, range 0.81 to 1.18) than in his sea-level controls (0.89, $N = 7$, range 0.75 to 1.01). Note, also, that the standard deviations increase with hematocrit, confirming the earlier studies of Hurtado (1932b).

The ratio HB/HV may be more important at altitude than at sea level. It is well known that the capillary hematocrit is less than the large-vessel venous hematocrit (Cokelet 1982). Because of the Farheaus effect,[9] the capillary hematocrit also may be markedly different in different organs (Riegel 1980), and the ratio HB/HV seems to be higher in subjects with polycythemia. Capillary proliferation at high altitudes (Valdivia 1959) may cause the ratio

Table 3.6. A comparison of the Means for HB, HV, PLV, RCV, and HB/HV measurements

	HB	HV	PLV	RCV	HB/HV	Source
Normal ($N = 40$)						
Mean	40.2	46.3	39.9	26.8	.867	(1)
SD	±3.7	±3.1	±5.0	±4.0	±.061	
P. vera ($N = 20$)						
Mean	53.3	58.8	39.5	46.7	.913	(2)
SD	±7.4	±8.8	±5.5	±14.0	±.107	
Lung disease ($N = 18$)						
Mean	47.3	52.8	39.2	36.1	.896	(3)
SD	±7.5	±7.6	±7.8	±11.2	±.033	
High-Altitude ($N = 13$)						
Mean	60.1	62.0	33.4	51.7	.963	(4)
SD	±12.4	±9.9	±9.4	±16.6	±.113	

Sources: (1) Retzlaff et al. 1969; (2) Lertzman et al. 1964; (3) Vanier et al. 1963; and (4) Sánchez, Merino and Figally 1970.

Note: HV = venous hematocrit, HB/HV = body-to-venous hematocrit ratio.

to vary more than it does at sea level. Furthermore, a wider discrepancy between the venous and capillary hematocrits may protect the high-altitude native from the effects of increased viscosity.

There is an apparent decrease in plasma volume with increasing venous hematocrit in subjects with polycythemia vera and chronic obstructive lung disease, and also in high-altitude natives (table 3.7). Contraction of the plasma volume may, therefore, be an important component of chronic mountain sickness. One study of the variation of plasma volume in poly-cythemic states concluded that there is little variation of plasma volume as red cell volume increases either in subjects with polycythemia vera and chronic lung disease or in high-altitude natives (Vanier et al. 1963). Howev-er, only simultaneous measurements of red cell and plasma volumes are accurate enough to allow such conclusions to be drawn. The only available simultaneous measurements in high-altitude natives are those by Sánchez, Merino, and Figallo (1970), who showed that red cell and plasma volume are negatively correlated only in the high-altitude subjects (table 3.7). Thus, there is a tendency for high-altitude natives to have contracted plasma volumes when red cell volume increases.

These seemingly abstruse arguments force consideration of the pos-sibility that contracted plasma volume may be a part, at least, of the etiology of symptoms in chronic mountain sickness. In support of this hypothesis, it has been demonstrated in patients with relative polycythemia[10] that repeated venesection raises the plasma volume (Humphrey, Michael, and Pearson 1980). In sea-level polycythemia, increased blood volume increases cardiac output (Sjöstrand 1953), which can compensate somewhat for the increased viscosity caused by polycythemia. However, if the high-altitude subject, for whatever reason, cannot completely compensate, then both hyperviscosity and reduced cardiac output will result, contributing to the symptoms of chronic mountain sickness.

In summary, it appears that the classic measurements of Hurtado, Me-rino, and Delgado (1945) severely overestimate total blood volume in chron-ic mountain sickness because of errors arising from assuming a unit ratio of body-to-venous hematocrit. The few direct measurements available for red

Table 3.7. Correlation coefficients for VH, PLV, and RCV measurements

	VH and PLV				RCV and PLV			
	r	SE	r/SE	N	r	SE	r/SE	N
P. vera	−.11	±.23	.52	20	.21	±.23	.90	20
COPD	−.54	±.24	2.21	18	.25	±.24	1.03	18
High-Altitude	−.70	±.29	2.44	13	−.58	±.29	2.01	13

Note: COPD = chronic obstructive pulmonary disease.
Data derived from table 3.6.

cell volume in chronic mountain sickness subjects agree with known relationships between red cell volume and hematocrit in other types of polycythemia occurring at sea level. Although simultaneous measurements of red cell and plasma volume are few, the available data suggest that subjects with chronic mountain sickness may have a contracted plasma volume. The methods used for these measurements are extremely important.

3.8   The Regulation of Red Cell and Plasma Volumes

Although an absolute increase in the red cell volume is believed to be the hallmark of chronic mountain sickness, understanding is needed of what part in its etiology may be played by contracted plasma volume. Very little is known about the regulation of the plasma volume in high-altitude natives. Chapter 7 describes severely reduced plasma flow in the kidney in high-altitude subjects with polycythemia. This reduction in critical organs such as the kidney and the brain undoubtedly is important for various blood transport functions.

CHAPTER FOUR

The Structure and Function of Hemoglobin at High Altitudes

About 97 percent of the oxygen in the blood is physically bound to hemoglobin. Estimates of the amount of oxygen in the blood, however, are obtained by measuring the amount of oxygen physically dissolved in plasma (PO_2), which represents only about 3 percent of the total. In order for PO_2 measurements to accurately reflect the total oxygen in the blood, the relationship between PO_2 and the degree of hemoglobin saturation must be known. This relationship is the oxygen equilibrium curve (OEC), and its regulation is the subject of this chapter.

A "shift to the right" of the hemoglobin OEC is frequently cited as an adaptive mechanism in high-altitude natives and sojourners. That is, it is widely believed that in adapted humans the affinity of hemoglobin for oxygen decreases to facilitate the release of O_2 in the tissues. However, it was argued by Barcroft (1934) and recently shown with data from extreme altitude (Winslow, Samaja, and West 1984) that just the opposite may be true: an increase in affinity is probably advantageous, because O_2 can be taken up better in the lungs. These two views have not been reconciled because until recently the mechanism of hemoglobin action has not been clearly understood, nor have the methods needed for accurate measurements been available.

4.1 The Blood Oxygen Equilibrium Curve

The relationship between the amount of oxygen bound to hemoglobin (saturation) and the oxygen physically dissolved in solution (oxygen tension, PO_2) under equilibrium conditions is the familiar oxygen equilibrium curve (OEC) of hemoglobin (fig. 4.1). Its position is often represented by the value P50, the PO_2 at which saturation is 50 percent. If oxygen affinity increases, the OEC shifts left and P50 is reduced. If oxygen affinity decreases, the OEC shifts right, and P50 is increased. The principal physiologic effectors of hemoglobin function, H^+, 2,3-diphosphoglycerate (2,3-DPG), and CO_2, all shift the OEC to the right, as does an additional effector, temperature.

Early in this century a fundamental difference between the oxygenation properties of myoglobin and hemoglobin was recognized. The former curve is hyperbolic, and the latter is sigmoid (Hill 1910). As demonstrated in figure 4.2, this peculiar sigmoid shape permits efficient transport of oxygen. At arterial PO_2 (90 torr) myoglobin is 95.4 percent saturated, and hemoglobin saturation is 93.5 percent. If mixed venous blood has a PO_2 of 40 torr,

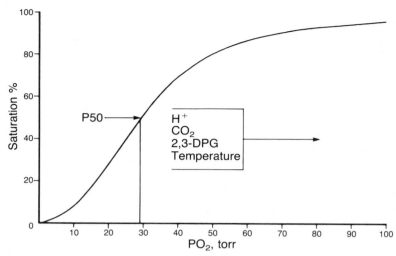

Figure 4.1. The normal whole-blood-oxygen equilibrium curve. P50 is the PO_2 at which hemoglobin is half-saturated with oxygen. The principal effectors that alter the position and shape of the curve under physiologic conditions are indicated.

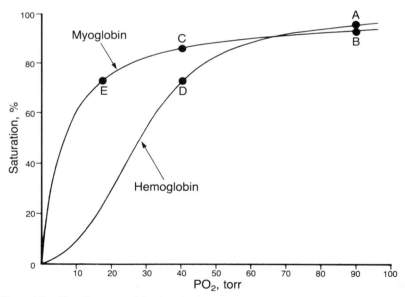

Figure 4.2. The advantages of the sigmoid shape of the oxygen equilibrium curve. Note that while both curves allow a saturation of about 95 percent at a sea-level PaO_2 of 90 torr (points A and B), the hemoglobin curve allows unloading of about 23 percent of its O_2 at $P\bar{v}O_2$ of 40 torr (point D), compared to only about 7 percent (point C) for myoglobin. In order for myoglobin to deliver the same amount of O_2 as hemoglobin (point E), $P\bar{v}O_2$ (and therefore tissue PO_2) would have to be about 15.5 torr in this example.

and saturation of the hemoglobin curve is about 72.9 percent, about 22.5 percent of the O_2 has been released. However, because the myoglobin curve is hyperbolic, only about 7.1 percent of the O_2 would be released at the same PO_2, and a mixed venous O_2 tension of about 15.5 torr would be necessary to supply as much O_2 as is supplied by hemoglobin. The physical basis for the sigmoid O_2 binding in hemoglobin was discovered long after its physiologic importance was appreciated. Because the binding of each oxygen molecule to hemoglobin apparently facilitates the binding of subsequent molecules, early biochemists used the term *cooperativity* to describe the sigmoid shape.

Over the past fifty to seventy-five years many scientists studying the regulatory role of hemoglobin in the oxygen transport process have presumed that shifts in the position and shape of the OEC adapt humans to hypoxia. However, heme-containing proteins are ubiquitous in the plant and animal kingdoms, and hemoglobin almost certainly evolved as an oxygen carrier before humans emerged from the evolutionary competition. There is no a priori reason to believe that the behavior of the OEC at high altitude is "good" or "bad," or even that it is a uniquely human property. To be objective, one must observe the in vivo properties of hemoglobin as accurately as possible, then try to understand these properties in the overall scheme of oxygen transport. Only then can the relative importance of shifts to the left or right of the OEC be assessed.

4.2   The Structure and Function of Hemoglobin

Hemoglobin is a protein molecule made up of four polypeptide subunits, each of which is linked to an iron-containing tetrapyrrole prosthetic group, heme. Because oxygen binds reversibly to the iron atom, each hemoglobin molecule can bind four molecules of oxygen. The protein subunits have a molecular weight of approximately 16,100 daltons, and each one is structurally very similar to myoglobin.

In the normal adult human, approximately 97 percent of the red cell protein is hemoglobin A, which contains two alpha and two beta chains in a tetrameric structure. As X-ray crystallographic studies show, hemoglobin can take one of two conformations, the difference between them being the strength of the intersubunit chemical bonds (Bolton and Perutz 1970). Although certain details of the mechanism of oxygen binding to hemoglobin are still unclear, the most useful current model is based on these two conformations. In one, the subunits are maximally bonded and the structure is "tense," or T. In the other conformation, some of the intersubunit bonds are ruptured and the structure is "relaxed," or R. That molecular oxygen more easily enters the region of the heme in the R conformation explains its higher affinity.

At all stages of oxygenation, an equilibrium exists between the T and the R conformations. However, the position of the equilibrium curve is strongly influenced by the number of oxygen molecules bound. Nearly all the deoxygenated hemoglobin is in the T conformation, whereas nearly all the oxyhemoglobin is in the R conformation. The OEC has a sigmoid shape because the molecule in the R state has a much higher affinity for oxygen than it does in the T state.

To visualize this interaction, consider the successive binding of oxygen to hemoglobin. Deoxyhemoglobin is in the T state. As the first oxygen molecule is bound, the hemoglobin molecule is forced open a bit, rupturing one or more of the intersubunit bonds, and some of the molecules change to the R conformation. This increases their oxygen affinity; the second oxygen molecule is bound more easily; and so on. On the average, most of the molecules switch from T to R between the second and third oxygen molecules, causing the OEC to be steepest in its central portion. This is extremely important because small changes in PO_2 in this steep portion lead to large changes in oxygen saturation (fig. 4.2).

The position of the OEC under physiologic conditions is regulated almost entirely by three effectors: H^+, 2,3-DPG, and CO_2. Each of these small molecules stabilizes the T conformation by strengthening the intersubunit bonds. In the presence of H^+, for example, the deoxy conformation is stabilized and overall O_2 affinity is reduced (the Bohr effect). To further stabilize the T structure, 2,3-DPG binds between beta-chains, as does CO_2 to a smaller extent. Increasing the number of these bonds decreases oxygen affinity and contributes further to the Bohr effect. Thus, depending on the pH, increases in 2,3-DPG or CO_2 tension (PCO_2) shift the OEC to the right.

Early writings on the physiologic effects of hemoglobin-O_2 interactions use the terms *Bohr effect* and *Haldane effect*. These terms came into use before the details of hemoglobin function were known, so some confusion exists as to their current definition. As originally used, the Bohr effect described the decreased O_2 affinity caused by CO_2. The Haldane effect described the increased CO_2 capacity of the blood when O_2 was given up. A modern explanation of these effects can now be provided on the basis of the mechanisms outlined above.

Both the Bohr and Haldane effects are explained by the separate reactions of H^+ and CO_2. CO_2 has two effects on hemoglobin function: a direct effect as it binds to hemoglobin, stabilizing the T conformation and lowering O_2 affinity, and an indirect effect of decreasing pH and further stabilizing deoxyhemoglobin. The pH effect is due to the fact that H^+ is liberated when CO_2 is rapidly hydrated to the acid H_2CO_3 in the plasma, a reaction catalyzed by carbonic anhydrase. Thus, as blood enters the tissue capillary circulation, O_2 diffuses into tissues and CO_2 diffuses into blood. These reactions are driven by the gradients between tissue and blood for each of the gases. The two effects of CO_2, direct and indirect, decrease O_2 affinity of hemoglobin and facilitate O_2 release.

Most modern authors reserve the term *Bohr effect* to define the O_2-linked reversible binding of H^+ to hemoglobin. The log of the P50 bears a linear relationship to pH over the physiologic range of pH (7.0–7.8), and its slope, the "Bohr factor," is about -0.4 at constant PCO_2 (Wranne, Woodson, and Detter 1972). Although the term *Haldane effect* is still used in the physiologic literature, it is not usually used by biochemists, because it really describes the combined effects of H^+ and CO_2 on hemoglobin function. We prefer the current definition of the Bohr effect and do not use *Haldane effect*, because it no longer describes a unique biochemical reaction.

4.3   Older Studies of Blood Oxygen Affinity

Paul Bert (1878) was the first to construct an oxygen equilibrium curve relating fractional hemoglobin saturation with oxygen partial pressure. The knowledge of the structure and function of hemoglobin was refined enormously by the group at Cambridge University, primarily under Barcroft. This group, throughout Barcroft's life and that of his student, Roughton, laid the groundwork for our present understanding.

Blood oxygen affinity was an important part of Barcroft's 1921–22 expedition, although his studies focused on acclimatization of his colleagues rather than of natives. Barcroft obtained measurements of arterial saturation and PO_2 in three high-altitude natives, four high-altitude Caucasian permanent residents, and expedition members (table 4.1). The main purpose of the measurements was to settle a controversy about oxygen secretion in the lung, a theory of Haldane's that Barcroft proved invalid. The most remarkable feature of these data is the "high degree of unsaturation of the arterial bloods of those native to the mountains" (Barcroft et al. 1923). In fact, the arterial saturation in natives was only slightly decreased (mean, 84.6 percent), while the arterial PO_2 (PaO_2) was markedly reduced (mean, 46.7 torr). The net result (fig. 4.3) appeared to be that the OEC was shifted to the left (P50 24.4 torr, compared with 29.7 torr for the expedition members).

Barcroft also measured the in vitro oxygen affinity of the blood of these three natives of Cerro de Pasco. He exposed samples to different mixtures of oxygen, at partial pressures of CO_2 similar to those found in the alveolar air. The results (fig. 4.3) show that, compared with sea-level controls measured in the same way, the curves are clearly shifted to the left (P50s of 18, 22, and 23 torr, compared with 25, 27, and 23 torr). Barcroft regarded this alteration as favorable for the uptake of oxygen in the lung.

Barcroft suspected the explanation for a left-shifted OEC in high-altitude natives lay in the acid-base regulation of the interior of the red cell. He believed the polycythemia observed in these subjects provided buffering by

Table 4.1.   Arterial measurements, Cerro de Pasco, 1921–22

Name	PAO$_2$ (torr)	PaO$_2$ (torr)	SaO$_2$ (%)	P50 (torr)
Expedition members (sea level)				
Meakins	100	99	95	
Redfield	—	—	97	
Bock	—	—	95	
Harrop	—	—	95	
Mean	100	99	95.6	30.6
Expedition Members (4,300 m)				
Meakins	55.6	58	91	
Redfield	59	—	87.5	
Binger	47	—	84	
Bock	50	—	81.5	
Harrop	50	—	82	
Mean	52.3	58	85.2	29.7
Caucasian Residents (4,300 m)				
McQueen	59	57	86	
Philpotts	55	48	91	
McLaughlan	56	47	86	
Cuthbertson	54	55	87	
Mean	56	51.2	87.5	24.4
Indian Natives (4,300 m)				
Zelada	51	50	86	
Villareal	—	40	82.5	
Baracoyle	62	50	82.3	
Mean	56.5	46.7	84.6	24.4

Source: Barcroft et al. 1923.

hemoglobin, which could be at least as important as the increased O$_2$ carrying capacity: "It allows of a more alkaline corpuscle at a given CO$_2$ pressure of 25 mm, a higher dissociation curve, and therefore a corpuscle which is more acquisitive of oxygen in the lung . . . That concentration of corpuscles, coupled with alteration of the CO$_2$ tension, could give the blood a highly satisfactory oxygen dissociation curve greatly enhances the importance of the polycythemia" (Barcroft et al. 1923, 379).

The existence of the intracellular alkalosis, however, remained to be demonstrated. Barcroft rejected, correctly, specific effects of bicarbonate and CO$_2$ on hemoglobin itself as accounting for this effect and finally concluded that the cause was the buffering capacity of the increased number of red cells. To demonstrate this, he obtained a sample of venous blood from one of the expedition members and attempted to reconstruct the conditions of native polycythemic blood. He centrifuged the samples and reconstituted them at three different hematocrits (table 4.2). The pH was calculated from the PCO$_2$ and the Henderson-Hasselbalch formula:[1]

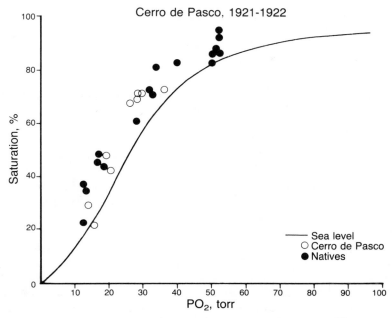

Figure 4.3. Barcroft's data on oxygen equilibrium. The solid line is the mean of curves obtained in expedition members at sea level. Open circles are the data obtained in the same subjects in Cerro de Pasco, and closed circles are the values for natives. (Data from Barcroft et al. 1923).

$$pH = pK' + \log \frac{(HCO_3^-)}{(PCO_2 \times \alpha)} \qquad (4.1)$$

where α is the coefficient of solubility of CO_2 in plasma. The calculations suggested that an increased hematocrit was responsible for the paradoxically higher O_2 saturation in the face of decreased pH.

Table 4.2. Barcroft's in vitro experiment, Cerro de Pasco, 1921–22

	Hemoglobin (% of normal)		
	154	108	65
Observed PCO_2 (torr)	27	19	26.5
Observed PO_2 (torr)	17	19	17
Observed saturation (%)	65	40	36
Saturation extrapolated to $PCO_2 = 27$, $PO_2 = 19$ torr	74	37	33
pH, wire	7.41	7.37	7.33
pH, extrapolated to $PCO_2 = 27$ torr	7.39	7.36	7.31
pH calculated from Henderson-Hasselbalch, $pK' = 6.1$	7.30	7.42	7.34

Source: Barcroft et al. 1923.

The only explanation offered for these results was that the pK', 6.1, was not correct when the hematocrit was abnormally elevated. In a note added in proof, Barcroft stated that Warburg, who had sent him a copy of his latest book, had increased the value of pK' and included a correction for hemoglobin concentration. However, when he applied Warburg's new formulas, the plasma pH tended to be more acid at any ratio of bound/free CO_2, in conflict with his initial results. Unfortunately, Barcroft never settled the controversy and instead turned his attention to fetal-maternal O_2 transfer and hemoglobin physichochemical properties.

In the 1935 expedition to Chile, Keys, Hall, and Barron studied three residents of 3,600 meters. They reported a P50 value 1.7 millimeters higher than the sea-level values of the expedition members but found no difference between the group and eight residents of 5,340 meters (Keys 1936; Dill, Talbott, and Consolazio 1937). Why these results differed from Barcroft's was not discussed in print by either group.

In 1944, Aste-Salazar and Hurtado reported a series of measurements made in twelve natives of Morococha, altitude 4,500 meters. This study, also showing a right shift (lower O_2 affinity) of the OEC, is widely cited as showing that reduced hemoglobin oxygen affinity is adaptive in hypoxia, since it would theoretically lead to increased tissue PO_2 (Hurtado 1964). Although it challenged Barcroft's belief in the benefit of a left shift, it did not indicate why Barcroft's data might have been wrong. Nor does it address an important question: how can a right shift be beneficial in hypoxia, when it is agreed that a left shift in the fetus is beneficial? (The fetus faces an O_2 supply problem similar to that of high-altitude natives.)

Perhaps some of these conflicts can be appreciated from an understanding of the experimental methods used at that time. In the work reported by Aste-Salazar and Hurtado, arterial blood was drawn in Morococha, stored under mercury, and transported, cold, to Lima. There, after a period of three to seven hours, O_2 and CO_2 contents were measured in the VanSlyke apparatus[2] (see Keys 1936 for methods). Repeated measurements were made on blood equilibrated at pCO_2 of 40 torr and 200 torr to get two points on the CO_2 dissociation curve, and $PaCO_2$ could be read using the measured CO_2 content. Samples of the same blood were equilibrated at PO_2s of 25, 35, 40, 55, and 65 torr, and arterial PCO_2 was equilibrated (determined as above) in the range 34–38 torr to obtain the points on the oxygen equilibrium curve. In all cases, pH was calculated by the Henderson-Hasselbalch equation, which requires PCO_2 and $[HCO_3{}^-]$. The pH corrections were made by Bohr factor ($\Delta \log PCO_2/\Delta \log pH$) of -0.48. Finally, the points were plotted according to the logarithmic form of the Hill equation

$$\log (Y/1 - Y) = n \log (PO_2) + k, \qquad (4.2)$$

and the best straight line was drawn, probably by eye.

Table 4.3. Blood oxygenation data of Aste-Salazar and Hurtado

	N	HbO$_2$ cap (ml/dl)	pH	Arterial P50 (torr)	P50 pH 7.4 (torr)
Sea-level controls	17	21.86	7.39	24.73	24.39
		± .93	± .04	± .75	± .81
Natives of 4,540 m	12	29.48	7.36	27.39	26.13
		± 2.16	± .03	± 1.50	± 1.68

Source: Aste-Salazar and Hurtado 1945.
Note: Means are ± 1 SD.

The results indicate that the P50 under standard conditions (i.e., pH 7.4, PCO$_2$ 40 torr) is slightly higher in the high-altitude natives than in sea-level controls (table 4.3). However, the estimated pH in these natives was slightly lower, and, therefore, the in vivo P50 was felt to be significantly higher than in the controls. These authors concluded that "the slight decrease in the affinity of hemoglobin for oxygen, observed at high altitudes, may be interpreted as a favorable compensatory adjustment to the low pressure environment. It appears that under this condition the basic problem relates to the delivery of oxygen to the tissues, and a right deviation of the oxygen dissociation curve, even if slight, would be of appreciable benefit to this process, especially when we consider the increased quantity of blood hemoglobin present" (Aste-Salazar and Hurtado 1944).

In summary, these pioneering works on the role of blood oxygen affinity in adaptation of natives to high altitudes all seem to show a decreased affinity under standard conditions of pH and pCO$_2$ compared with controls measured the same way, if the calculation methods were identical. Only Barcroft's initial observations of unexpectedly increased arterial saturation at a given PO$_2$ (left shift of the OEC) remained unexplained. Subsequent workers found a right shift under standard conditions, and the rationale developed that this right shift allowed improved O$_2$ unloading in the tissue capillary beds. At the time these studies were reported, many deficiencies in the state of knowledge of hemoglobin and blood chemistry precluded their full interpretation. Some later clarifications are:

1. The relationship between pH and pCO$_2$ was clarified by Singer and Hastings (1948).

2. The solubility coefficient of CO$_2$ in plasma is temperature dependent, and pK' depends not only on temperature, but also on pH (Thomas 1972).

3. The partition of intracellular and extracellular CO$_2$ depends on pH and hemoglobin saturation, as shown by Van Slyke, et al. (1928).

4. The effect of 2,3-DPG was not appreciated until recently (Chanutin and Curnish 1967; Benesch and Benesch 1969).

5. The Hill plot describes the OEC only in its middle portion. More refined mathematical models are more accurate in the extremes (Winslow et al. 1977). Furthermore, the shape of the OEC is dependent on pH and the 2,3-DPG/hemoglobin molar ratio (Samaja and Winslow 1979, Winslow et al. 1983).

4.4   The Role of 2,3-DPG

Lenfant and co-workers (Lenfant et al. 1969) confirmed that the in vitro OEC of high-altitude natives is shifted to the right. They reported that "low oxygen saturation in the venous blood appears to be the regulating factor, and changes occurring in the concentration of some intracellular constituents seem to be the mechanism of action." Publication of this work coincided almost exactly with the demonstration that the red cell constituent, 2,3-DPG, strongly influences the position of the OEC (Chanutin and Curnish 1967; Benesch and Benesch 1969), and in a later publication, Lenfant and co-workers used this mechanism to explain their results (Lenfant, Torrance, and Reynafarje 1971). Following these papers, a large number of reports seemed to show that this important cellular constituent was a potent regulator of red cell oxygen affinity, and all previous data had to be reevaluated in light of this discovery. The main problem with their earlier work is that after venous blood is sampled, the concentration of 2,3-DPG rapidly decreases. The decrease is also temperature dependent, although keeping the sample on ice does not prevent its disappearance altogether.

2,3-DPG is a normal constituent of the glycolytic pathway (fig. 4.4). Its synthesis seems to be most closely regulated by the enzyme phosphofructokinase, whose activity is markedly stimulated by alkalosis (Espinos, Alvarez-Sala, and Villegas 1982). Initial observations of its increase in hypoxia led to the hypothesis that its concentration is dependent on hemoglobin saturation. However, Lenfant showed convincingly that pH is the principal controlling factor at altitude. To do this, he treated several sojourners with acetazolamide, a carbonic anhydrase inhibitor that prevents the alkalosis that normally occurs with exposure to hypoxia. In these subjects 2,3-DPG did not increase, and their OECs did not shift rightward, as did those of the controls (Lenfant, Torrance, and Reynafarje 1971).

Recent studies by the authors found red cell 2,3-DPG to be increased in natives of Morococha (fig. 4.5), but the degree of increase was not correlated with either arterial saturation, PO_2, or hematocrit (Winslow et al. 1981). Paradoxically, when several subjects underwent staged phlebotomy,

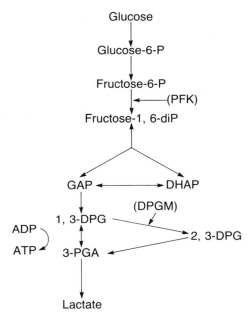

Figure 4.4. The metabolism of glucose by erythrocytes. The concentration of 2,3-DPG is profoundly influenced by the activity of phosphofructokinase (*PFK*), an enzyme whose activity is strongly pH-dependent.

2,3-DPG decreased, suggesting that its control is not dependent on arterial O_2 content. It must also be remembered that the concentration of 2,3-DPG is higher in younger red cells. Therefore, when the erythropoietic stress is great, the mean age of the circulating red cell mass is less, which of itself will increase the blood concentration of 2,3-DPG.

The question of whether 2,3-DPG plays an important physiologic role in O_2 transport in high-altitude humans still is not settled. Arguments based on theory have been advanced that it does (Neville 1977), and some animal experiments seem to confirm this idea (Moore and Brewer 1981). Computer models of O_2 uptake in the lung, however, suggest that when O_2 uptake is limited by diffusion, as it is at high altitudes, a right shift of the OEC is detrimental (Turek and Kreuzer 1981; Bencowitz, Wagner, and West 1982). This is intuitively apparent upon examination of the normal OEC (fig. 4.1). If arterial PO_2 is on the steep descending portion (50–55 torr), a right shift will decrease arterial O_2 saturation and content. If venous PO_2 is very low, as it would be during exercise, however, a right shift would affect venous PO_2 very little, because the curve is flat below about 15 torr.

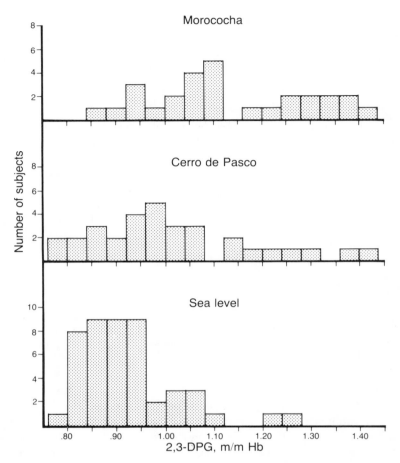

Figure 4.5. The distributions of 2,3-DPG concentration at sea level and at high altitude. (Winslow and Monge, unpublished data.)

4.5 The Blood Oxygen Affinity in vivo

All studies carried out in Cerro de Pasco, with the exception of Barcroft's, agreed that the position of the OEC in high-altitude natives is shifted to the right, either absolutely or in relation to sea-level controls, and the adaptive value of a right-shifted curve was all but established as dogma. However, experimental work began to suggest that increased O_2 affinity may be protective in animals exposed to very high altitude (Eaton, Skelton, and Berger 1974; Turek, Kreuzer, and Hoofd 1973; Turek and Kreuzer 1976, 1982). Moreover, a subject with a rare, inherited, abnormal hemoglobin with high O_2 affinity seemed to tolerate exercise better than did a normal sibling at high altitude (Hebbel, Kronenberg, and Eaton 1977; Hebbel et al. 1978). Monge C. and Whittembury (1974) pointed out that in animals native to high altitude, increased, rather than decreased, O_2 affinity was the rule. Computer simulations also suggest that increased O_2 affinity may aid O_2 uptake in the lung (Bencowitz, Wagner, and West 1981). Finally, climbers on Mt. Everest have an OEC that is severely left-shifted (P50 = 19.5 torr) because of striking respiratory alkalosis; this shift is probably crucial for adequate blood oxygenation at extreme altitude (Winslow, Samaja, and West 1984).

Why, after sixty-two years of expeditions and experimentation, is the position of the in vivo OEC in high-altitude natives still controversial? The problem is that to estimate the in vivo OEC one of two procedures must be followed. Either the curve can be measured in vitro under known conditions and extrapolated to the in vivo conditions (if the relationships are known) or, preferably, immediate measurements of saturation and PO_2 can be made on blood drawn from an artery or a vein. Both have advantages but in the first, an array of PO_2-saturation pairs can be obtained, whereas in the second, only single points are measured.

Work by the authors in Morococha in 1979 attempted both the above approaches (Winslow et al. 1981). Through collaboration with a group in Milan directed by Luigi Rossi-Bernardi and another at the National Institutes of Health directed by Robert Berger, an automated device was developed that could record the entire continuous OEC from 0 torr to 150 torr under specified conditions of pH, pCO_2, and a known 2,3-DPG/hemoglobin ratio (Winslow et al. 1977). The measurement could be made automatically within about 30 minutes after venipuncture, and the results agreed favorably with the best measurements available by conventional methods (Winslow et al. 1977).

The experimental subjects who participated in these studies were slightly older than those studied by Aste-Salazar and Hurtado, but they represented a broader cross section of the population of Morococha. All the subjects had been born at altitudes above 3,000 meters, and none had visited sea level during the three months prior to the tests. Their hematocrits ranged from 48 percent to 82 percent, mean 61 ± 8 percent. The hematocrit and hemoglobin values did not correlate with age.

The OEC data were fit to the Adair equation[3] (Winslow et al. 1977). This mathematical model has the advantage that no assumptions need be made about the final saturation after the blood sample is oxygenated, but the technique yields P50 values slightly higher than some of the older data. In the authors' study, the in vitro P50 determined in this way was again noted to be slightly above the values measured in sea-level controls when expressed at pH 7.4 (fig. 4.6). This increase is explained by increased red cell 2,3-DPG (fig. 4.5). Both the P50 values and 2,3-DPG concentrations fell in rather wide distributions and were not correlated with each other. Therefore, there

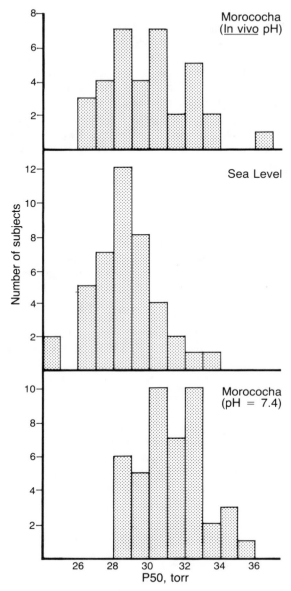

Figure 4.6.   The distributions of P50 at sea level and at high altitude. In the top panel, values are expressed at in vivo pH; in the bottom, at pH 7.4. (Winslow et al. 1981.)

must be many factors that control the precise position of the OEC in an individual.

The problem with this approach is in estimating the in vivo position of the OEC. In an attempt to make the in vitro conditions as close to in vivo conditions as possible, samples were equilibrated with 8 percent CO_2, which, at a barometric pressure of 455 torr and 37 °C, gives a CO_2 partial pressure of about 35 torr, a value a little higher than that found in most subjects' arterial blood. To relate the results to in vivo conditions, knowledge of the arterial pH and PCO_2 is required. While the effect of PCO_2 on P50 in this range is minimal, the estimation of pH is critical.

It had been noted previously that the measured pH of blood samples with elevated hematocrit could be significantly lower than plasma pH, and the explanation was thought to be an interaction between the red cells and the surface of the glass electrode (Whittembury et al. 1968). Severinghaus also found this discrepancy but attributed it to metabolic changes in the red cells during the time required to make the appropriate measurements (Severinghaus, Stupfel, and Bradley 1956). To check this possibility in our subjects, samples of blood were adjusted to various hematocrits, equilibrated with gas of known composition, layered under mineral oil, and quickly centrifuged in a minicentrifuge (about one minute was required for the procedure). The pH of both plasma and whole blood then was measured. The results confirmed the previous studies showing that the difference in plasma and blood pH increases with increasing hematocrit (fig. 4.7).

When the data in figure 4.7 were used to correct pH to in vivo plasma pH, the result was an estimate of the position of the OEC that was not significantly different from that of the sea-level controls (fig. 4.6). This result has the following significant implications: (1) the in vivo position of the OEC is not different in high-altitude natives; (2) the effect of elevation of 2,3-DPG in these subjects in shifting the OEC to the right is offset by respiratory alkalosis; and (3) the existence of respiratory alkalosis suggests a lack of full acclimatization in the natives studied.

A proper interpretation of the position of the in vivo OEC, if the estimation is based on in vitro data, depends on accurate knowledge of in vivo pH. This value has been reported as being anywhere from 7.36 to 7.431 (table 4.4). This range corresponds to a difference in P50 of about 1.1 torr, if a Bohr factor of -0.4 is used.[4] (The actual value of the Bohr factor depends on PCO_2 and 2,3-DPG/Hb molar ratio; Samaja and Winslow 1979.) However, the in vivo P50 could be in error by several times this value, since such corrections may be used more than once in some of the older methods of measurement. The pH measurements on separated plasma shown in Table 4.4 are significantly higher than those on whole blood in natives of similar altitude. This difference is consistent with the argument that polycythemia leads to a spuriously low pH measurement.

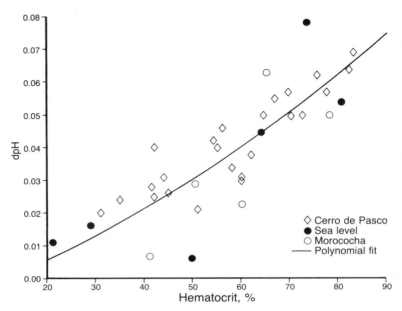

Figure 4.7.   The suspension effect of red cells on apparent blood pH. The difference between plasma and blood pH (*dpH*) is shown as a function of hematocrit. Data are from natives of Cerro de Pasco, Morococha, and sea level. (Winslow et al. 1981.)

The best approach to the estimation of the in vivo OEC would be to measure saturation and PO_2 independently and simultaneously in arterial and venous blood, allowing the body to be its own tonometer. Such data are reminiscent of Barcroft's 1921–22 Cerro de Pasco results (fig. 4.8, cf. fig. 4.3). The actual arterial values at in vivo pH are above and to the left of the observed in vitro OEC. These data constitute the most reliable estimate of in vivo OEC, because no corrections are made for pH. They are the only measurements we know of in which simultaneous PO_2 and saturation pairs were obtained. Regardless of the actual value of pH, the data suggest strongly that the O_2 affinity of high-altitude natives is increased, as originally proposed by Barcroft, and the effect of increased 2,3-DPG is more than offset by chronic respiratory alkalosis (Winslow et al. 1981).

4.6   The Bohr Effect

An interesting study that arrived at novel conclusions was carried out by Morpurgo et al. (1970), who reported an increased Bohr effect in Peruvian high-altitude natives of Morococha. That is, that the position of their blood oxygen equilibrium curve was more sensitive to changes in pH than was that

Table 4.4.   Blood-gas and pH values in high-altitude natives

Altitude (m)	N	Hct (Hb)[a]	PaO$_2$ (torr)	SaO$_2$ (%)	PaCO$_2$ (torr)	pH	Source
4,300	3	—	46.7	84.6	—	—	(1)
4,300	12	—	—	—	—	7.360	(2)
4,500	40	(20.6)	45.1	80.1	33.3	7.370	(3)
4,515	22	(19.5)	—	82.8	33.8	7.400	(4)
4,300	6	56.0	—	—	32.5	7.431[b]	(5)
4,300	5	73.8	—	—	39.0	7.429[b]	(5)
3,700	—	—	—	—	3.0	7.431[b]	(6)
4,545	—	—	—	—	—	7.424[b]	(6)
4,820	—	—	—	—	—	7.426[b]	(6)
3,960	3	—	—	—	—	—	(7)[c]
4,880	4	—	—	—	—	7.399	(7)[c]
4,500	6	73.4	—	—	—	—	(8)
4,500	10	65.5	—	—	—	—	(8)
4,300	6	54.4	45.2	74.7	31.6	7.414	(9)
4,500	4	63.3	44.1	73.3	32.2	7.405	(9)
4,300	4	—	50.8	—	32.9	7.405	(10)
4,500	35	61.0	51.7	85.7	34.0	7.395	(11)

Sources: (1) Barcroft et al. 1923; (2) Aste-Salazar and Hurtado 1944; (3) Hurtado, Velászuez, Reynafarje et al. 1956; (4) Chiodi 1957; (5) Monge, Lozano and Carcelén 1964; (6) Severinghaus and Carcelén 1964; (7) Lahiri et al. 1967; (8) Lenfant et al. 1969; (9) Torrance 1970; (10) Rennie 1971; and (11) Winslow et al. 1981.
[a]Numbers in parentheses are Hb (g/dl).
[b]Plasma pH.
[c]Himalayan subjects.

of lowlanders. In these studies, P50 was measured at two pH values, 6.7 and 7.4. The results were identical to those with blood from Europeans at pH 6.7, but the high-altitude natives showed relatively decreased affinity at pH 7.4. In a later publication Morpurgo et al. concluded that the effect was not due to 2,3-DPG, and similar results were found in diabetic patients (Battaglia, Morpurgo, and Passi 1971). They suggested that a small molecule, as yet unidentified, may explain the observations (none has been identified).

Morpurgo and co-workers suggested that this increased Bohr effect might represent a genetic adaptation to high altitudes (Morpurgo et al. 1970) and might be an important difference between Andean and Himalayan natives, because they could not repeat the findings in Nepalese natives (Morpurgo et al. 1972). They also claimed that Sherpas have increased O$_2$ affinity compared with Peruvian natives (Morpurgo et al. 1976). However, the Nepalese data were refuted when newer techniques demonstrated that the Bohr effect and O$_2$ affinity in Nepalese natives could be explained on the basis of known effectors of hemoglobin function (Samaja, Veicsteinas, and Cerretelli 1979).

Detailed studies demonstrated that the O$_2$ affinity of normal red cells can be completely accounted for by the known allosteric effectors of hemoglobin

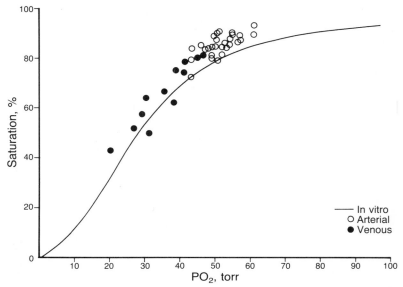

Figure 4.8.   The in vivo oxygen equilibrium curve at Morococha. The solid line represents the mean of the continuously measured in vitro curves, corrected to pH 7.4. Open and closed points are the saturation-PO_2 pairs for arterial and venous samples, respectively. (Winslow, Monge, and Winslow, unpublished data.)

function: H^+, 2,3-DPG, and CO_2, with minor contributions from Mg^{++}, Cl^-, and ATP (Horvath et al. 1977).

Because Morpurgo's data suggested that some other effector could participate in the regulation of O_2 affinity at high altitudes, the authors reopened the question of the Bohr effect in Peruvian high-altitude natives by a series of measurements on natives of Morococha (Winslow, Monge, Winslow, et al. 1985). The ΔlogP50/ΔpH slope in fresh whole blood titrated with either NaOH or lactic acid was found to be −0.387 for the natives of Morococha, and −0.416 for persons at sea level. The difference between these slopes is not statistically significant, but it could be explained by an increased 2,3-DPG/Hb molar ratio in the Morococha subjects. These slopes, the "fixed acid Bohr effect," agree well with values of −0.37 reported by Wranne, Woodson, and Detter (1972) and of −0.40 reported by Naeraa et al. (1966) for fresh sea-level blood, but titrated at fixed PCO_2 with HCl and NaOH. Our findings did not substantiate the earlier report that Peruvian high-altitude natives have an increased Bohr effect (Morpurgo et al. 1970).

It is difficult to explain the previous data of Morpurgo and co-workers, because the methods and conditions of their experiments differed significantly from ours, as did their physiologic conditions. Their measurements were made with hemolysates diluted in CO_2-free 0.1 M phosphate buffers of known pH. This technique would cause some distortions in physiologic interpretation, because the effects of H^+, 2,3-DPG, and CO_2 are interrelated. That is, these effectors compete for certain binding sites on the hemoglobin molecule, and alteration of any one of them will alter the effects of the others. In addition, hemoglobin concentration itself is an important determinant of hemoglobin function, since dissociation of tetramers to dimers may become significant at low concentration, and the O_2 affinity of dimers is considerably higher than that of tetrameters.

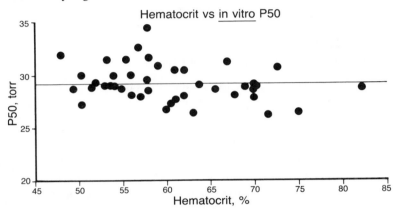

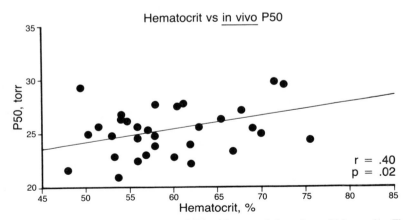

Figure 4.9. The relationship between P50 and hematocrit in natives of Morococha. The correlation is significant under in vivo conditions of pH and PCO_2. This is consistent with the lower pH and higher PCO_2 in polycythemic subjects, and it argues against the hypothesis that high oxygen affinity could contribute to erythropoietic stimulation. (Winslow, Monge, and Winslow, unpublished data.)

An additional effector of hemoglobin usually not considered in red cell and whole blood studies is the chloride ion. The concentration of intracellular Cl^- increases when HCO_3^- decreases (the chloride shift). Thus, in compensated respiratory alkalosis, it is possible that intracellular Cl^- concentration could be altered to a degree to affect hemoglobin oxygenation. Indeed, in 1937 Dill and co-workers reported a slight shift of the red cell–to–plasma Cl^- ratio in a number of Chilean high-altitude natives (Dill, Talbott, and Consolazio 1937). Whether the choride shift has important physiologic consequences for hemoglobin oxygenation at high altitudes remains to be seen.

4.7   The Blood Oxygen Affinity and Chronic Mountain Sickness

An intriguing idea that occurred to the authors was that subjects with highest hemoglobin concentrations or hematocrits may have increased whole blood oxygen affinity. This idea came from the fact that at sea level, subjects with increased oxygen affinity due to either (1) a genetically altered hemoglobin molecule or (2) increased carboxyhemoglobin from industrial or smoking exposure have increased hemoglobin concentration, apparently as a compensatory mechanism. The idea was tested in Morococha in 1978 by selecting a group of subjects with a broad range of hematocrits. No correlation was found between in vitro P50 (i.e., measured at PCO_2 35 torr) and hematocrit (fig. 4.9). When expressed under in vivo conditions, the correlation is significant. However, the reverse of the expected result was found: a decrease in O_2 affinity is associated with a higher hematocrit, possibly because of a lower tissue PO_2.

CHAPTER FIVE

Circulation

The circulation is a key link in the O_2 transport chain. Its regulation is complex and deeply integrated with ventilation, exercise, and tissue metabolism; it is influenced by training, body habitus, and body composition and age, to name just a few of the related variables. Consideration of the heart and other components of the circulatory system without frequent reference to these effectors would be impossible. Therefore, separation into chapters of information about these different areas is somewhat arbitrary. Central to the purpose here is consideration of the effects of polycythemia on the circulation, keeping in mind the well-known increase of blood viscosity with hematocrit (fig. 5.1).

This chapter reviews information about the performance of the heart and the effects of long-term hypoxia on its role in the circulation. It discusses circulation in organs whose functions are integrated with blood flow: the brain, the lung, and muscle mass. Subsequent chapters on ventilation (chap. 6), the kidney (chap. 7), and exercise (chap. 8) overlap with this one. Observations on removal of blood by phlebotomy provide useful insights into the physiologic effects of polycythemia.

The amount of O_2 transferred to tissues from the blood is the product of the arterial-venous O_2 content difference and the cardiac output. If pulmonary oxygenation is normal, the O_2 content of arterial blood will vary directly with hemoglobin concentration. In hypoxia, however, deficient arterial O_2 content could be compensated for by an appropriate change in cardiac output, but in fact, such compensations are never complete. Thus, in patients with severe anemia, tissue PO_2 is low because increased cardiac output is not sufficient to compensate for the decreased O_2 capacity. This chapter and subsequent ones examine the hypothesis that, in patients with chronic mountain sickness, O_2 delivery to tissues is reduced because increased O_2 capacity does not compensate for decreased cardiac output.

5.1 Physiologic Considerations

The effects of hematocrit variation on the regulation of the circulation have been studied in detail by Guyton and colleagues (Guyton, Jones, and Coleman 1973). Their work, mainly with dogs, has probed into the intricate interrelations between polycythemia, cardiac output, and blood pressure and flow. Some studies have been carried out of humans with polycythemia vera (Goldsmith 1936; Altschule, Volk, and Henstell 1940), and a greater number have involved patients with cyanotic congenital heart disease. These

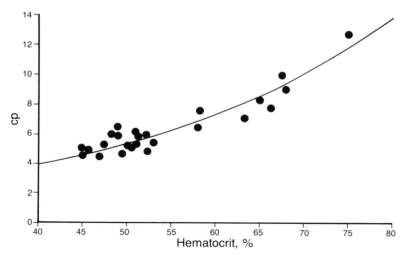

Figure 5.1.   The dependence of blood viscosity on hematocrit in natives of Cerro de Pasco.
(Winslow, Monge, and Dixon, unpublished data.)

latter subjects, however, cannot be used as a model for the effects of polycythemia because they have altered circulatory dynamics as a result of their
congenital malformations. The normal control of the cardiac output is very
complex, and the regulation in high-altitude natives is likely to be even more
so because of the effects of hypoxia, altered ventilation, blood volume, and,
possibly, autonomic control. One can approach this problem by first outlin-
ing a few of the principles that seem to apply to the effect of polycythemia on
cardiac output in the highly controlled laboratory setting, then asking
whether they are consistent with the fragmentary data available for high-
altitude natives.

Guyton and Richardson (1961) studied venous return to the hearts of dogs
as a function of right atrial pressure. In these animals, blood was pumped
externally from the right atrium into the pulmonary artery. By regulating the
rate of pumping in this way, the right atrial pressure could be controlled, and
the venous return could be measured with a flow meter. They found a very
predictable relationship between right atrial pressure and venous return, and
that the hematocrit had a profound effect (fig. 5.2a). That is, in polycythemia, a given right atrial pressure results in a lowered venous return.
Since cardiac output must equal venous return in the steady state, this means
that cardiac output was profoundly reduced by increases in hematocrit. Note
that this experimental design does not account for any regulation that may
occur in the peripheral circulation, or in the neural control of the heart.

Castle and Jandl (1966) drew attention to the fact that blood volume
increases in polycythemic states, and that it is necessary to consider the

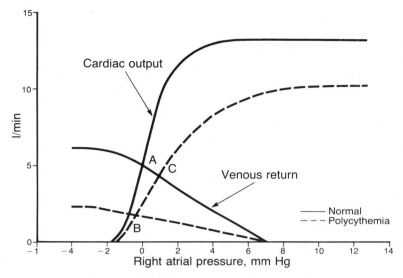

Figure 5.2. The relationships of pressure, venous return, and cardiac output. Normally, venous return decreases and cardiac output increases as right atrial pressure increases (*solid lines*). The equilibrium (point *A*), shown as the intersection of these two lines, represents the normal condition. Acute polycythemia decreases venous return and cardiac output because of increased systemic resistance to flow (*dashed lines*), establishing a new equilibrium (point *B*). Compensation may be achieved by peripheral vascularization, expanded blood volume, and increased systemic pressure. In theory, the cardiac output could return almost to its normal value (point *C*). (Modified, with permission from Guyton, Jones, and Coleman 1973.)

combined effect of multiple variables on the control of cardiac output. Very few experimental observations are available to draw a significant parallel between laboratory models and the in vivo effects of polycythemia on cardiac output. Guyton, Jones, and Coleman (1973) pointed out that polycythemic subjects need not have reduced cardiac output if systemic pressure is increased. This is illustrated in figure 5.2, in which the solid curves represent the normal circulation, with *A* as the equilibrium point. If the hematocrit increases suddenly, the viscosity and resistance to venous return increase, and the venous return curve falls; since systemic pressure does not increase immediately, cardiac output also falls, and a new equilibrium point, *B,* is reached. This is almost exactly the finding in dogs made acutely polycythemic (Richardson and Guyton 1959). In chronic polycythemia, blood volume increases, increasing venous return and systemic pressure. If, in addition to this change, the peripheral resistance decreases due to vascularization, the venous return can be restored to its normal value, point *C* in figure 5.2. In fact, with cardiac hypertrophy and a lessened resistive load on the heart, the cardiac output curve may actually return to normal. Unfortunately, no measurements of this degree of sophistication have been made in high-altitude natives, and one must look to circumstantial evidence to try to evaluate this model for the relationship between hematocrit, viscosity, and cardiac output.

Normal lowland subjects taken to a simulated altitude of 4,000 meters (barometric pressure 462 torr) do not show a reduced cardiac output within the first hour of exposure (Stenberg, Ekblom, and Messin 1966). However, Hoon and co-workers showed, in studies on lowlanders transported to similar altitudes for longer periods, that the cardiac output fell, reaching a minimum three days after arrival; reduced stroke volume in these subjects was not compensated by tachycardia (Hoon et al. 1977). Pugh (1964) showed that reduced cardiac output remains depressed even after several months of high-altitude exposure. In high-altitude natives, however, cardiac output has been reported to be the same as it is at sea level (Peñaloza et al. 1963; Moret et al. 1972). An important difference between sojourners and natives is that the latter tend to be more polycythemic.

The heart of the high-altitude native increases in size, muscle mass, and metabolism, and its failure is often considered as part of the clinical picture of chronic mountain sickness. In addition, adjustments of the regional distribution of the cardiac output affect all organ systems and their functions. Sometimes the interactions between blood perfusion and organ function are exceedingly complex, as in those of the brain and the lung, and they may involve complicated feedback regulatory loops.

5.2   Systemic Circulation

It is commonly believed that the incidence of coronary artery disease and systemic hypertension is lower in high-altitude natives than it is in persons at sea level. This is obviously a complex matter, because we now know that these properties are governed by many factors, including diet, exercise, age, genetic makeup, and smoking habits, just to mention the common ones. Nevertheless, the clinical impression of lower systemic blood pressure in high-altitude natives was substantiated in epidemiologic studies in Peru (Ruiz et al. 1968). The results of these studies, summarized by Peñaloza Durand and Martineaud 1971), were believed to be due to increased vascularization of the capillary beds and diminished peripheral resistance in response to hypoxia. However, Peñaloza pointed out that the difference in blood pressures was only in the systolic value, and, in fact, diastolic pressures were found by Ruiz and co-workers to be slightly higher in high-altitude natives. These authors attributed the increase to polycythemia, because they claimed the values significantly decreased after bleeding (Ruiz and Peñaloza 1970). Unfortunately, no blood volume measurements are available for these studies.

No case of myocardial infarction or significant coronary artery disease was reported in a series of 300 autopsies performed in Cerro de Pasco (Ramos et al. 1967). Moreover, further epidemiologic studies by Ruiz and co-workers showed that electrocardiographic signs of ischemic coronary disease were less frequent than in sea-level controls (Ruiz et al. 1969). Because of these provocative facts, Arias-Stella and co-workers performed postmortem studies of the coronary trees of the hearts of ten natives of Cerro de Pasco; these were compared with those of ten sea-level controls (Arias-Stella and Topilsky 1971). They found increased branching of the coronary circulation at several levels and concluded that increased vascularization could explain the decreased incidence of myocardial disease.

In spite of this increased vascularization of the myocardium in high-altitude natives, Moret (1971) and Grover (Grover, Lufchanowski, and Alexander 1971) showed that coronary blood flow was reduced compared with that of sea-level controls. Thus, it would seem that at high altitudes there may be an increased volume of myocardial blood and, perhaps, of O_2 reserve. Moret also measured coronary blood flow and O_2 transport parameters in four subjects with chronic mountain sickness. The results indicated increased coronary blood flow (probably because of increased left ventricular work), normal O_2 content of coronary sinus blood, and an indication of underperfusion of some areas of the myocardium. Moret calculated the O_2 consumption for the hearts of patients with chronic mountain sickness to be 9.7 milliliters per 100 milligrams of tissue, compared with 7 milliliters per 100 milligrams for high-altitude controls.

5.3 Cor Pulmonale and Chronic Mountain Sickness

Detailed studies of cardiovascular hemodynamics in chronic mountain sickness were carried out by Peñaloza and co-workers in the Peruvian Andes (Peñaloza and Sime 1971). They selected ten subjects with chronic mountain sickness and compared them with appropriate high-altitude and sea-level controls (table 5.1). The results showed that subjects with chronic mountain sickness had elevated right ventricular, pulmonary artery, and systemic vascular pressures, thereby suggesting similarities between this clinical entity and Brisket disease of cattle (Hecht et al. 1962). Peñaloza and colleagues went on to show that the signs of cor pulmonale (right heart failure) could be reversed by descent to sea level (fig. 5.3). In a later publication, Peñaloza distinguished two causes for pulmonary hypertension: hypoxia and polycythemia (Peñaloza, Sime, and Ruiz 1971). Hypoxia is relieved immediately after descent, while the reduction of pulmonary artery pressure is much slower (fig. 5.3).

Drawing on the anatomic data of Arias-Stella (see chap. 2), Peñaloza concluded that chronic mountain sickness is due primarily to alveolar hypo-

Table 5.1.   Cardiovascular findings in high-altitude natives

	CMS Subjects	High-Altitude Controls	Sea-Level Controls	Difference (p)[a]
	$N = 20$	$N = 12$	$N = 25$	
Age (yr)	38 ± 9	24 ± 6	21 ± 1	<.001
Heart rate (min$^-$)	83 ± 15	72 ± 10	68 ± 9	ns
Hematocrit (%)	79.3 ± 4.2	59.4 ± 5.4	44.1 ± 2.6	<.001
SaO$_2$ (%)	69.6 ± 4.9	81.4 ± 4.6	95.7 ± 2.1	<.001
Mean pressures (mm Hg)				
Right atrium	3.9 ± 1.8	2.9 ± 1.4	2.6 ± 1.3	ns
Right ventricle	29 ± 13.6	15 ± 3.4	9.0 ± 1.5	<.01
Pulmonary artery	47 ± 18	23 ± 5	12 ± 2	<.001
Pa wedge	5.7 ± 2.3	6.9 ± 1.4	6.2 ± 1.7	ns
Systemic	105 ± 18	91 ± 9.6	95 ± 8	<.05

Source: Peñaloza and Sime 1971.
[a]Significance level for difference between CMS and high-altitude subjects.

ventilation, which in turn leads to muscularization of the pulmonary vessels and pulmonary hypertension. When these data and conclusions were presented at the 1971 Ciba symposium, the discussion pointed out a potential flaw in this hypothesis: removal of blood by phlebotomy was known in some

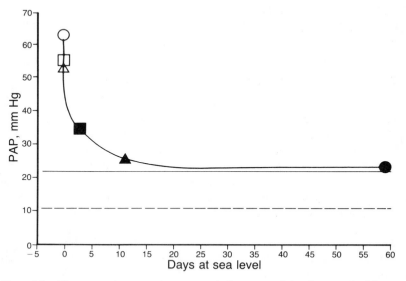

Figure 5.3.   The mean pulmonary-artery pressure in three cases of chronic mountain sickness, as a function of time of residence at sea level. The horizontal solid and dashed lines represent normal values for highlanders and lowlanders, respectively. The initial rapid drop after descent to sea level is due to relief of hypoxia, while the longer decrease is due to reversal of chronic polycythemia. (Modified, with permission from Peñaloza and Sime 1971.)

cases to reverse the apparent hypoventilation (Peñaloza, Sime, and Ruiz 1971). In other words, PaO_2, and SaO_2 increased, while $PaCO_2$ decreased; this seems to indicate that even if hypoventilation is the primary cause of chronic mountain sickness, it is at least partly reversible by hemotocrit reduction.

5.4 Electrocardiographic Findings

Cor pulmonale is a condition of right heart failure attributable to pulmonary arterial hypertension. It is associated with characteristic ECG signs. Peñaloza described the electrocardiographic findings of right heart strain in high-altitude natives of all ages (Peñaloza and Echevarria 1957; Peñaloza et al. 1960; Peñaloza 1962). Ten normal sea-level residents who lived for one year at Morococha (4,500 m) demonstrated similar changes: posterior rightward rotation of the mean QRS axis, increased amplitude of the R wave in aVR, and a deepened S wave in V_1. These changes, however, were still not as striking as those found in natives of the same altitude, and the authors concluded that more than one year of exposure to altitude would be required to cause clinical cor pulmonale.

To determine whether such electrocardiographic changes (and, presumably, cor pulmonale) correlate with hematocrit in lifelong residents of Cerro de Pasco (4,300 m), the authors recorded twelve-lead scalar electrocardiograms in forty-seven subjects (table 5.2). They had generally lower hematocrits (mean 55.0 ± 8.5 percent) than those selected by Peñaloza and co-workers but constituted a

Table 5.2.   Electrocardiographic findings in natives of Cerro de Pasco

	Polycythemic subjects	High-altitude controls	Difference (p)
	N = 10	*N = 25*	
QRS			
Axis (deg)	63 ± 49	14 ± 103	ns
Ampl (mv)	1.130 ± .570	1.160 ± .540	ns
P			
Axis (deg)	56 ± 19	53 ± 18	ns
T			
Axis (deg)	38 ± 19	37 ± 5	ns
Ampl (mv)	.539 ± .199	.410 ± .150	.05
R/S(V5) + R/S(V1)	5.75 ± 4.26	3.46 ± 2.29	.05
HR	71 ± 11	72 ± 13	ns
PR(sec)	.18 ± .02	.16 ± .02	.05
QRS(sec)	.07 ± .01	.06 ± .01	ns
QTc(sec)[a]	.406 ± .039	.423 ± .029	ns

Source: Winslow and Monge, unpublished data.
[a] $QTc = QT/\sqrt{R - R}$.

larger group and represented a spectrum of hematocrit values. A continuum of symptoms was observed, and subjects were not easily classified into chronic mountain sickness groups and normal groups. Therefore, to compare high- and low-hematocrit groups, an arbitrary cutoff of 60 percent hematocrit was used to distinguish polycythemic and "normal" subjects.

In contrast to the report of Peñaloza and Sime (1971), no significant difference was found between the polycythemic and normal groups in mean QRS amplitude or vector, but there was a large variation in both groups (fig. 5.4). In one subject (3780), the mean QRS vector shifted toward normal, and its amplitude almost doubled after reduction of the hematocrit by hemodilu-

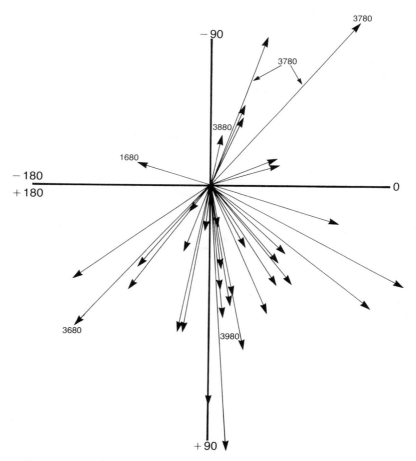

Figure 5.4. Mean QRS vectors for a sample of native residents of Cerro de Pasco. The excessively polycythemic subjects are noted by their case numbers. The mean vector for subject 3780 shifted to the left after hemodilution. (Winslow and Monge, unpublished data.)

tion. This shift, which probably occurred because of reduced pulmonary artery pressure, suggests an immediate relief of the work the heart must perform in overcoming the resistive effect of polycythemia.

Similar patterns emerged among P and T wave amplitudes and vectors. No differences between polycythemic and normal groups could be detected, and a large variation was again noted. With few exceptions, the resting heart rate, PR, QRS, and QT intervals were within the range of sea-level normal (Katz 1977). Normal ranges for these values at high altitudes have not been established by large population studies, however. In the groups studied, only the PR interval was significantly longer ($p = .05$) in the high-hematocrit group.

Peñaloza et al. (1960) classified ECG patterns by tabulating various combinations of R and S wave amplitudes in high- and low-hematocrit groups. Following their analysis with the authors' data, only the sum $R/S(V5) + R/S(V1)$ was significantly different for the two groups. Again, the large variation in these measurements is striking. One must question, however, the usefulness of such arbitrary parameters.

The lack of a strict correlation between ECG changes suggestive of cor pulmonale and chronic mountain sickness raises doubt of the value of those changes in identifying the increased pressures and venous return predicted by Guyton, Jones, and Coleman (1973). R wave morphology is an indirect indicator of cardiac volume (Brody 1956), and its amplitude correlates with acute blood loss (Manoach et al. 1971; Scherf and Bornemann 1968). It has been used to monitor the cardiac response to exercise (Battler et al. 1979) and to predict the presence of coronary artery disease at sea level (Baron et al. 1980; Kentala, Heikkila, and Pyorala 1973). In our subjects, the mean QRS amplitude increased in the left chest leads after phlebotomy, and, in one, the R wave upslope increased dramatically, suggesting increased venous return.

Peñaloza proposed that chronic mountain sickness is a form of chronic cor pulmonale, similar to that seen at sea level resulting from parenchymal lung disease. The authors' studies suggest that, while cor pulmonale may be a feature of advanced chronic mountain sickness, the two are not necessarily etiologically linked. That is, if Peñaloza's hypothesis was correct, a continuum of electrocardiographic evidence of right heart enlargement and strain should have been seen in the subjects, and ECG signs of cor pulmonale would be a consistent finding in all cases of chronic mountain sickness. Instead, tremendous variability in both hematocrit and ECG findings was found. One must conclude that there is no compelling evidence against the simpler hypothesis that cor pulmonale is simply a late manifestation of long-term hypoxic exposure, coupled with an increased pulmonary resistance to flow.

5.5   Cardiac Output

5.5.1   Normal Control of Cardiac Output

The major adjustment in the O_2 delivery system when tissue demand increases is an increase in cardiac output. In normal sea-level humans, the cardiac output can increase by about fourfold; this increase is mediated primarily by increased heart rate and secondarily by increased stroke volume. During exercise, most of the increased cardiac output is directed to exercising muscle.

The heart rate increase during exercise is under the general control of the autonomic nervous system, either by a decrease in parasympathetic restraint or by a sympathetic stimulation. The latter can occur either by neural stimulation or by an increase in circulating catecholamines. In normal, resting sea-level humans, the baseline heart rate is about 60 per minute and can increase to about 200 per minute. The actual value for a person is age-dependent, and the maximum decreases with age.

Starling (1918) claimed that stroke volume played the central role in determining the cardiac output. That conclusion, however, was derived from in vitro experiments with a heart-lung preparation; later work by Rushmer (1959) showed the constancy of stroke volume in exercise. It is now known, however, that under severe stress the stroke volume does increase somewhat in exercise (Horwitz, Atkins, and Leshin 1972). Furthermore, stroke volume is higher in the supine posture than in the erect (Chapman, Fisher, and Sproule 1960), and it increases after physical training (Saltin and Åstrand 1967). The mechanism of stroke volume increase is either by reduction of afterload (resistance to flow), an increase in preload (venous return to the heart), or an increase in the myocardial contractile state (Vatner 1976).

5.5.2   The Measurement of Cardiac Output

A few technical points are important in consideration of cardiac output data, particularly in high-altitude natives. There are two commonly used methods, indicator dilution and the direct Fick technique. In the first, the currently preferred method, a bolus of material is injected into the pulmonary artery and detected downstream from the site of injection. The result is obtained by integrating the curve relating concentration of the substance with time. The material injected is usually iced saline (thermodilution); older studies used various dyes. In the thermodilution method, the sensor is a thermistor located on the catheter distal from the site of injection. Implicit in this method is the assumption that equilibration of the cold material is complete by the time the blood reaches the sensor, and that all components of the blood are at equilibrium. To the authors' knowledge, these assumptions have not been verified adequately in polycythemic persons.

The second method is the calculation of the cardiac output directly from the Fick equation. This equation relates cardiac output, O_2 uptake, and the arterial-mixed venous O_2 content difference:

$$\dot{Q} = \dot{V}O_2/(a - \bar{v})O_2 \qquad (5.1)$$

where $\dot{Q}$ is the cardiac output, $\dot{V}O_2$ is the O_2 uptake, and $(a - \bar{v})O_2$ is the arterial-venous O_2 content difference. More assumptions are required when this method is used. First, the subject must be in the "steady state"; that is, the O_2 taken up in the lungs must equal the O_2 utilized in the body. The steady state is usually verified by observation of the gas exchange ratio, $\dot{V}CO_2/\dot{V}O_2$, to be about 0.8. The second assumption is that the difference between arterial and mixed venous O_2 must be known accurately, either from direct measurements of O_2 contents of the blood or from measurements of PO_2 and calculation of the SaO_2 by a known O_2 dissociation curve or by direct measurement of SaO_2. Other methods are available for measuring cardiac output,[1] and some are noninvasive. However, these require even more assumptions, and data obtained by them will not be discussed here.

5.5.3   Cardiac Output in High-Altitude Natives

The first determination of cardiac output in high-altitude natives was carried out in Morococha in 1938 by Rotta and co-workers (cited in Rotta et al. 1956). They used the acetylene technique[2] (Grollman 1932) and found a slight increase in resting cardiac output in the Morococha natives as compared with that of the sea-level controls. Interestingly, Theilen, together with Gregg and Rotta, later using the dye dilution technique and found a large increase in the cardiac output in the Morococha natives (Theilen 1954). When Rotta and co-workers used the Fick technique in the same population, however, they found no differences in cardiac output. Peñaloza and his group and Monge C. and co-workers, also using the dye dilution technique, found normal values or slight increases in Morococha natives (Peñaloza et al. 1963, Monge C. et al. 1955). In measurements in Cerro de Pasco, the authors observed that thermodilution gave results higher than those of direct Fick when both techniques were measured simultaneously (Winslow, Monge, Brown, et al. 1985). This unsettling result lends uncertainty to the measurements that depend on the steady-state assumption.

Contradictory results were found using Fick calculations in four natives of Leadville, Colorado, 3,100 meters (Hartley et al. 1967). These studies showed a slight decrease in cardiac output compared with that of sea-level controls, but they had an increased $(a - \bar{v})O_2$ difference, at a given rate of O_2

uptake. The decrease in cardiac output was mediated by decreased stroke volume and was not reversed by administration of supplemental O_2 at altitude. Cardiac output and stroke volume both increased after descent to sea level. The subjects of this study had been born at a high altitude, but their parents were lowlanders, in contrast to studies in Andean natives. Their mean hematocrit was 48.5 percent, body weight 71.2 kilograms, and surface area 1.87 m^2, all of which are not typical of high-altitude natives (see chap. 2).

Banchero and colleagues also used the O_2-Fick technique to study thirty-five male natives of Cerro de Pasco, Peru (Banchero et al. 1966). Although individual data were not given in their paper, these workers found a mean cardiac output and $(a - \bar{v})O_2$ difference that was not different from a sea-level control group of twenty-two subjects. In their high-altitude group, the mean body surface area was 1.55 meters^2 (1.63 m^2 for the sea-level controls), and the mean hematocrit was 58.7 percent. They noted that the increased cardiac output with exercise was mediated almost exclusively by an increase in heart rate, while the stroke volume remained almost constant.

The cardiac output determinations in high-altitude Andean natives show contradictory results, despite having been done by the same groups of investigators in similar populations. Studies in North American high-altitude residents may not be strictly comparable, inasmuch as the two groups of subjects—Andeans and North Americans—are different sizes. Nevertheless, the results suggest that the cardiac output is higher in the Andean resident, and they compare favorably with expected sea-level values. Another important difference between the natives of the two areas is that the hematocrits in the Andeans are higher, and a satisfactory description of the effect of hematocrit on cardiac output in humans is still incomplete. In chapter 10, detailed measurements are presented in one subject in Cerro de Pasco, Peru, whose cardiovascular hemodynamics at rest and in exercise were studied using both thermodilution and direct Fick methods. In this subject, elevated hematocrit lowered the cardiac output, an effect that could be reversed (at least temporarily) by hemodilution.

All the data reviewed above are consistent with the view that the lifelong high-altitude native does not have increased cardiac output. In view of Peñaloza's findings of increased pulmonary artery pressures, one may postulate that Guyton's predictions for chronic polycythemia may be correct: a high-pressure, low-velocity type of circulation develops, with expanded blood volume in systemic, pulmonary, and coronary vascular beds. Furthermore, one can suggest that this type of circulation, while serving as a reservoir of O_2, responds sluggishly to sudden increases in metabolic demand (such as during exercise), lowers tissue PO_2, and increases the O_2 debt that must be paid on exertion (see chap. 8). This hypothesis will recur, particularly in relation to exercise and the physiologic consequences of bloodletting in polycythemic high-altitude natives.

5.5.4   Cardiac Response to Exercise

In addition to venous return, the cardiac output is controlled by heart rate. The authors have studied the heart rate response to cycle ergometer exercise in a number of natives of Cerro de Pasco to try to determine the effects of hematocrit. In general, all the subjects performed well in these tests, after they were familiarized with the apparatus and procedures. Exact comparison of these subjects with controls must take into account the mean ages of the subjects. To make such a comparison, age-adjusted values were predicted for maximal heart rate (HR_{max}) and work ($WORK_{max}$). Sea-level formulas were used (Altman and Dittmer 1971), because data for high-altitude natives are not available. $WORK_{max}$ was calculated from HR_{max} and the slope $dHR/dWORK$. Plots of HR versus work were made, and linear regression was used to project the HR_{max}.

Table 5.3 shows that members of the polycythemic group were slightly older than the controls, and that the predicted HR_{max} and $WORK_{max}$ are also less. However, the heart rate and work achieved by both groups, as percentages of those predicted, are similar: no significance could be attributed to the small differences observed in HR_{max} or $WORK_{max}$ when a t test for small samples was used. These results suggested that polycythemia in the subjects was not associated with any exercise restriction.

The ECG was monitored with a modified V5 lead (*RA*, right midaxillary line; *LA*, left midaxillary line; *LL*, scapular tip). When the heart rate appeared to be constant, the work rate was abruptly increased while the subject

Table 5.3.   Maximal work and heart rate in natives of Cerro de Pasco

	Polycythemic Subjects	High-altitude Controls
	N = 11	*N = 27*
Age (yr)	50.5 ± 10.9	38.0 ± 18.5
Hct (%)	65.6 ± 5.2	49.9 ± 3.2
Heart rate		
Max	146 ± 28	158 ± 30
% predicted	82 ± 15	84 ± 14
Work		
Max	622 ± 217	78 ± 17
% predicted	822 ± 330	74 ± 27

Source: Winslow and Monge, unpublished data.
Note: Values are ±1 SD.

continued to pedal at the same rate. The rise in heart rate was found to follow an exponential function, and the methods used to evaluate the time course of change are discussed in detail by Whipp and Wasserman (1972).

The heart rate also was measured at rest in the recumbent position (taken from the scalar ECG recording) and during constant work rate exercise at two work levels and at two hematocrits, before and after bloodletting (table 5.3). The heart rates were fit to equation 5.2 to evaluate the time constant (τ) for a response to the imposition of a square wave increase in work. An example of the data from one subject and of the curve fit is shown in figure 5.5.

Of the four subjects studied in this way, three had increased heart rate at rest and during unloaded cycle pedaling. The fourth, subject 3780, behaved differently from the others in many ways and perhaps should be considered as a special case. This subject was older than the others (seventy-three years) and was the only subject with symptoms and physical signs of congestive heart failure.

Subject 3680 had an apparent increase in heart rate and τ, but because the exercise test had to be terminated in the second minute of the 300-kpm level, it is questionable whether a true steady-state heart rate was ever reached.

Subjects 3880 and 3980 both displayed increased heart rates at rest and at both levels of exercise. Furthermore, the time constants for a change in heart rate decreased in both. Thus, the increased heart rate in the incremental tests

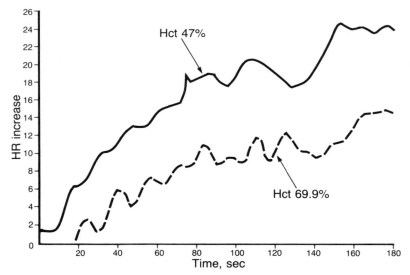

Figure 5.5.   The heart-rate response to imposition of a square-wave work load. Note that after hemodilution, the response is faster and a higher heart rate is achieved. (Winslow and Monge, unpublished data.)

observed in these two subjects seems to be a result of brisker responsiveness to increased work, in addition to the other factors that normally control steady-state heart rate.

5.6 Pulmonary Circulation

Monge C. and co-workers made direct measurements of the pulmonary circulation in a group of ten high-altitude natives, then compared the results with those of twenty sea-level controls obtained by the same techniques (Monge C. et al. 1955). Using their own method, they injected Evans blue dye into an antecubital vein, then monitored its appearance in the femoral artery. The appearance of the dye in the arterial blood and its buildup time and disappearance time were all delayed in the high-altitude group (see fig. 5.6). Curves such as the ones in figure 5.6 were used to calculate the cardiac output and volume of blood in the chest (table 5.4). These authors concluded that high-altitude natives have a greater volume of blood in the lungs than do sea-level controls, either expressed as an absolute value, corrected for body size, or as a percentage of total blood volume. The cardiac output of the natives was, however, slightly higher than that of the sea-level controls. This means that the pulmonary circulation is characterized as a high-pressure,

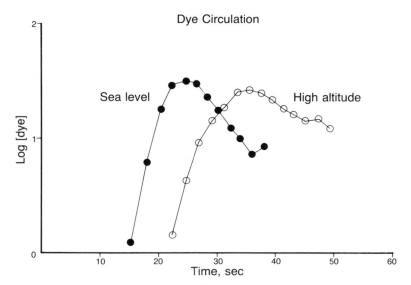

Figure 5.6.   Sea-level and high-altitude curves for appearance of dye in the femoral artery after injection into the antecubital vein. The high-altitude native shows a delayed appearance, a longer buildup time, and longer disappearance, corresponding to a longer mean circulation time. (Modified from Monge C., et al. 1955.)

Table 5.4.   Pulmonary circulatory measurements of subjects at low and high altitudes

	Sea-Level Controls	High-Altitude Natives	Difference (p)
	N = 20	N = 10	
Age (yrs)			
Hematocrit (%)			
Surface area (m²)	1.72	1.55	
Appearance time (sec)			
Circulation time (sec/m²)			
Cardiac index (1/min/m²)			.04
Central blood volume (1/m², as % of total)			<.01
			.02
Thoracic blood volume (1/m², as % of total)			

Source: Monge C. et al. 1955.

large-volume, low-velocity system, similar to the coronary circulation. Whether this increased volume of blood in the lungs may act as a reservoir for O_2 in some circumstances is considered in chapter 10 ("Bloodletting").

Monge's data also provide information about the relationship between hematocrit and hemodynamics. The mean circulation time is correlated with hematocrit when both high- and low-altitude populations are considered together (fig. 5.7).

The cardiac index (cardiac output/body surface area) values deserve special comment. Figure 5.7 shows that there is no relationship between the cardiac index and hematocrit for the sea-level group. However, the altitude data taken alone (excluding one case) show a strong negative correlation ($r = -.80$, $p = .01$). An extrapolation of the regression line suggests that the high-altitude native with a sea-level hematocrit will have a high cardiac index, but the cardiac index sharply decreases with polycythemia. These results are relevant to our discussion in chapter 10 of the optimal hematocrit and are generally supported by the experimental work in dogs (Guyton, Jones, and Coleman, 1973) and the authors' own experience with bloodletting (Winslow, Monge, Brown, et al. 1985).

To the authors' knowledge, this study has never been repeated using radioisotopic methods, so that allowances for unknown capillary hematocrit could be a problem in the strict quantitative interpretation of Monge et al. However, it is likely that the results are qualitatively correct and may have important implications, inasmuch as increased blood volume could decrease the vital capacity (Glaser and McMichael 1940). These results are also in agreement with an apparent reduction in functional residual volume in the lungs of one subject studied in detail before and after hemodilution (see chap. 10).

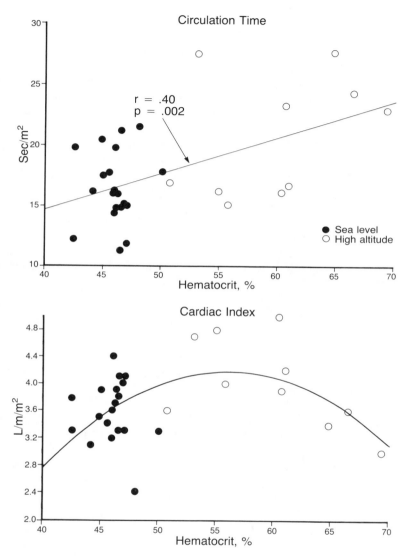

Figure 5.7. The mean circulation time and cardiac index as a function of hematocrit. Data from sea level and high altitude are shown. The hematocrit dependence of circulation time appears to fall on a continuous line, while the cardiac output values show a maximum at about 55 percent hematocrit. (Data from Monge C. et al. 1955.)

5.7   Cerebral Circulation

The supply of O_2 to the brain is of obvious importance, because the brain controls many of the integrative functions of acclimatization. Furthermore, the most prominent complaints of subjects with chronic mountain sickness are related to cerebral function: confusion, lethargy, and sleep disturbances.

Not surprisingly, the cerebral circulation is subject to tight coupling with other physiologic functions, such as ventilation and acid-base status. A brisk increase in brain blood flow occurs in response to acute hypoxia or hypercapnia. This hypoxic response seems to be mediated by O_2 unavailability, whether it is due to anemia, hypoxia, or increased hemoglobin O_2 affinity (Doblar, Santiago, and Edleman 1977; Wade et al. 1980). That these reflexes are mediated by central chemoreceptors, not peripheral ones, is indicated by the fact that they are intact even in the absence of the carotid bodies (Heistad et al. 1976; Traystman, Fitzgerald, and Loscutaff 1978).

In addition to the chemical stimuli that affect the cerebral circulation, blood viscosity per se is a potent effector. This has been demonstrated convincingly by recent studies in sea-level subjects with even marginally elevated hematocrits (Thomas et al. 1977a, 1977b). In these studies, Thomas and co-workers found that lowering the hematocrit from 53.6 percent to 45.5 percent was associated with a decrease in blood viscosity of 30 percent and an increase in brain blood flow of 73 percent. They recommend that hematocrits greater than 46 percent should be viewed as an indication for treatment by phlebotomy, particularly in patients who are at risk for vascular occlusive disease.

The importance of blood viscosity in cerebral function has been underscored by additional recent data. The Framingham study, in which cardiovascular risk factors in 5,185 North American men and women were studied for sixteen years, showed that the risk of a cerebrovascular event was proportional to hemoglobin concentration and was doubled when the hemoglobin was greater than 15 grams/deciliter in men or 14 grams/deciliter in women (Kannel et al. 1972). This study found, however, that cigarette smoking and hypertension also were risk factors, and these effects were not easily distinguishable from those of polycythemia alone. In a more recent study, Tohgi and co-workers found a direct relationship between hematocrit and the incidence of stroke in 432 autopsied subjects with a mean age of 77.1 years (Tohgi et al. 1978). They found a significantly higher risk of stroke when the hematocrit was greater than 46 percent, but in subjects whose age was greater than seventy-eight years, a hematocrit greater than 41 percent was associated with increased risk.

Results such as the Framingham study may not be clearly applicable to high-altitude natives in that there are many cultural, behavioral, and environmental differences between the two. For example, cigarette smoking is not common in high-altitude natives of Peru, and their diets are much lower in fat. It would be of considerable interest to carry out similar epidemiological studies in isolated populations such as those in Peru, Chile, or Asia to perhaps better understand the lack of many "Western" diseases such as atherosclerosis.

The end result of reduced cerebral oxygen supply should be compromised cerebral function, but cerebral function is difficult to quantify. The effects of chronic exposure to hypoxia of various degrees can be measured by careful psychologic and psychomotor testing, however, and may be long-lasting, as demonstrated by studies done in the members of the 1981 American Medical Expedition to Everest (Townes 1984). These subjects, studied at various altitudes up to 8,000 meters, still had measurable abnormalities when studied one year after the expedition.

Conclusive psychologic testing in high-altitude natives of the Andes or the Himalayas has been impossible because of cultural and language problems. However, Willison and co-workers claimed that sea-level subjects with mild polycythemia have measurable disturbances of alertness when the hematocrit is elevated only slightly (Willison et al. 1980). They administered psychologic tests and measured cerebral blood flow in a group of subjects whose mean hematocrit was 53.4 percent, then compared the results with those in a control group of subjects whose hematocrits were less than 46 percent. They found significantly poorer cerebral function in the polycythemic group, but the results in a subset, after reduction of the hematocrit from 53.7 percent to 47.9 percent by simple phlebotomy, did not differ from those of the controls. Performance in the psychologic tests correlated significantly with improvement in cerebral blood flow.

If the reduced psychomotor function in polycythemic subjects is mediated by reduced O_2 delivery to the brain, then hypoxia and polycythemia may have additive effects. This matter is of great importance in natives of high altitudes, and the above studies indicate that even moderate altitudes may have significant effects.

In sojourners to altitude, blood flow in the brain returns to normal sea-level values within a few days of ascent, in a manner parallel to ventilatory acclimatization (Severinghaus et al. 1966). High-altitude natives appear to have cerebral blood flows similar to those of sea-level natives with equivalent hematocrits. However, there is a linear decrease in blood flow with increasing hematocrit in high-altitude natives (Milledge and Sørensen 1972; McVergnes 1973; Sørensen et al. 1974). In these natives, the cerebrovascular response to hypoxia seems to be intact, since breathing O_2 decreases cerebral blood flow (fig. 5.8). Thus, the polycythemic high-altitude native is left with the detrimental effect of viscosity on cerebral blood flow, without the stimulating effect of hypoxia or hypercapnia.

The relationship between blood flow to the brain and sleep ventilation is

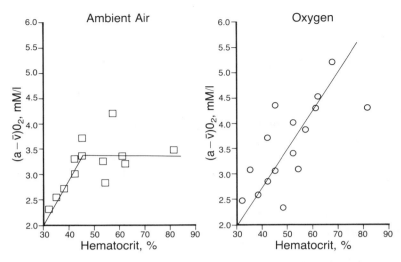

Figure 5.8. The relationship between the hematocrit and measured arteriovenous oxygen difference across the brain in high-altitude residents breathing either ambient air or oxygen. Note that relief of hypoxia seems to result in a higher $(a - \bar{v})O_2$ difference. If O_2 uptake is constant, this suggests reduced blood flow. (Modified from Sørensen et al. 1974.)

of considerable importance in chronic mountain sickness, and it may provide a link between the circulation and ventilatory effects of polycythemia. (This is discussed in detail in chap. 6, "Ventilation.") Patients with excessive polycythemia seem to desaturate more during sleep than do controls, a phenomenon that can be reversed by respiratory stimulants. At the same time, evidence suggests that high-altitude natives do not display periodic breathing during sleep, as do sea-level sojourners. This loss of periodic breathing is thought to be related to "blunted" hypoxic respiratory drive. Isolated case reports suggest that sleep desaturation may be a result, not a cause, of polycythemia in sea-level subjects (Neil et al. 1980; Stradling and Lane 1980), and it would be of great interest to see whether the same is true of subjects with chronic mountain sickness.

5.8 Circulation in Skeletal Muscles

Many investigators of high-altitude physiology have been impressed by the physical capabilities of high-altitude natives. As investigations gradually showed that these remarkable persons ventilated less and that their cardiac output was not greater than sea-level persons, it seemed that "tissue adaptation" might be likely, that is, that O_2 utilization by the tissues might be more efficient. Possible ways in which this could occur would be increased capillary density, increased myoglobin content of muscles, or more efficient energy metabolism by tissue mitochondria.

5.8.1 The Capillarity of Skeletal Muscles

In theory, a decrease in the diameter of muscle fibers and an increase in the number of capillaries per unit mass of muscle should facilitate the transfer of O_2 from red cells to sites of metabolism because the distance for diffusion would be smaller (see Forster 1964 for a general discussion of gas diffusion in tissues). The authors know of no studies of human muscle biopsies that confirm such a mechanism, but Valdivia (1959) reported a denser micro-vascularity in the skeletal muscle of the Andean guinea pig as compared with that of sea-level controls, suggesting that this mechanism is possible. These studies have been confirmed in rats (Tenney and Ou 1970; Cassin et al. 1971; Turek, Grandtner, and Kreuzer 1972) and in cattle (Ou and Tenney 1970).

Although increased capillarity probably does increase the efficiency of O_2 transfer in high-altitude animals, Banchero (1983) has challenged the concept that this is an adaptation to hypoxia. He presented convincing evidence in guinea pigs to suggest that the capillary-to-fiber ratio is a linear function of growth. He pointed out that in the earlier studies of Cassin, the high-altitude animals were smaller than the sea-level controls and that this, not hypoxic exposure, explained the increased ratio. Banchero's recent work suggests that cold is an additional factor in determining the capillary-to-fiber ratio in guinea pigs (Banchero, Kayer, and Lechner 1985). The diffusion distance for O_2 in rats also may be regulated by the degree of activity of the specific muscle (Snyder, Wilcox, and Burnham 1985). In any event, it seems that high-altitude animals do have increased capillary-to-fiber ratios, but whether this is a mechanism of adaptation in human natives remains to be seen.

5.8.2 Myoglobin

Myoglobin is a muscle protein structure that is very similar to one of the subunit polypeptide chains of hemoglobin. Because it is monomeric, it has a very high affinity for O_2 and is devoid of cooperativity. Its P50, the PO_2 at which it is half-saturated with O_2, is about 6 torr (Rossi-Fanelli and Antonini 1958; Gayeski and Honig 1978), which means that it remains nearly saturated under normal resting conditions, because the normal $P\bar{v}O_2$ at sea level is about 40 torr.

Animals such as diving mammals, which experience severe O_2 deprivation, accumulate tremendous stores of myoglobin, which presumably act as a reservoir of O_2. In addition, it can be argued that myoglobin facilitates the diffusion of O_2 from red cells to muscle cells (for example, see Artigue and Hyman 1976). In high-altitude environments, the tissue PO_2 may reach very low values, particularly during exercise, and the temperature of exercising muscle increases. Both of these will lead to unloading of O_2 from myoglobin. For example, it is argued in chapter 10 that during exercise the femoral vein PO_2 of one of our subjects must have reached nearly 0 torr. If this is true, myoglobin could have been an important source of O_2.

Valdivia (1956) obtained muscle biopsies from the sartorius muscles of nine healthy young natives of Cerro de Pasco for the measurement of myoglobin content. He found $7.03 \pm .73$ milligrams/gram tissue in the natives, compared with $6.07 \pm .70$ milligrams/gram in the controls. The difference was significant, with a p value of less than .02. There are many pitfalls in interpreting data of this type since diet, muscle mass, and state of hydration may all influence the myoglobin content. However, the studies were done carefully; these problems were considered; and the author concluded that the myoglobin content of muscles of high-altitude natives is increased. To the authors' knowledge, these studies have not been confirmed by other observers, and no data are available for sojourners or for high-altitude natives of other geographic regions or other genetic backgrounds.

5.8.3   Mitochondria

Another possible tissue adaptation to hypoxia is greater efficiency of energy utilization in the mitochondria. This subject was reviewed by Mela and Wagner (1983), who concluded that hypoxia does induce an increase in the respiratory capacity and cytochrome turnover during electron transfer reactions in rats. The concentrations of the cytochromes do not appear to be rate limiting, because enhanced electron transfer occurs even when the concentrations are low. This area of research is still developing and may yield important new information about adaptation to hypoxia.

CHAPTER SIX
Ventilation

Of all the changes that occur during *acute* exposure to high altitude, hyperventilation is perhaps the most significant. Breathing at a higher rate causes a number of advantageous interacting physiologic events to occur. The alveolar PO_2 (PAO_2) increases, $PACO_2$ decreases, blood pH increases, and the hemoglobin-oxygen equilibrium curve is shifted to the left (increased affinity) to facilitate uptake of O_2 in the lung. The net result is that arterial O_2 saturation is protected. These mechanisms were demonstrated clearly during the American Medical Research Expedition to Everest, where gas exchange measurements were obtained at the highest point on earth (West et al. 1983; Winslow, Samaja, and West 1984). The drop in $PACO_2$ due to hyperventilation correlates with preserved PAO_2 at extreme altitudes (fig. 6.1).

Patterns of permanent residents of high altitudes are in contrast to this apparently clear picture. Chiodi (1957) discovered that natives of the Argentinean Andes ventilated less at rest than did recently acclimatized lowlanders, and these observations were extended to natives of the Peruvian Andes (Severinghaus, Bainton, and Carcelén 1966). Thus, it appears that the hyperventilatory response to hypoxia is "blunted" in the high-altitude native, who must take advantage of other mechanisms to compensate for decreased O_2 availability. The evidence that ventilatory blunting in high-altitude natives is an acquired, not genetic, phenomenon is convincing (Sørensen and Severinghaus 1968a, 1968b; Weil et al. 1971; Lahiri et al. 1976).

Unfortunately, the control of respiration in normal humans and natives of high-altitudes is not yet completely clear. Related issues are periodic breathing and sleep apnea, both of which may contribute to decreased arterial saturation and, perhaps, stimulated erythropoiesis. Furthermore, a decreased ventilatory rate is normal in the aging process.

The hypothesis that chronic mountain sickness is related to the control of ventilation is advocated by some pulmonary physiologists. However, the supporting data have been accumulated over many years from diverse geographic locations (Andes, Rockies, Himalayas) and altitudes in subjects of varying ages and physical condition, who have been exposed to different altitudes for different periods of time. Therefore, the literature is understandably confusing. This chapter attempts to summarize the major concepts and data pertinent to the control of ventilation in permanent high-altitude residents. A subsequent chapter will consider the related subject, ventilation during exercise.

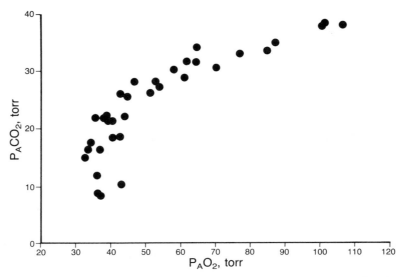

Figure 6.1. An O_2-CO_2 diagram, showing the composition of alveolar gas in acclimatized subjects at high altitude. At extreme altitude the marked hyperventilation maintains alveolar PO_2 at approximately 35 torr. (Modified, with permission, from West et al. 1983.)

6.1 Morphometry

Hurtado's early work in the Peruvian Andes gave rise to the widespread belief that the chest of the high-altitude native is greatly enlarged: "Since early childhood there is a definite appearance of a prominent and large chest as proportionally compared with the rest of the body dimensions, and at this age it is often continuous in front with a prominent abdomen" (Hurtado 1932a). Monge M. and Monge C. (1966) compared data obtained in high-altitude natives with those in sea-level controls and confirmed an increase in the anterioposterior distance of about 10 millimeters and an increase in the sternal height of about 16 millimeters, but they noted no difference in the transverse diameter of the chest, indicating a more rounded chest cavity with a greater capacity.

In a recent review of the chest dimensions of various high-altitude natives, Hackett (Hackett et al. 1984) concluded that Sherpas and Tibetans do not seem to have the large chest dimensions that typify Quechua Indians, particularly when the shorter stature of the Andeans is taken into consideration (table 6.1). Heath and Williams (1981, 30–31) pointed out that the real importance of these dimensions, in regard to adaptation and gas exchange, is the internal surface area of the lung and its effect on O_2 diffusion. For example, in normal humans there seems to be a positive correlation between body height and the internal surface area (Haselton 1972), but the effect of

Table 6.1.   Anthropometric data in high-altitude natives

Altitude (m)	N	Age (yr)	Height (cm)	Weight (kg)	Chest measurement Circumference (cm)	Width (cm)	Depth (cm)
				Sherpa			
3,500	61		162.2	54.6	84.6 (0.52)	—	—
2,880	25	26	164.7	51.1	88.5 (0.54)	—	—
2,600	109	18–85	163.1	56.3	—	28.8 (.177)	19.7 (.120)
				Tibetan			
3,800	28	25–35	160.1	—	—	26.6 (.166)	20.4 (.127)
4,000	40	30	158.9	55.2	89.7 (0.56)	27.6 (.174)	20.6 (.129)
—	52	25–35	160.0	—	—	28.2 (.176)	20.5 (.128)

Source: Hackett et al. 1984.
Note: Numbers in parentheses are circumferences divided by height.

the rounded configuration of the Quechua Indian chest on this relationship is unknown. Unfortunately, no adequate methods exist to quantitate the surface area of the lung in vivo.

In a survey of forty-five residents of Morococha, Peru, the authors found no correlation between hematocrit or hemoglobin concentration and either inspired or expired chest circumference, regardless of whether the measurement was corrected for height. Unexpectedly, the mean circumference/height in the subjects (0.578 ± 0.040) correlated with age (fig. 6.2). The significance of this finding is difficult to estimate, but it is well known that vital capacity decreases with age in normal humans at sea level. In high-altitude natives of Morococha, Velásquez (1972) has also shown a diminishing vital capacity with age. Figure 6.2 shows a similar drop in subjects from the authors' studies in Morococha and Cerro de Pasco. Therefore, if total lung capacity increases but vital capacity decreases, one may infer that the residual volume must also decrease.[1] The data in table 6.1 do suggest that the differences between natives of different geographic areas may be related to their length of hypoxic exposure, inasmuch as Peruvian natives are known to migrate vertically less than do Sherpas, and they tend to reside more permanently at higher altitudes.

6.2   Lung Capacities

It is commonly believed that Peruvian natives of high altitudes have increased vital capacities. This concept, initially suggested by Hurtado (1932a), has been supported by many other observers. Frisancho (1975), who has studied pulmonary adaptation in humans of various ages, has suggested that the vital capacity of high-altitude residents depends on the

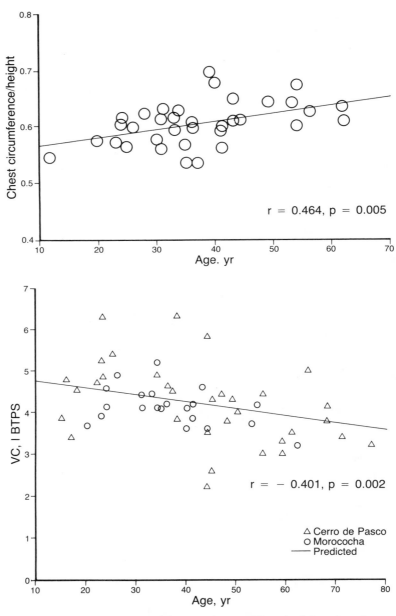

Figure 6.2. The age dependence of chest morphometry. The ratio of chest circumference to height increases significantly with age. Vital capacity decreases slightly wih age but is the same as predicted from sea-level standards. Measurements are pooled from a study of male subjects of Morococha and Cerro de Pasco. (Winslow and Monge, unpublished data.)

time of life when acclimatization began. Frisancho and colleagues showed that if acclimatization begins early enough in life, the vital capacity of lowlanders transplanted to high altitudes is as great as it is in the high-altitude native. Lahiri et al. (1976) studied vital capacities and hypoxic ventilatory response in subjects of various ages at Puno, Peru (altitude 3,800 m) (table 6.2), where they found that the normal pattern of development seems to be an increase in vital capacity and a decrease in hypoxic ventilatory response[2] with age.

These studies suggest that the first years in life are very important in determining lung function in later life. Indeed, recent work with beagles raised at sea level compared with others taken to 3,100 meters as puppies or as adults confirms this idea (Johnson et al. 1985). Johnson and co-workers showed that the animals taken to altitude as puppies have increased lung distensability, diffusing capacity ($D_L CO$), and lung tissue volume.

In contrast to Peruvian Indians, Sherpas have been studied much less intensively. Hackett and co-workers compared Sherpa porters in the Khumbu region of Nepal with lowland trekkers and found that the vital capacities of the Sherpas were 102.7 ± 2.6 percent of predicted values and of trekkers 104 ± 2.2 percent (Hackett et al. 1980). When plotted against body height, the vital capacities of Sherpas and trekkers do not appear to be different. In figure 6.3 data from native residents of Morococha (4,500 m) and Cerro de Pasco (4,300 m), Peru, have been added to those of Hackett et al. The means for the different groups in figure 6.3 are compared in table 6.3. It can be seen that the Quechua Indians are shorter than either Westerners or Sherpas, they are somewhat older, and their vital capacities are smaller. However, a typical sea-level predictive formula indicates that these values are not different from those of either of the other two groups. Thus, perhaps the different morphometry of these diverse racial groups requires that different standards be established for their predicted vital capacities. These data also show that the large variation in vital capacities that occurs in high-altitude natives makes careful selection of subjects very important in comparative studies.

Table 6.2. Respiratory adaptation to high altitudes

Duration of Hypoxia	Ventilatory Response to Acute Hypoxia[a]	Vital Capacity Increase[a]
Birth to 1 week	1	0
2–6 months	+++	0
5–8 years	++++	+
8–12 years	+++	++
12–20 years	++	+++
20–25 years	+	+++

Source: Lahiri et al. 1976.
Note: Based on sea-level predictive formulas.
[a]Symbols denote relative quantities.

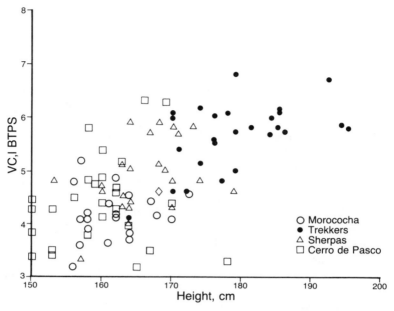

Figure 6.3. The relationship between vital capacity and height in Sherpas, western trekkers, and Quechua Indians in Morococha and Cerro de Pasco. Although the Peruvian subjects are somewhat older than the trekkers and Sherpas (see table 6.3), the relationship of vital capacity and height appears to be about the same. (Sherpa and trekker data from Hackett, Reeves, Reeves et al. 1980.)

6.3 Pulmonary Diffusing Capacity

The uptake of O_2 into pulmonary capillary blood ($\dot{V}O_2$) is described by the Fick diffusion equation:

$$\dot{V}O_2 = D_L O_2 \, (PAO_2 - PcO_2) \tag{6.1}$$

Table 6.3. Vital capacity of high-altitude populations

	Trekkers	Sherpas	Natives of Morococha	Natives of Cerro de Pasco
	$N = 25$	$N = 25$	$N = 21$	$N = 34$
Age (yr)	30 ± 1	28 ± 2	36 ± 2	42.4 ± 3.0
Height (cm)	178.5 ± 1.5	166 ± 1	161.6 ± 1.0	159.4 ± 1.4
Weight (kg)	69.4 ± 1.5	58 ± 2	64.6 ± 2.1	$4.207 \pm .165$
Vital Capacity (lBTPS)	$5.65 \pm .13$	$4.9 \pm .13$	$4.160 \pm .101$	105.3
Percent predicted[a]	107.1	106.2	98.2	

Source: Data for Sherpas and trekkers are from Hackett et al. 1980.

Note: Errors are ±1 SE.

[a]Vital capacity = 0.056 (height) − 0.017 (age) − 4.21 (Altman and Dittmer 1971).

where D_LO_2 is the diffusing capacity of O_2, PAO_2 is alveolar O_2 tension, and PcO_2 is the mean pulmonary capillary O_2 tension. The same equation also describes the diffusion of CO_2 in the lung, except that the solubility of CO_2 in tissue is twenty times that of O_2 and its rate of change is therefore much faster. The diffusing capacity for any gas is defined as the amount of gas that passes across the alveolar membrane per minute per millimeter Hg difference in gas pressure on the two sides of the membrane.[3] Roughton and Forster (1957) further defined the membrane and blood components of D_LO_2:

$$1/D_LO_2 = 1/D_MO_2 + 1/\varnothing Vc \qquad (6.2)$$

where D_MO_2 is the diffusing capacity of the pulmonary membrane, $\varnothing$ is the reaction rate constant for hemoglobin with O_2, and Vc is the volume of capillary blood. In practice, the overall diffusion capacity for O_2 (D_LO_2) is measured, values for $\varnothing$ and Vc are assumed, and D_MO_2 is calculated from equation 6.2.

The main driving force for the uptake of O_2 in the lung is the difference between PAO_2 and PcO_2 (eq. 6.1). At high altitude, this difference in the pressure gradient of O_2 is diminished, and the other factors in equation 6.1 play a relatively more important role. These various quantities interact, particularly in exercise when cardiac output changes as well. This chapter discusses only the membrane component of diffusion.

In normal sea-level humans, the gradient between alveolar and arterial blood is 6–17 torr (Harris and Heath 1977). The mechanisms for this gradient are: (1) the inherent diffusion properties in the membrane itself, (2) uneven perfusion/ventilation, and (3) right-to-left shunts as some of the blood in the pulmonary capillaries is mixed with venous blood from bronchial or Thebesian veins. Velásquez (1956) and Hurtado (1964) noted that in Morococha natives this gradient is reduced to about 1 torr, but other workers have found gradients more like those in sea-level natives (Kreuzer et al. 1964).

Careful measurements of the various components of the diffusing capacity in highland natives have been carried out by Remmers and Mithoefer (1969) and DeGraff et al. (1970) in Indian natives of La Paz, Bolivia (3,700 m), and in Leadville, Colorado (3,100 m), respectively. Both studies found increased overall diffusion of O_2 (D_LO_2), which could be attributed to increased volume of pulmonary blood and increased hemoglobin concentration. However, both studies also concluded that the membrane component (D_MO_2) is increased in these natives, probably because of increased surface area for diffusion. Heath and Williams (1981) also speculated that pulmonary arterial hypertension could have the additional beneficial effect of increasing the uniformity of pulmonary vascular perfusion.

Pulmonary diffusion was studied in a twenty-eight-year-old man, a native of 3,033 meters, in Colorado by Hecht and McClement (1958). This subject had a hematocrit of 81 percent; his symptoms of chronic mountain sickness decreased when he descended to 1,463 meters but recurred at about 1,676 meters. At sea level he was found to have a mild diffusion block. Hecht and McClement suggested that mild pulmonary abnormalities could underlie all cases of chronic mountain sickness. Unfortunately, similar studies in high-altitude natives with chronic mountain sickness have not been systematically performed. This would be very important, but must be done carefully inasmuch as several variables need to be quantified. For example, the reaction rate of O_2 with hemoglobin ($\emptyset$) should not be assumed to be constant, and the effect of 2,3-DPG and pH variation should be considered (see chap. 4). In addition, the volume of pulmonary blood needs to be measured, not assumed, since in chronic mountain sickness the usual relationships between red cell mass and plasma volume, not to mention capillary hematocrit, may be deranged (see chap. 3). Finally, extreme polycythemia has a strong hemodynamic effect (see chap. 5), which will alter pulmonary capillary transit time for red cells.

6.4   Normal Control of Ventilation

The membrane for gas exchange in the human is located deep within the thorax. While this arrangement protects the very delicate interface between the environment and the body fluids, it requires a constant rhythmic movement of the chest wall to exchange gas. Regulation of this movement must be very precise to maintain not only PO_2 and PCO_2, but pH as well, inasmuch as bicarbonate is the chief buffering system of the plasma. Therefore, either inappropriate hyper- or hypoventilation could have adverse consequences.

The portions of the central nervous system that control the automatic bellows action of the chest are located within the upper medulla and the pons. They are influenced by neurons in the cerebral cortex for such activities as talking, laughing, and so on, but are remote from contact with either the environment or the sites of metabolic need of the body. Therefore, they depend upon peripheral chemoreceptors to sense environmental alterations and are subject to superimposed voluntary (cortical) control. Weil and co-workers have shown evidence that the overall control of ventilation may have a genetic component (Collins et al. 1978). This intriguing finding supports a possible physiologic basis for differences between the ability of different racial groups to acclimatize to high altitudes (Cruz and Zeballos 1975).

6.4.1   Central Chemoreceptors

The cells of the central chemoreceptors are bathed in cerebrospinal fluid (CSF), separated from the blood by the blood-brain barrier. The chemoreceptor cells respond directly to H^+ and CO_2 concentrations by increasing ventilation. The blood-brain barrier is impermeable to H^+ and HCO_3^-, but it is freely permeable to CO_2. Because CO_2–HCO_3^- is the main buffering system in the CSF, as it is in the blood, this impermeability means that the CSF will be very responsive to changes in CO_2, because its low protein concentration gives it much less buffering capacity than that of the blood. With time, the kidney can compensate for disturbances in acid-base balance and return the CSF pH to normal values (about 7.32) by movement of HCO_3^- across the blood-brain barrier.

Although the central chemoreceptor cells respond mainly to CO_2 and H^+, their sensitivity must be modulated by the effect of O_2, inasmuch as central sensitivity is diminished in some chronically hypoxic individuals. This is illustrated by the fact that sojourners to high altitude decrease their ventilation when they breath O_2, while both Andean natives and Sherpas hyperventilate (Hurtado 1964; Hackett et al. 1980). These observations indicate that in the high-altitude native the neural regulatory components of ventilation are normally depressed by hypoxia.

6.4.2   Peripheral Chemoreceptors

In humans, the main peripheral chemoreceptors are located in the carotid bodies at the bifurcation of the common carotid arteries. These small structures have a rich blood supply and a very high blood flow for their size. Therefore, in spite of a high metabolic rate, their arterial-venous O_2 difference is low, which means that they are essentially sensitive to PaO_2. (It is of interest to compare this situation with that of the kidney, another organ that has a high blood flow and low $(a - \bar{v})O_2$. Both are regulatory centers in hypoxia; one for ventilation, the other for erythropoiesis; see also chap. 7.)

In chronic hypoxia the carotid body chemoreceptors stimulate ventilation in response to the hypoxia, although the details of this important reflex are not completely known. In high-altitude natives, the size of the carotid bodies may be greatly increased, and chemodectomas are common. Many of these natives lack a normal hypoxic ventilatory drive; and their sensitivity to hypoxia is similar to that of patients with bilateral carotid body resections. The peripheral chemoreceptors also respond to CO_2 and H^+, but they respond much less than do the central chemoreceptors.

6.4.3   Ventilatory Reflexes

In normal sea-level humans, $PaCO_2$ plays the most important role in regulating ventilation. The CO_2 response is normally characterized by measuring the minute ventilation $(\dot{V}_E)^4$ of a subject who rebreathes from a closed anesthesia bag to which O_2 is added to replace that consumed. Usually, the end-tidal O_2 and CO_2 are monitored to give an estimation of the arterial concentrations of these gases. Increasing the inspired CO_2 $(FICO_2)$ to about 15 percent can stimulate ventilation to greater than 100 liters/minute, but further increases may actually inhibit ventilation. Most of the stimulus to increase ventilation in such a procedure comes from the central chemoreceptors.

The hypoxic ventilatory drive can be quantitated by a similar maneuver; that is, a subject rebreathes from a closed bag with the CO_2 scrubbed or replenished to keep $PACO_2$ constant, while PAO_2 steadily decreases. Figure 6.4 shows such measurements on a young Peruvian man compared with a healthy acclimatized lowlander. The absence of a ventilatory response in this case is apparent, and the effect on heart rate is impressive (fig. 6.5). The hypoxic ventilatory drive is completely mediated by the peripheral chem-

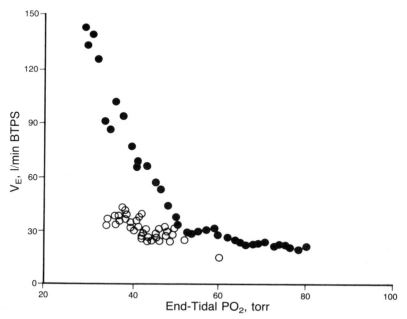

Figure 6.4. The ventilatory response to hypoxia (HVR). An acclimatized lowlander (*filled circles*) is compared with a lifelong native of Cerro de Pasco (*open circles*). Note that there is no significant increase in V_E.

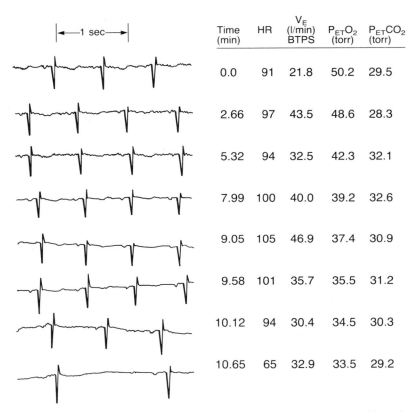

Time (min)	HR	V_E (l/min) BTPS	$P_{ET}O_2$ (torr)	$P_{ET}CO_2$ (torr)
0.0	91	21.8	50.2	29.5
2.66	97	43.5	48.6	28.3
5.32	94	32.5	42.3	32.1
7.99	100	40.0	39.2	32.6
9.05	105	46.9	37.4	30.9
9.58	101	35.7	35.5	31.2
10.12	94	30.4	34.5	30.3
10.65	65	32.9	33.5	29.2

Figure 6.5. Cardiac conduction in a high-altitude native during measurement of hypoxic ventilatory drive (fig. 6.4). Note progressive bradycardia as $P_{ET}O_2$ decreases, due to failure to increase V_E. (Winslow and Monge, unpublished data.)

oreceptors. Indeed, in the absence of peripheral chemoreceptors, oxygen has a depressive effect on ventilation and as such it may explain the paradoxical response to hypoxia seen in some native subjects of high altitude (see below).

It is well known that exercise is a potent stimulus to ventilation. In heavy exercise, lactic acid accumulates and H^+ stimulates ventilation. However, the nature of the chemoreceptor response during light to moderate exercise has not been studied as carefully. In normal sea-level humans performing submaximal exercise, the drop in pH or PO_2 or rise in $PaCO_2$ is very slight or nonexistent, although ventilation increases dramatically. At high altitude the matter is still more complex; O_2 uptake is limited by diffusion (see eq. 6.1) and PaO_2 decreases during exercise. Therefore, the hypoxic drive is superimposed on whatever other stimuli exist. Thus, strict comparisons of data collected at sea-level and high altitude must be done with these considerations taken into account.

6.4.4   Development and Control of Ventilation

The ventilatory peripheral chemoreflex in response to hypoxia is not fully developed in newborns, regardless of altitude of birth, although the hypercapnia response seems to be intact (Lahiri et al. 1978). As noted earlier, the work of Sørensen indicated that the reflexes for hypoxic ventilatory drive are established early in life (Sørensen 1968a, 1968b), and Lahiri has shown that the reflex increases from birth to about ten years, then steadily declines in high-altitude natives (table 6.2). Hypoxic ventilatory drives were also found to be important in natives in Leadville, Colorado (Byrne-Quinn, Sodal, and Weil 1972).

These observations are important in several respects. First, they mean that in any study of O_2 transport in high-altitude natives it is important to specify the altitude of birth of the subjects and the history of exposure to high altitudes. Unfortunately, many early studies cannot be interpreted because of this problem. Second, lifelong natives of high altitudes and sojourners, even with nearly equal exposure to hypoxia, may have different ventilatory drives if the early years of their lives were spent at different altitudes. Hackett et al. (1984) pointed out (correctly, the authors believe) that hypoxia should be viewed as the product of years and altitude. In view of the pattern of the chemoreflexes, however, perhaps weight should be given to the first decade of life. Finally, the observation that chronic mountain sickness is more common in Tibetan sojourners than in high-altitude natives (Huang et al. 1984) has special significance if one believes in the hypoventilatory etiology of chronic mountain sickness. That is, the sojourners would be expected to have drives that are more intact.

6.5   Ventilation in High-Altitude Natives

Haldane and Priestley were probably the first to clearly understand that increased ventilation occurred in sojourners at high altitudes (West 1981). They stated, "Oxygen hyperpnœa is met with at greatly diminished atmospheric pressure, as in mountain climbing and balloon journeys at very high altitudes. It is also observed in mines, etc., in air containing less than 12% of oxygen and no corresponding excess of CO_2, as, for instance, in mixtures of fire-damp (CH_4) and air . . . the hyperpnœa is undoubtedly produced by deficiency of oxygen in the blood" (Haldane and Priestley 1905, 259). Hurtado found that residents of Morococha exhibited about 20 percent increased ventilation compared with controls in Lima, and that this increase amounted to about 40 percent when the smaller body size was accounted for (Hurtado 1964). He attributed this increased ventilation to increased sensitivity of the respiratory center to CO_2 and hypoxia, but he also noted that high-altitude residents are capable of longer breath-holding times (Velásquez 1956) than are lowlanders.

The critical observation, however, made by Chiodi at 3,990 meters and 4,515 meters in the Argentinian Andes, was that, while natives do hyperventilate, the degree of hyperventilation is less than it is either in newcomers or in acclimatized lowlanders, and that they have a diminished responsiveness to inhaled CO_2 (Chiodi 1957). Furthermore, during pure oxygen breathing, ventilation was depressed more in either newcomers or acclimatized lowlanders than it was in native residents. Chiodi interpreted these results as indicating a decreased chemoreceptor activity in high-altitude natives. Thus, removal of the hypoxic stimulus had little effect on their ventilation. In fact, the increased breath-holding time in high-altitude natives is probably due to decreased sensitivity of the peripheral chemoreceptors.

Severinghaus and co-workers studied six high-altitude natives with chronic mountain sickness and compared them with five normal residents of Cerro de Pasco and six lowlanders acclimatized to the same altitude (fig. 6.6) (Severinghaus, Bainton, and Carcelén 1966). They found that the chronic mountain sickness cases, in general, had CO_2 ventilatory responses similar to those of the two other groups. However, their hypoxic responses were lower. These investigators also suggested that chronic hypoxia leads to desensitization of the carotid bodies, resulting in reduced ventilation, increased $PaCO_2$, and decreased PaO_2. Although the small number of subjects did not permit convincing statistical analysis, they suggested the possibility that decreased hypoxic ventilatory response could be the etiology of chronic mountain sickness (fig. 6.6). These authors also considered the possibility that carotid body insensitivity could be the result of polycythemia, not its cause, but they believed this unlikely. Although this latter possibility seems remote, it needs to be disproved with a clear experimental approach.

6.6 The Effect of Age on Ventilation

Age is an important factor influencing respiration, particularly during exercise. Lung volume, maximal capacity for ventilation, and the O_2-diffusing capacity all decline with age in men (Cohn et al. 1954; Robinson 1938). However, most of the available information about the aging process comes from the comparison of persons in different age groups, not from those studied longitudinally over time. The effect of age on the O_2 transport system is of particular interest in chronic mountain sickness, inasmuch as

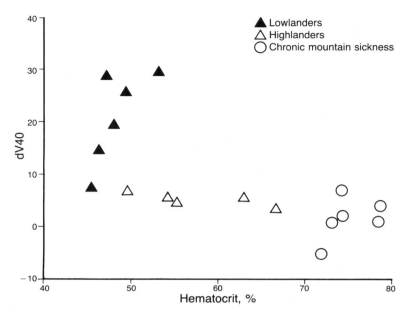

Figure 6.6. Hypoxic ventilatory sensitivity in acclimatized lowlanders and Quechua Indians with and without chronic mountain sickness. dV40 is the increase in minute ventilation when the PaO$_2$ is 40 torr, breathing air at rest. Note that the sensitivities for the subjects with chronic mountain sickness are more scattered, but are not significantly different from those for controls without chronic mountain sickness. Also note the wide variability in sensitivities for the lowlanders. (Modified, with permission from Severinghaus, Bainton, and Carcelén 1966.)

many of those affected are in the older age groups. In fact, Whittembury and Monge C. (1972) suggested that perhaps this illness is simply an exaggeration of the normal aging process, caused by life at high altitude.

The age-dependent decrease of arterial PO$_2$ was first noted by Loew and Thews (1962), who studied 390 normal, sedentary office workers. A decrease of several torr is to be expected in each decade of life (fig. 6.7). Dill noted that PAO$_2$, however, remains high or even increases slightly with age (Dill et al. 1963). This widening of the $(A - a)O_2$ gradient was attributed to changes in lung elasticity, ventilation-perfusion dynamics, and posture.

Many other changes were recently reviewed by Horvath and Borgia (1984), including a decrease in the lung diffusing capacity (D$_L$O$_2$), an increase in body fat, decreased strength, and decreased vital capacity. The changes in ventilatory drive are complicated by the expected hypoxia, but Horvath concluded that they were minimal and that the observed differences in ventilation were probably due to mechanical, not neural, factors. Resting cardiac output decreases by about 1 percent per year from the third to the ninth decades of life (Brandfobrener, Landowne, and Shock 1955), and the

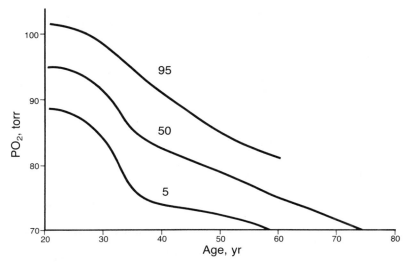

Figure 6.7.   The normal decrease of PaO_2 with age. Lines for the 95th, 50th, and 5th percentiles are shown. (Modified, with permission from Loew and Thews 1962.)

exercise maximum cardiac output, heart rate, and O_2 uptake also decrease (Horvath and Borgia 1984).

The hypothesis that age was a major contributing factor in chronic mountain sickness was supported by studies of Sime and co-workers, who found a correlation between resting ventilation, hematocrit, and age (Sime, Monge, and Whittembury 1975). Several cases of chronic mountain sickness studied by these workers had very low resting ventilation (fig. 6.8). Hurtado also presented data from several cases of chronic mountain sickness to support this conclusion (see chap. 8). Further, Weil and co-workers have found a correlation between the red cell mass and arterial O_2 content in normal humans (Weil et al. 1968). In spite of these data, however, the hypothesis that hypoventilation brought on by the aging process is the etiology of chronic mountain sickness remains unproved. Longitudinal studies on the normal hematologic and respiratory response to chronic hypoxia are badly needed to settle this important point.

6.7   The Control of Ventilation during Sleep

Anyone who has spent a night at a high altitude is aware of the problem of periodic breathing. Mosso was the first to note this phenomenon at the Canpanna Margherita in the Alps in 1898: "While we were at Gnifetti Hut (alt., 3,620 metres), my brother and I noticed that our breathing had become periodic, not only during sleep but also when awake. . . . A species of

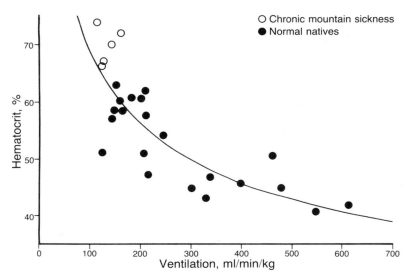

Figure 6.8.   The hematocrit and the resting ventilatory rate. All subjects were residents of 4,500 m. The line is the regression calculated by the authors. (Modified from Sime, Monge C., and Whittembury 1975.)

waves are formed, an indication of the periods which we shall see very markedly in other persons" (West 1981, 363–65). The periodic breathing can be annoying and extremely unpleasant in the sojourner, who may be abruptly awakened from sleep by the sensation of suffocation and must sometimes deliberately breathe during the apneic periods.

Douglas and Haldane (1909) showed that periodic breathing at high altitude could be reversed by administration of O_2 and that it was a normal physiologic occurrence. Feedback theory underlies current models of periodic breathing (Strohl and Fouke 1983). It is postulated that the control loop that includes the peripheral chemoreceptor sensors and the pulmonary musculature effectors is "underdamped." That is, decreases in O_2 and increases in CO_2 tensions are overcorrected, leading to periods of apnea, much as occurs after voluntary hyperventilation at sea level. Why the system should be underdamped is not clear and is in need of further study, but it may be explained by the difference in equilibration rates of the blood and cerebrospinal fluid pH and PCO_2.

In any event, periodic breathing during sleep leads to a gas exchange rate lower than that in regular breathing during wakefulness. Some of the reasons for this are the decreases during sleep in lung volume, cardiac output, and, perhaps, ventilatory drive. The ventilatory response to hypercapnia during sleep, however, is normally decreased (Bulow 1963), as is the response to hypoxia (Douglas et al. 1982), and both these alterations are particularly pronounced during rapid eye movement (REM) sleep. In sojourners to high altitudes, the degree of sleep hypoxia does not correlate with these drives as measured during wakefulness (Powles et al. 1978).

It is a seeming paradox that high-altitude natives appear to exhibit less periodic breathing during sleep than do lowland sojourners. Lahiri studied several Sherpa natives of both high and low altitudes, along with several acclimatized sojourners, during the 1981 American Medical Expedition to Everest (Lahiri, Maret, and Sherpa 1983). The persons with the highest hypoxic ventilatory response, whether they were Sherpas or Caucasians, displayed the most apneic episodes during sleep, whereas those with blunted hypoxic drives had the fewest (fig. 6.9). Perhaps the results can be rationalized under the hypothesis of the feedback loop, if the persons with the blunted drives have dampened the normal oscillations in pH and PCO_2. However, this idea is not consistent with the notion that blunted drives, apneas, and hypoxemia are etiologically linked to chronic mountain sickness. Similar studies in Andean natives and in subjects with chronic mountain sickness are sorely needed.

The consensus of opinion is that polycythemia is not a cause of blunted ventilatory drive in high-altitude natives. To support this position, Lahiri noted that sea-level natives who migrate to high altitude and develop polycythemia show a normal hypoxic drive (Lahiri et al. 1984). He also noted

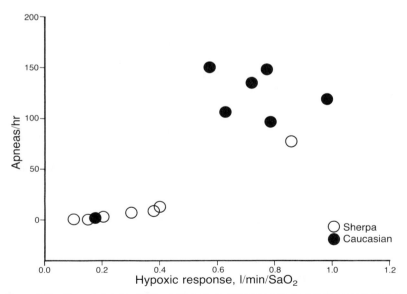

Figure 6.9. The relationship between hypoxic ventilatory response and frequency of sleep apnea in Caucasian lowlanders and Sherpas at 5,400 m. Apparently a low hypoxic drive reduces the number of apneas. (Modified, with permission from Lahiri, Maret, and Sherpa 1983.)

that young high-altitude natives who do not have ventilatory blunting also may have polycythemia. It is perhaps relevant, however, that some sea-level subjects with polycythemia vera may have sleep apnea that can be reversed by therapeutic lowering of hematocrit (Neil et al. 1980), and increased PaO_2 and decreased $PaCO_2$ has been noted in Andean subjects after phlebotomy or hemodilution (see chap. 10).

6.8 Ventilation and Chronic Mountain Sickness

Sime (1973) carried out early studies of ventilation during sleep in high-altitude natives of Morococha. He showed sleep ventilation decreasing with age in subjects between ages four and sixty years. Furthermore, both children and adults without excessive polycythemia had a small ventilatory response to isocapnic hypoxia, but no response to hyperoxia (table 6.4). His subjects with chronic mountain sickness showed no response to either stimulus.

Kryger and co-workers carried out a series of studies at Leadville, Colorado (Kryger et al. 1978a; Kryger et al. 1978b; Kryger et al. 1978c; Kryger and Grover 1983). They studied ten native male residents with hematocrits averaging 59.3 percent and found that their hypoxic ventilatory responses were similar to those of nonpolycythemic residents of Leadville with similar exposure (fig. 6.10). However, the polycythemic subjects showed hypoxic ventilatory depression; that is, when given supplemental O_2 to breathe, they increased their ventilation. There was no change in the controls. Kryger et al. noted that the polycythemic subjects dropped their SaO_2 during sleep more than did the controls (fig. 6.11), and they postulated that this added hypoxemia could provide the stimulus to increase erythropoiesis. As discussed earlier, this response is indicative of attenuated central chemoreceptor sensitivity, but it could also be a consequence of polycythemia in that increased viscosity is known to decrease cerebral blood flow.

Further evidence for the etiologic role of hypoventilation in chronic mountain sickness is the response to administration of medroxyprogesterone acetate (MPA), a respirataory stimulant. These workers administered this drug to seventeen persons with chronic mountain sickness in Leadville and

Table 6.4. Isocapnic hypoxic responses in natives of Morococha

| | | Age | hct | Ventilation (cc/min/kg at FIO_2) | | |
	N	(yr)	(%)	20.9%	16.7%	35.0%
Normal subjects	10	27	59	165 ± 27	191 ± 21	157 ± 21
CMS subjects	5	44	70	129 ± 18	130 ± 15	120 ± 11
Children	3	9	46	345	432	365

Source: Sime 1973.

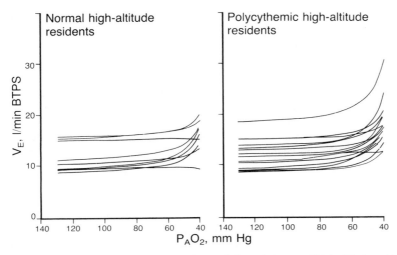

Figure 6.10.   The ventilatory response to isocapnic hypoxia in normal high-altitude residents and in those with chronic mountain sickness. Both responses are subnormal, but there is no difference between the two groups. (Modified, with permission from Kryger and Grover 1983.)

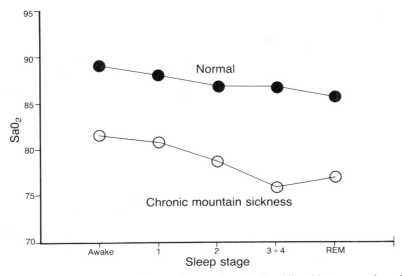

Figure 6.11.   The relationship between hematocrit and SaO₂ while subjects are awake and during various stages of sleep. Desaturation in the subjects with chronic mountain sickness is more pronounced than in the controls. The sleep desaturation does not correlate with the hypoxic ventilatory response when awake. (Modified, with permission from Kryger and Grover 1983.)

demonstrated convincingly that hematocrit decreased, while SaO_2 increased and $PaCO_2$ decreased (Kryger et al. 1978a, 1978b). They concluded that the primary action of the drug was to increase ventilation, thereby removing the stimulus to erythropoiesis. Although this conclusion may be correct, no controls were included in the studies to test whether a decrease in hematocrit alone could have stimulated ventilation. (Cerebral blood flow would be expected to increase, regardless of the mechanism of hematocrit reduction.) The authors' phlebotomy experience in Cerro de Pasco suggests that improved gas exchange can indeed be expected after the hematocrit is reduced (Winslow 1983, and chap. 10).

6.9   Excessive Polycythemia in Lowlander Sojourners

Observations in Tibet have shown that chronic mountain sickness is not limited to high-altitude natives. Huang and co-workers pointed out that this illness is actually more common in lowlanders who have migrated to high altitude than it is in natives (Huang et al. 1984). They found that 67 of 166 male sojourners, primarily government workers from low altitudes, had hemoglobin concentrations in excess of 20 grams/deciliter, compared with only 26 of 159 native Tibetans in one survey. They found 1 of 37 female sojourners and none of 74 female natives who met this criterion.

In studies of pulmonary gas exchange in their subjects, Huang and co-workers found that the sojourners with excessive polycythemia had lower resting ventilation, tidal volume, arterial pH, SaO_2, and diffusing capacity than did either acclimatized sojourner controls or high-altitude Tibetan natives (table 6.5). Their conclusion, that chronic mountain sickness is more common in Tibetan sojourners than in natives, is opposite to current views about Andean natives, and it suggests that the etiology of polycythemia maybe different in the two regions.

Xu-Chu and co-workers compared a group of Tibetan subjects with chronic mountain sickness with acclimatized lowlanders (Xu-Chu et al.

Table 6.5.   Ventilatory measurements, Tibetans at 3,890 meters

	Acclimatized Sojourners	Tibetan Highlanders	CMS Subjects
	$N = 20$	$N = 12$	$N = 14$
VE (l/min) BTPS	15.9 ± 0.9	16.9 ± 0.9	12.5 ± 0.8
Tidal volume, (lBTPS)	.914 ± .060	1.041 ± .100	.565 ± .013
$PaCO_2$ (torr)	28.2 ± 0.4	30.7 ± 1.9	35.5 ± 0.7
SaO_2 (%)	84.8 ± 0.8	83.1 ± 1.6	77.6 ± 1.1
D_LCO (ml/min/torr)	25.3 ± 1.6	27.6 ± 2.0	14.4 ± 1.1

Source: Huang et al. 1984.
Note: Values are ±1 SE.

1981). They found that tidal volume, minute ventilation, alveolar ventilation, arterial saturation, PCO_2, pH, and diffusing capacity all were reduced in the chronic mountain sickness subjects as compared to controls. They also found 2,3-DPG to be reduced in their subjects, and they suggested all of their data are consistent with a hypoventilatory etiology of chronic mountain sickness. In these studies, like those of Huang, the chronic mountain sickness subjects were not long-term residents of altitude, and their altitude of birth cannot be determined from the published reports.

These two Asian studies bring to mind that Monge M. and Monge C. (1966) described as "subacute mountain sickness" some cases they observed of newcomers who never truly acclimatized to high altitudes and who eventually developed excessive polycythemia. The newcomers to Tibet with excessive polycythemia would be examples of this clinical entity.

These results are particularly important in that they contradict the line of reasoning developed earlier in relation to the hypoventilatory etiology of chronic mountain sickness. Sojourners from low altitudes would not be expected to develop depressed ventilatory drives at high altitudes as do natives. No similar data are available from either the Andes or Leadville, and it will be extremely important to perform further studies with these fascinating subjects to understand their mechanism of O_2 transport and how they may differ from those of other racial or geographic groups. It is frustrating that measurements of drives, periodic breathing, and sleep desaturation are not available to correlate with individual erythropoietic responses to hypoxia, especially in comparisons among Andean, Tibetan, Nepalese, and lowland natives. Any or all of these physiological responses to hypoxia may be related to chronic mountain sickness, but the fact remains that each one is, in itself, a "normal" response.

6.10 Pregnancy

It is well known that ventilation increases in pregnancy, presumably because progesterone is a respiratory stimulant. Thus, the study of pregnant women, particularly in high altitudes, has provided important information about the relationships among ventilation, O_2 transport, and red cell mass. At low altitude, the increased ventilation of pregnancy does not increase arterial SaO_2 because of the shape of the hemoglobin O_2 dissociation curve (see chap. 4). However, at the altitude of Cerro de Pasco, the normal SaO_2 is on the steep part of the Oxygen Equilibrium Curve, and even small changes in PO_2 may have a large affect on SaO_2.

Although infant birth weight is reduced (Lichty et al. 1957) and infant mortality is increased (McCullough, Reeves, and Liljegren 1977) at high altitude compared with sea level, so many environmental considerations and other health considerations determine these factors that it is difficult to distinguish cause-and-effect relationships. Moore et al. (1982) provided the first evidence of a correlation between maternal ventilation and infant birth weight: apparently women with lower hypoxic ventilatory drive had smaller infants, and these authors concluded that fetal hypoxia could be the cause. To test their hypothesis, they studied twenty-one women at Cerro de Pasco during their thirty-sixth week of pregnancy and again at thirteen weeks postpartum (Moore et al. 1986). They found markedly reduced hypoxic drive when the women were not pregnant, but an increase when pregnant, leading to a 25 percent rise in resting ventilation and increased arterial O_2 saturation. A slight drop in hemoglobin concentration and unchanged cardiac output resulted in unchanged total O_2 transport in their patients.

These results provide an interesting link between ventilation and O_2 transport to the fetus. However, whether they shed any light on erythropoiesis is less clear. The subjects all decreased their ventilation when breathing supplemental O_2, distinguishing them from typical high-altitude residents with chronic mountain sickness. The drop in hemoglobin concentration is probably not related to erythropoiesis, inasmuch as expansion of the plasma volume in pregnancy is a normal occurrence. It would be of obvious interest to measure erythropoietin concentrations and red cell mass in these subjects to better understand the relationship between ventilation and red cell production.

CHAPTER SEVEN
Renal Function in High-Altitude Polycythemia

The kidney is a homeostatic organ whose functions defend blood volume, electrolytes, osmotic pressure, acid-base balance, and blood pressure. In addition, the kidney is the site of erythropoietin production, a hormone that is sensitive to oxygen lack and that stimulates bone marrow production of red cells. This organ is therefore of central importance in understanding the physiology of high-altitude natives. Fundamental questions such as the kidney's plasma blood flow, its level of oxygenation, its oxygen consumption, and its tubular function in the hypoxemic-polycythemic conditions of high altitude are discussed in this chapter.

Because of the small dimensions of the kidney and its large blood flow, its arterial-venous O_2 difference $((a - v)O_2)$ is small and its PvO_2 is high at sea level. In natives of high altitudes, however, the kidney experiences more tissue hypoxia than do other tissues whose PvO_2 is normally low. Despite the severe degree of tissue hypoxia, the kidney of high-altitude natives consumes a normal amount of oxygen and displays intact tubular function. In addition to these unique characteristics, the reduced plasma flow, with high filtration fraction and normal total renal blood flow, found in the high-altitude native constitutes an ideal model for the study of renal physiology.

7.1 Renal Functions

The kidney is a vascular organ that accounts for about 25 percent of the total cardiac output. This is an extraordinary flow (about 1,200 ml/min) with respect to kidney weight (about 300 g in man), and it underscores the importance of the organ in regulation of extracellular fluid. Three discrete renal processes are known to be involved in the elaboration of urine: glomerular ultrafiltration, tubular reabsorption, and tubular secretion. These are modulated by blood flow, tubular cell metabolism, and a system of hormonal regulation.

7.1.1 Renal Circulation

Blood flow to the kidney is derived from the renal arteries (fig. 7.1). This vessel branches into interlobar arteries that are distributed over the surface of the kidney and descend into the renal cortex. The arcuate arteries follow the longitudinal axis of the kidney and feed the interlobular arteries, which ascend in the cortex and feed the glomerular capillary beds. Thus, arterial

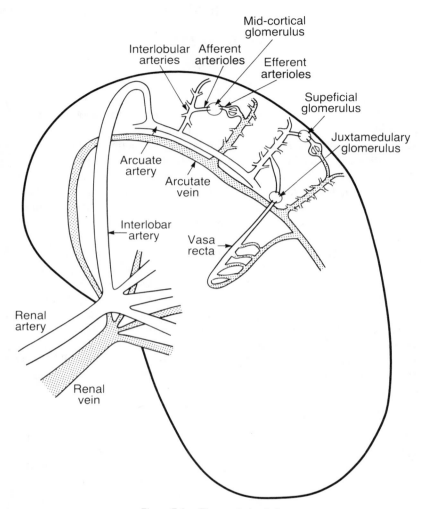

Figure 7.1.   The renal circulation.

blood is supplied only to the cortex; the medulla receives blood only from the efferent arterioles of the juxtamedullary capillary beds.

As shown in figure 7.1, a distinction can be made between the cortical and juxtamedullary glomeruli with regard to their blood supply. The efferent arterioles of the cortical glomeruli break up into capillary beds that perfuse cortical tubules and then return blood to the arcuate veins. The efferent arterioles of the juxtamedullary glomeruli instead descend into the medulla (vasa recta). This provides an anatomic basis for functional heterogeneity of nephrons, and a possible basis for the expectation that alteration in blood flow distribution could affect renal function.

Afferent arteriolar blood passes into the small glomerular capillaries, where plasma is ultrafiltered into the glomerulus, and the cell-rich blood is then collected in the efferent arterioles. The driving force for the ultrafiltration process is hydrostatic pressure within the glomerular capillary bed. This pressure is created by the arterial pressure itself, the relative states of vasoconstriction of the afferent and efferent arterioles, and the difference in viscosities of the blood as it enters and as it leaves the capillaries. The last point is particularly important in polycythemia, in that at higher hematocrits a change in hematocrit will have a more dramatic effect on blood viscosity and resistance to flow (see fig. 5.1).

The afferent arterioles contain cells that are a part of the juxtaglomerular apparatus (JGA). This structure, in addition to epithelial cells, contains the macula densa and Goormantigh cells. The epithelial cells are rich in glycogen, suggesting vigorous metabolic activity, and their shape and number of cytoplasmic contents are affected by the state of the renin-angiotensin system. Moreover, both the afferent and the efferent arterioles have rich (vasoconstriction only) nerve supplies. Thus, the glomerular circulation, with all its components, is an ideal target for close regulation of glomerular function.

Although the total renal blood flow (RBF) is very high with respect to other organs, the distribution of flow within the kidney strongly favors the cortex: cortical flow is about ten times that of the flow to the medulla. Nevertheless, medullary flow is still about the same as blood flow to the brain (Auckland 1974). In most physiologic conditions, RBF is very constant, varying only by a factor of about two. It is believed that all renal blood passes through glomeruli; that is, that no intrarenal shunts exist. The average red cell transit time in the renal cortex is about two to three seconds, while in the medulla it can be as much as one minute.

Smith (1951) stated that the basal renal nervous tone is so low as not to affect RBF. That is, that the anatomic system can regulate in only one direction: vasoconstriction. Many studies in the years since his statement have shown it to be generally true, although much more is known now about the nature of the various reflex mechanisms. Some of the stimuli known to cause renal vasoconstriction are hypoxia, hypercarbia, increased intracranial pressure, and strong emotions. Particularly interesting are the recently discovered atrial peptide hormones, whose actions provide a long-sought link between atrial pressure, renal arteriolar tone, and Na^+ reabsorption (see 7.1.5, Hormonal Control of Renal Function).

7.1.2 Glomerular Filtration

The rate of glomerular filtration (GFR) is usually measured using inert materials that are filtered in the glomerulus but are neither secreted nor reabsorbed by the tubules. Inulin, a commonly used example, is a large polysaccharide derived from Dahlia roots and Jerusalem artichokes. Its appearance in the urine is proportional to its plasma concentration and therefore is a direct function of the GFR. The formula for calculating the clearance of Inulin is the general clearance formula used for any substance:

$$\text{Clearance} = \text{extraction rate/plasma concentration} \qquad (7.1)$$

The normal GFR in man is 100–150 milliliters/minute.

7.1.3 Renal Plasma Flow

The classic measurement of renal plasma flow (or affective renal plasma flow, ERPF) is the clearance of paraaminohippurate, PAH. This substance, like inulin, is filtered in the glomerulus, but the small amount remaining in the efferent plasma is efficiently secreted into the tubules by the tubular epithelium. The efficiency of this process, at low PAH concentration, is such that it is about 90 percent complete. Thus, the balance between plasma and urine PAH is

$$U_{PAH} \times V = ERPF \times (A_{PAH} - V_{PAH}) \qquad (7.2)$$

where U_{PAH} is the urine concentration, V is the urine flow, and A_{PAH} and V_{PAH} are the renal arterial and venous PAH concentrations, respectively. However, since clearance by the kidney is essentially complete, V_{PAH} is zero, and equation 7.2 reduces to

$$RPF = (U_{PAH} \times V)/A_{PAH} \qquad (7.3)$$

In practice, a low concentration of PAH is infused intravenously while the urine flow and PAH concentration are measured. It is important to understand that the efficiency of PAH excretion is less than 90 percent in diseased kidneys and in anemia, but for abnormal states the efficiency must be checked by actual measurements of renal vein PAH concentration.

7.1.4 Active Tubular Transport

In addition to passive removal of various substances by ultrafiltration, active secretion and reabsorption of other substances occurs in the tubular cells. For example, Na^+, glucose, Ca^{++}, K^+, phosphate, and water are all actively reabsorbed by tubular epithelial cells. Some substances, including H^+, K^+, and water are also actively secreted into the tubules.

A detailed discussion of the mechanisms of these processes would be a diversion from the main theme of this book. Of critical importance, however, is the fact that most of the oxygen-requiring metabolism of the kidney is directed at reabsorption of Na^+, and the amount of Na^+ that must be reabsorbed is proportional to the amount filtered, or to the renal blood flow.

7.1.5 Hormonal Control of Renal Function

Both blood pressure and Na^+ reabsorption are influenced by a system of interacting hormones, shown in figure 7.2. Renin is secreted in response to reduced renal artery pressure or reduced Na^+ in the tubules. Renin stimulates the release of angiotensin II, a compound that raises blood pressure and stimulates aldosterone secretion. Aldosterone leads to Na^+ retention and improved flow. These effects have a negative-feedback influence on further renin production.

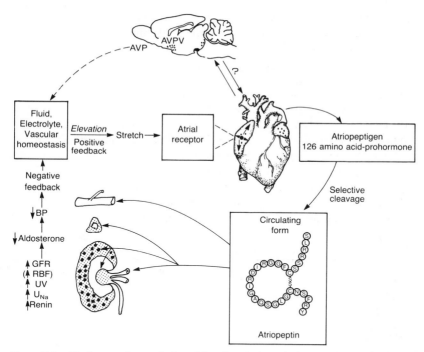

Figure 7.2. The hormonal control of renal function. Atriopeptin is stored in granules in the perinuclear atrial cardiocytes. Elevated vascular volume releases atriopeptin, which acts on the kidney to increase the glomerular filtration rate *(GFR)*, renal blood flow *(RBF)*, urine volume *(UV)*, and sodium excretion *(U_{Na})* and to decrease plasma renin activity. Natriuresis and diuresis are also facilitated by suppression of aldosterone and the release of arginine vasopressin *(AVP)*. Decreased vascular volume provides a negative feedback that suppresses circulating levels of atriopeptin (with permission, from Needleman and Greenwald 1986.)

Recently, a new group of polypeptide hormones that appear to be produced in the atria of the heart has been described and characterized. These atrial peptides have many effects that oppose the renin-angiotensin-aldosterone system, as shown in figure 7.2. These hormones increase GFR without increasing renal blood flow, even when arterial pressure is low. They also increase the filtration fraction (FF), suggesting a selective constriction of the efferent arterioles, or dilation of afferent arterioles. Although their exact mechanisms of action are not yet known, they could act directly on the glomerular membrane, or they could alter the flow distribution pattern within the kidney.

Because the atrial peptides were discovered so recently, no information has been collected yet on what role, if any, they might play in acclimatization (or non-acclimatization) to hypoxia. They are mentioned here only because they could provide a link between venous return to the heart (atrial stretch) and the regulation of fluid balance. Thus, the system could be very important in understanding the late stages of chronic mountain sickness, in which congestive heart failure is a prominent feature.

7.2   Renal Hemodynamics in High-Altitude Natives

The ability of the kidney to extract PAH was measured by renal vein catheterization in natives of Cerro de Pasco (altitude 4,300m) Rennie et al. 1971. The extraction of PAH was found to be normal at high altitudes, indicating that the measurement of renal plasma flow with this substance is valid in the hypoxemic-polycythemic conditions of the high mountains (table 7.1). Becker, Schilling, and Harvey (1957) were the first to demonstrate that the kidney of Peruvian high-altitude natives had a diminished plasma flow and an increased filtration fraction (FF).

Becker's results were confirmed and extended in 1965 (Lozano and

Table 7.1.   Renal oxygen-transport values in subjects at low and high altitudes

	Lima	Cerro de Pasco
	$N = 2$	$N = 4$
PaO_2	96.6	50.8
Hematocrit (%)	45	68
ERBF (ml/min/1.73 m^2)	1,480	1,322
ERPF (%)	91.5	91.8
CaO_2 (ml/dl)	20.2	23.9
CvO_2 (ml/dl)	19.2	22.7
$(a - \bar{v})O_2$ (ml/dl)	1.07	1.19
$\dot{V}O_2$ (delivery, ml/min/1.73 m^2)	300	315
$\dot{V}O_2$ (uptake, ml/min/1.73 m^2)	15.9	15.7

Source: Rennie et al. 1971, "Renal Oxygenation."
Note: Altitudes are Lima, sea level, and Cerro de Pasco, 4,300 m.

Monge 1965). A comparative study was carried out with fifteen sea-level residents and ten high-altitude native residents of Morococha (altitude 4,500 m) in the Peruvian Andes (fig. 7.3). Included in the study were three patients with chronic mountain sickness, also residents of Morococha. Inulin and PAH clearances were used to evaluate GFR and ERPF. The differences in total blood flow were not significant. There was a reduction in ERPF and GFR, with increased FF in the high-altitude natives; the reduction was more marked in the patients with chronic mountain sickness. If the FF had remained constant at high altitude, the GFR would have been reduced to levels of clinical significance. This study also showed a positive correlation between hematocrit and FF (fig. 7.4).

Because the increase in hematocrit increases blood viscosity and this in turn may alter renal hemodynamics, the correlation between these two variables was examined in a study of Peruvian high-altitude natives (Whit-

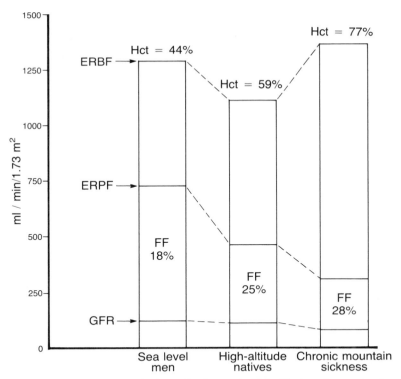

Figure 7.3.   Renal hemodynamics in sea-level controls, high-altitude natives, and natives with chronic mountain sickness. *ERBF* = effective renal blood flow; *ERPF* = effective renal plasma flow; *GFR*, = glomerular filtration rate; and *FF* = filtration fraction. (Lozano and Monge C. 1965.)

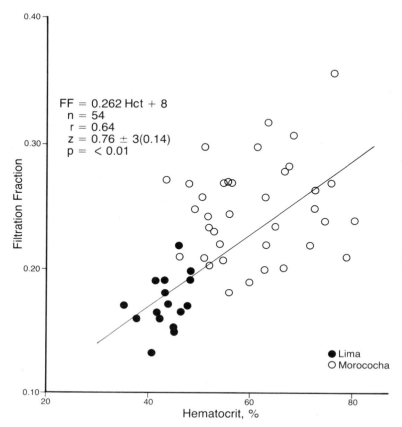

Figure 7.4. The dependence of the filtration fraction on the hematocrit. The Morococha subjects are natives of high altitude. (With permission, from Gonzales 1971.)

tembury et al. 1968). Samples were taken at different altitudes in normal male and female volunteers to obtain a large range of values. Viscosity was measured in a plate-cone viscometer (fig. 7.5). The regression equation was used to convert the hematocrit values determined during renal studies into viscosities and to plot the renal hemodynamic parameters as functions of viscosity (fig. 7.6). The calculated viscosities are shown at two shear rates. Blood flow does not correlate with viscosity, and ERPF and GFR diminish as viscosity increases. Filtration fraction increases as a function of viscosity up to a value of about 10 cp and then levels off.

Two natives of Morococha who were studied two years apart both showed a marked increase in viscosity in the second study. Despite this increase, FF varied little, which was expected since the two studies were done when the viscosities were already high. The half-shadowed circles on

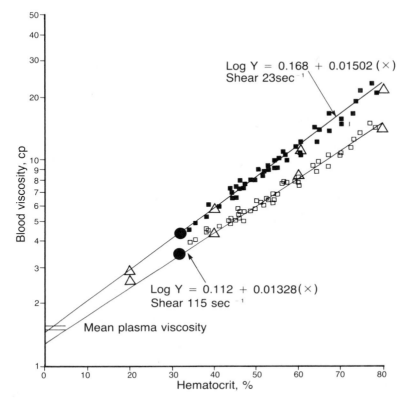

Log Y = 0.168 + 0.01502 (×)
Shear 23sec⁻¹

Log Y = 0.112 + 0.01328(×)
Shear 115 sec⁻¹

Mean plasma viscosity

Figure 7.5. The relationship between the logarithm of blood viscosity and the hematocrit in humans at two shear rates (*open* and *closed squares*). Triangles correspond to hematocrits obtained in vitro by varying the red cell concentration of human blood. Circles correspond to the average values for alpaca (high-altitude camelid) blood. (Whittembury et al. 1968.)

the right side of figure 7.6 correspond to cases of anemia studied by Bradley and Bradley (1945). Glomerular filtration drops both in anemia and polycythemia; the maximal value for this fundamental renal parameter seems to correspond to the normal hematocrit at sea level.

The mechanism by which the hypoxemic-polycythemic condition of high altitudes alters renal hemodynamics is far from understood. Intravascular pressures and resistances were found to be normal in Cerro de Pasco natives studied by renal vein catheterization (Rennie et al. 1971). Although both the afferent and the efferent resistances were normal, the possibility of changes in the intraglomerular pressure as the cause of renal hemodynamic alterations is not disproved by these rather imprecise measurements. Although difficult to explain in terms of physiologic mechanisms, the fact remains that an increased hematocrit negatively correlates with renal plasma flow (fig.

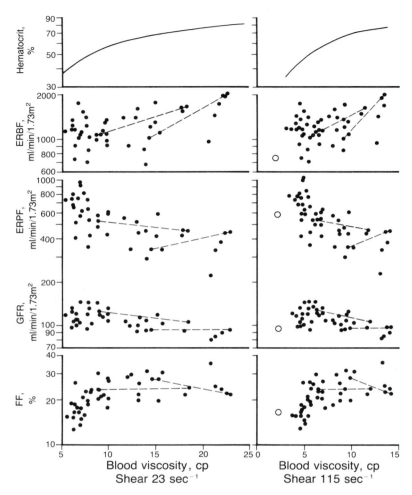

Figure 7.6.   The relationship between the parameters of renal function and blood viscosity at two shear rates. Abbreviations are as in the legend for fig. 7.3. The connected points are data measured from individuals at two-year intervals, demonstrating the progression with age. The closed circles represent cases of anemia. (Monge C, unpublished data.)

7.7). In persons with high hematocrits, ERPF can be reduced to less than half the sea-level average.

Recent studies using single-nephron techniques have demonstrated the dominant role that renal plasma flow plays in the formation of glomerular filtrate. As Blantz (1977) pointed out, "At a constant systemic protein concentration and at filtration pressure equilibrium, the major mediator of change and autoregulation of nephron filtration rate is the rate of nephron

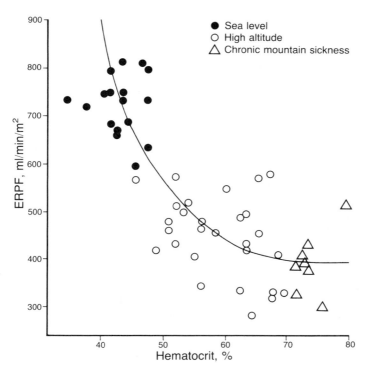

Figure 7.7. The dependence of effective renal plasma flow *(ERPF)* on the hematocrit. (Monge C. et al. 1969.)

plasma flow." Figure 7.8 shows the correlation between GFR and ERPF in Peruvian subjects studied at sea level and at high altitudes. Also shown is the same correlation taken from Blantz's review, using data obtained by the micropuncture technique. The similarity of the responses found in these two studies is striking.

To study the reversibility of renal hemodynamics, a study was undertaken in six high-altitude natives of Morococha. Five of them were normal subjects, and one had symptoms of chronic mountain sickness (Gonzales 1971). To distinguish the effects of hypoxemia from those of polycythemia, these subjects were studied first at Morococha, again at twenty-four hours after their arrival in Lima, and after thirty days of residence in Lima. Inulin and PAH clearances were used in the measurement of GFR and ERPF (table 7.2). The values found in Morococha were in agreement with those previously reported in a more extensive series (Lozano and Monge 1965). Previous experience indicated that hypoxemia in these subjects would have been partially or totally corrected by descent to sea level. Because their

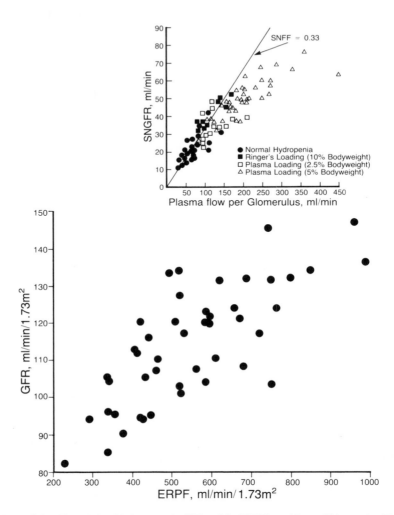

Figure 7.8.   The relationship between the GFR and the ERPF in residents of Morococha. The same correlation is shown in hydropenic (water-deprived) single-nephron studies done by micropuncture, with normal nephrons, nephrons perfused with Ringer's lactate, and plasma infused at 2.5 percent and 5 percent body weight. (Monge C., unpublished data; micropuncture data and insert with permission from Blantz 1977.)

polycythemia remained almost unmodified during the first twenty-four hours, the results were interpreted as indicating that the hypoxemia was not responsible for the hemodynamic changes found at high altitude. In contrast, after thirty days in Lima, the hemodynamic parameters decreased to almost sea-level values and so did the hematocrit.

Table 7.2.   Renal hemodynamics in high-altitude natives

| | In Morococha | After descent to Lima | |
		1 day	30 days
Age (yr)	38.5 ± 1.8	—	—
Height (cm)	159.3 ± 3.0	—	—
Weight (kg)	65.7 ± 4.3	—	—
Hematocrit (%)	60 ± 4	57 ± 5	49 ± 4
GFR (ml/min/1.73m^2)	100 ± 6	100 ± 3	114 ± 4
RPF (ml/min/1.73m^2)	417 ± 32	448 ± 26	630 ± 87
RBF (ml/min/1.73m^2)	1068 ± 94	1129 ± 156	1241 ± 154
FF (%)	24 ± 1	23 ± 1	19 ± 2

Source: Gonzales 1974.

Filtration fraction was plotted as a function of viscosity in these subjects (fig. 7.9). The individual points correspond to subjects studied in Peru both at sea level and at high altitude. The points joined by lines correspond to the subjects who descended to sea level. The subject with chronic mountain sickness was a severe hypoventilator even after descent to sea level. He underwent bloodletting of 1,000 milliliters a few days before the last study in Lima to lower his hematocrit. His GFR, ERPF, and FF showed insignifi-

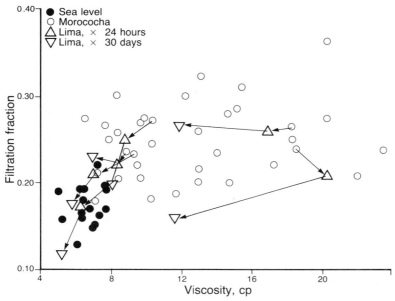

Figure 7.9.   The relationship between the filtration fraction (*FF*) and viscosity in Peruvian sea-level residents and high-altitude natives. Connected points represent individuals studied in Morococha, then after one day or thirty days in Lima. (With permission from Gonzales 1971.)

cant changes after twenty-four hours of residence in Lima. It can be seen that the results of the longitudinal study coincide well with individual determinations done in residents of either sea level or high altitude. The subject who shows a different path was the one with chronic mountain sickness. The conclusions of this study were that the modified renal hemodynamic properties of high altitude are in response to a high hematocrit, and that this modification is totally reversible when the hematocrit reaches sea-level values.

These results are in agreement with those reported in polycythemia vera, in which there is little or no hypoxemia (deWardener, McSwiney, and Miles 1951). In this condition, bloodletting reverses the hemodynamic changes. Moreover, hypoxemic and moderately polycythemic subjects with cor pulmonale increase FF with acute oxygenation.

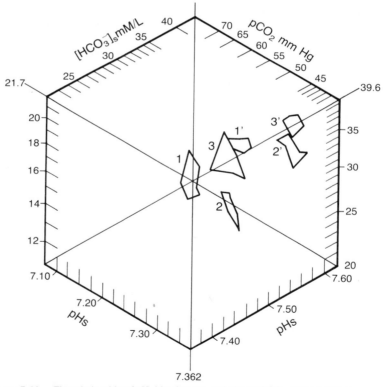

Figure 7.10.   The relationship of pH, bicarbonate, and plasma PCO_2. The triaxial nomogram was reconstructed to fit the intersection to the mean values at sea level. Areas *1, 2,* and *3* correspond to basal figures in sea-level residents, high-altitude natives, and natives with chronic mountain sickness, respectively. Areas *1', 2',* and *3'* correspond to figures after bicarbonate loading. (Monge C. 1964.)

Table 7.3.   Tubular reabsorption of sea-level and high-altitude subjects

Location	Subjects	HCO_3^- (mmol/min)	Cl^- (mmol/min)	Na^+ (mmol/min)
Lima	normal	2.39 ± .15	9.85 ± .25	12.9 ± .5
Cerro de Pasco	normal	2.58 ± .22	10.0 ± .15	13.1 ± .2
Cerro de Pasco	CMS	2.99 ± .08	9.74 ± .24	13.0 ± .4

Source: Monge, Lozano, and Carcelén 1964.

7.3   Renal Excretion of Bicarbonate

To study tubular function in high-altitude natives, Monge C. and co-workers induced metabolic alkalosis in seventeen volunteers: six were normal sea-level residents, six were normal high-altitude natives at Cerro de Pasco, and five were high-altitude natives with chronic mountain sickness, also residents of Cerro de Pasco (Monge C., Lozano, and Carcelén 1964). Blood acid-base studies and bicarbonate tubular maximum (Tm) were determined in all subjects (fig. 7.10). The normal high-altitude natives showed their typical low $PaCO_2$ and slightly alkaline plasma pH. The subjects with chronic mountain sickness showed a $PaCO_2$ that was no different from the sea-level values, indicating hypoventilation. These findings were supported by Sime (1973), who measured ventilatory rate directly.

After bicarbonate loading, the maximal reabsorption of HCO_3^-, Cl^-, and Na^+ were determined (table 7.3). There were no significant differences among the groups, with the exception that the bicarbonate reabsorption of the natives with chronic mountain sickness was significantly higher than that in the other two groups. These results suggest that the normal native is in a new steady state of acid-base equilibrium with low $PaCO_2$ and normal bicarbonate tubular reabsorption. Patients with chronic mountain sickness have a higher bicarbonate Tm because of their higher $PaCO_2$, which is known to act as a stimulus for the bicarbonate reabsorption. In summary, the tubular capacity to reabsorb bicarbonate is not impaired in high-altitude natives.

7.4   Renal Excretion of Acid

The ability of the kidney to excrete acid at high altitudes was studied by Lozano, who induced acidosis by intravenous infusion of ammonium chloride in six normal sea-level residents and six normal high-altitude natives of Cerro de Pasco (Lozano et al. 1969). Ten parameters related to the acid-base equilibrium were studied (fig. 7.11). The similarity of response between the two groups is remarkable. Bicarbonate, which is normally found at lower concentration in the high-altitude native's blood, changed in a parallel fashion to the changes in sea-level subjects, demonstrating that the natives are in

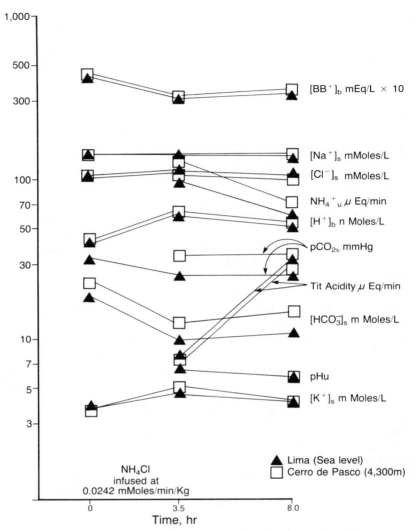

Figure 7.11.   A semilogarithmic plot of ten parameters of the acid-base equilibrium studied before and after a constant intravenous infusion of ammonium chloride. Control, postinfusion (3.5 hr post-control), and recovery (8 hr postinfusion) samples were obtained. Subscripts *u*, *b*, and *s* represent urine, blood, and serum. (with permission, from Lozano et al. 1969.)

a different state of acid-base equilibrium. If one considers the $PaCO_2$ values as an index of the respiratory control activity in the acid-loaded subject, the similar drop in $PaCO_2$ would also indicate that the respiratory control in this condition is not different from that observed in the sea-level subjects. The capacity of the tubule to acidify urine and to produce titratable acid was the same in both groups. Urine ammonium excretion also had a similar response in both groups. As in the case of bicarbonate, one may conclude that the hypoxic environment of the high mountains diminishes neither the renal defense nor the total body defense against metabolic acidosis.

7.5 Renal Excretion of Sodium in Response to Angiotensin

Small amounts of angiotensin infused intravenously are known to produce renal hemodynamic changes, as well as a specific tubular reabsorption of sodium. This technique was applied as a test of the renal capacity to handle sodium in high-altitude natives (Torres et al. 1970). Six normal sea-level residents were studied in Lima, and eight normal high-altitude natives were studied in Morococha. Basal, angiotensin infusion, and post-angiotensin infusion collections of blood and urine were obtained (fig. 7.12). The reduction of GFR and ERPF was observed in both groups, but reduction took place to a smaller degree in the high-altitude natives. The index, [Na]/[Inulin], appears at the extreme right of the figure. After angiotensin infusion, this index fell to 44 percent in the sea-level group and to 49 percent in the high-altitude group, but the difference was not significant. Recovery figures also were similar in both groups. The smaller hemodynamic response in the high-altitude group was attributed to an increased amount of blood in the polycythemic kidney, which would cause it to be less contractile. As in the reabsorption of bicarbonate and the secretion of H^+, the tubular capacity of the kidney of the high-altitude native to reabsorb sodium in the presence of angiotensin is not impaired.

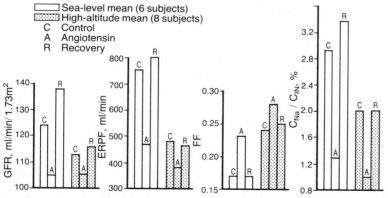

Figure 7.12.   The renal physiologic changes induced by angiotensin. Synthetic angiotensin was infused at 0.32 μg/min during 60 min. Urine and blood samples for clearance determinations were obtained before, during, and after angiotensin infusion. (With permission from Torres et al. 1970.)

7.6   Maximal Urinary Concentrating Capacity

Delgado (1969) studied fifteen sea-level men at Lima and fifteen high-altitude natives of Morococha. After water deprivation and pitressin tannate administration, the subjects' maximal urinary concentrating capacity was elevated (fig. 7.13). The maximal urine osmolarity (Uosm), although lower at high altitude than at sea level, was within normal sea-level limits. The solute output (Uosm × V) was lower in the high-altitude natives, which was believed to be due to their low-protein diet. If Uosm is corrected by (Uosm × V), then the index Uosm/(Uosm × V) shows no significant difference between the two groups. The results were interpreted as indicating that the renal concentrating mechanism in the high-altitude native is unimpaired.

7.7   Maximal Tubular Free-Water Reabsorption Capacity

Delgado (1969) also induced osmotic diuresis in five male sea-level subjects in Lima and in five male high-altitude natives in Morococha. The diuresis was induced by intravenous mannitol infusion in hydropenic conditions, and pitressin was administered (fig. 7.14). The maximal tubular free water reabsorption (T^cH_2O), when corrected for 100 ml of GFR, is very similar between the two groups. The urinary volume (V), the osmolar clearance (Cosm), and the slope of the linear portion of the functional relationship of (Cosm) and V also show no significant differences between the two groups. Figure 7.15 shows this functional study in one sea-level subject and one high-altitude native. The similarity of response is striking. As in the case of the maximal concentrating ability, these results were interpreted as indicat-

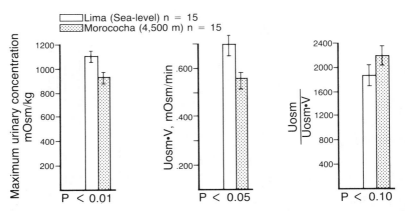

Figure 7.13.   The maximal urinary concentration after water deprivation and administration of pitressin in sea-level residents and high-altitude natives. When the maximal urine osmolarity ($Uosm_{max}$) was corrected for the solute output ($Uosm - V$), there were no statistically significant differences between the two populations. (With permission, from Delgado 1969.)

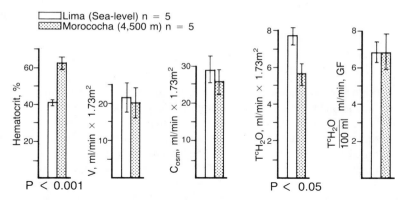

Figure 7.14. The maximal tubular reabsorption capacity studied in hydropenic conditions by mannitol infusion. Sea-level residents are compared with high-altitude natives. When corrected by the glomerular filtration rate, T^cH_2O showed no differences between the two populations. (With permission, from Delgado 1969.)

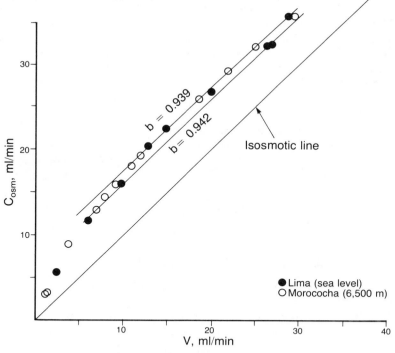

Figure 7.15. An example of the relationship between C_{osm} and urine volume (V) during osmotic diuresis. Closed circles correspond to an experiment conducted in a sea-level native. The similarity of response is evident. The slope (b) of the linear portion of the function relationship does not differ between the two sets of points. (With permission, from Delgado 1969.)

ing that maximal tubular free water reabsorption is unimpaired at high altitudes.

7.8 Renal Oxygenation

The kidney's small dimensions and large blood flow make possible a small arteriovenous O_2 difference and a high PvO_2 at sea level. Nevertheless, at high altitudes the kidney has more tissue hypoxia than do other tissues, despite the small drop in the arteriovenous PO_2 difference (Cerro de Pasco 4.4 torr, Lima 29.5 torr; table 7.1). The high renal PvO_2 at sea level, which is an indicator of tissue PO_2 (Tenney 1974), makes the kidney more sensitive to hypoxia than other organs whose PvO_2 is lower. Note that this situation is very similar to oxygen transport to the carotid body, another organ whose regulatory functions are critical in hypoxia (see chap. 6).

Monge C. (1983) presented a theoretical study of PvO_2 as a function of PaO_2 using the Fick oxygen transport equation, the oxygen equilibrium curve, and hemoglobin concentration from PaO_2 in Peruvian natives (Monge C. and Whittembury 1976a). Using this formulation and experimental values applicable to these populations, one can calculate PvO_2 as a function of PaO_2 for circulation of both the system and the kidney. When the calculations were applied to the kidney, renal blood flow ($\dot{Q}_b$) instead of systemic blood flow was the only changed parameter. It is assumed that the P50 and Hill's parameter, n, were not different in renal and systemic circulations.

The difference between the renal and the mixed venous PO_2 ($P\bar{v}O_2$) as a function of PaO_2 variation is shown in figure 7.16. Down to a PaO_2 of about 65 torr, there is an insignificant change in systemic $P\bar{v}O_2$. In contrast, the renal PvO_2 declines as the PaO_2 falls below sea-level values. These unique features of the O_2 uptake by the kidney make it uniquely sensitive to hypoxia. This is not surprising, because the kidney is the site of erythropoietin, the hormone responsible for regulating the size of the red cell mass.

7.9 Renal Abnormalities in High-altitude Natives

Early observations by Monge M. and Monge C. (1966) showed the presence of significant proteinuria in some cases of chronic mountain sickness. Also, physicians in Cerro de Pasco mention the common occurrence of "one to two plus" proteinuria in urinary samples of persons considered normal by clinical standards. Rennie (1969) reported similar proteinuria in cyanotic subjects with congenital heart disease. Because of these similarities, Rennie, Martecorena, Monge, et al. 1971) and Sirotzky (1947) carried out a systematic study in Peru of protein excretion at three different altitudes.

Thirty normal sea-level men were studied in Lima, along with nineteen

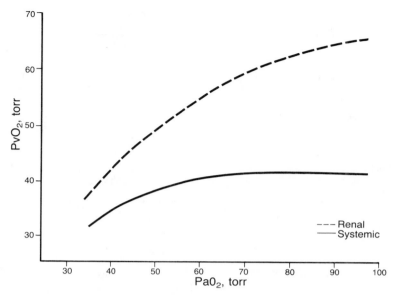

Figure 7.16. Renal PvO_2 as a function of PaO_2, calculated from a theoretical model that includes the polycythemic response to changes in PaO_2 in Peruvian natives. (Monge C., unpublished data.)

apparently normal high-altitude natives in Yauricocha (4,650 meters) and twenty-six in San Cristobal (4,710 meters). All were well-nourished. The study included the accurate measurement of protein excretion rate, proteinemia, creatinine clearance, hematocrit, and the excretion rate of strong electrolytes (table 7.4). The urinary protein excretion rate, although within normal clinical limits, was higher in the high-altitude natives. The creatinine clearance was lower at the highest altitude, and this population also showed the highest hematocrits. The proteinemia and the excretion of strong electrolytes were no different for the three populations, and the urea excretion rate was higher at high altitudes. The results, interpreted as indicating an increased rate of urinary protein excretion in the high-altitude population, could not be explained by starvation, because food intake was adequate in all subjects.

Out of eighty-one volunteers, six high-altitude natives were grouped separately because they had evidence of severe renal abnormalities (table 7.5). All members of this subgroup had reduced clearances with elevated serum creatinine, and they all showed hypoproteinemia in the absence of clinical proteinuria. Three of them had serum creatinines of approximately 14 milligrams/deciliter, indicating severe renal failure. None had anemia, but one had a hematocrit of 75 percent, despite a creatinine of 15 milli-

Table 7.4. Urinary protein excretion rates and creatinine clearances in residents of low and high altitudes

	Lima	Yauricocha	San Cristobal
	$N = 30$	$N = 19$	$N = 26$
Surface area (m^2)	$1.67 \pm .13$	$1.55 \pm .05$	$1.61 \pm .07$
Hematocrit (%)	43.6 ± 2.4	57.4 ± 4.8	64.7 ± 5.8
Serum protein (g/dl)	$7.2 \pm .4$	$7.3 \pm .3$	7.3 ± 1.1
Serum albumin (g/dl)	$4.1 \pm .3$	$4.2 \pm .2$	$4.2 \pm .5$
Serum creatinine (mg/dl)	$.83 \pm .10$	$.81 \pm .08$	$.94 \pm .5$
			($p < .02$)
Creatinine clearance	110 ± 17	114 ± 39	91 ± 23
(ml/min/1.73 m^2)			($p < .01$)
Urinary protein excretion	61.6 ± 20	105.7 ± 85.3	110.6 ± 49.7
(μg/min/1.73 m^2)			($p < .001$)

Source: Rennie et al. 1971, "Urinary Protein Excretion"; Sirotsky 1974.
Note: Values are ± 1 SD. Values of p are for differences with sea-level controls. Altitudes are Lima, sea level; Yauricocha, 4,654 m; and San Cristobal, 4,710 m.

grams/deciliter. The absence of hypertension, anemia, and proteinuria in the presence of severe renal failure and hypoproteinemia makes this entity a unique nephropathy. Although the researchers considered the hypoxemic-polycythemic condition of high-altitude natives as a possible cause of the nephropathy, because both the high-altitude towns studied are mining centers, mineral contaminants in the environment should also be considered as a possible cause of toxic nephropathy.

According to Naeye (1965), glomeruli of children who died accidentally in Leadville (3,100 m) resemble those found in children with cyanotic congenital heart malformations. Glomeruli enlarge after the first month of life because of a proliferation of glomerular elements. Possible causes cited

Table 7.5. Urinary protein excretion rates and creatinine clearances in high-altitude natives with a nephropathy of unknown origin

	Subject					
	1	2	3	4	5	6
Surface area (m^2)	1.68	1.61	1.58	1.53	1.44	1.64
Hematocrit (%)	51	55	59	75	50	62
Serum protein (g/dl)	5.9	4.6	5.9	2.7	4.0	4.9
Serum albumin (g/dl)	3.7	2.9	3.5	1.6	2.6	2.3
Serum creatinine (mg/dl)	6.7	13.6	3.4	15.1	14.6	1.3
Creatinine clearance						
(ml/min/1.73 m^2)	13	7	29	6	—	56
Urinary protein excretion						
(μg/min/1.73 m^2)	74	58	87	110	—	—

Sources: Rennie, Martecorena, Monge, et al. 1971; Sirotsky 1974.
Note: See table 7.4 for comparison with the normal population.

for this alteration are increased blood volume and viscosity, arterial hypoxemia, and reduced renal parenchymal oxygen tension.

7.10.   The Polycythemic Kidney as a Model

The reduced plasma flow found in the high-altitude native, together with
high filtration fraction and normal total renal blood flow and tubular function, comprises an interesting model for renal physiology. This combination
of hemodynamic changes in the presence of intact tubular function poses
challenging questions for the renal physiologist. For example, a hematocrit
of 80 percent combined with a filtration fraction of 30 percent should raise
the hematocrit in the efferent arteriole to 86 percent. The extremely viscous
blood and slow-circulating plasma will irrigate the tubules without altering
the enormous reabsorbate, secretion, and concentrating functions. Most
single-nephron studies are conducted in animals from hydropenic conditions
to those produced by plasma expansion with the use of albumin and/or saline
infusions (Blantz 1977), but a reduced plasma flow in the absence of ischemia has not been an experimental model so far. Such a model can be
produced by intermittent hypoxia, which produces polycythemia in the
absence of hypoxemia if the animals are studied at sea level (Whittembury
1983). Micropuncture studies of the nephrons of these experimental animals
should be carried out in future studies of renal function.

The high-altitude kidney is also a model for studies of renal bicarbonate
reabsorption in the presence of a permanent state of hyperventilation. It has
been shown that, despite a low $PaCO_2$ and $[HCO_3{}^-]$ in the blood plasma,
the bicarbonate Tm of normal natives remains within sea-level limits. This
new steady state of renal bicarbonate reabsorption remains sensitive to an
elevation of $PaCO_2$. This condition is found in natives with chronic mountain sickness in whom the bicarbonate Tm rises and the plasma bicarbonate
concentration approximates sea-level limits. In these cases the $PaCO_2$ also
approximates the values found at sea level.

CHAPTER EIGHT
Exercise Capacity

Many visitors to high-altitude communities have been impressed by the physical work capacity of high-altitude natives. Barcroft et al. (1923, 358) provided an early description of Peruvian miners at work:

> The greatest feats of exertion . . . were performed by the porters who carried metal from some of the old Spanish mines. We were fortunate enough to visit one of these. The mine was said to be 250 feet below the surface, and the staircase which led down to it 600 in length. The porters varied greatly in age and stature, some being mere boys. One such said he was 10 years of age, but looked older. The load which he brought up was about 40 lbs.; another porter of perhaps 19 years carried up a load of about 100 lbs. In every case the exercise was spasmodic. The respiration was of the most laboured description. It could be heard from far down the staircase before the man, or rather his light, came into view; the climb was very slow and consisted of the ascent of a few steps at a time, each spasmodic ascent being followed by a long pause.

The physical capacity for work of the Himalayan Sherpas is legendary. The description of the Sherpa porters with the Himalayan Scientific and Mountaineering Expedition of 1960–61 by Pugh et al. (1964, 436) is an example:

> The Sherpa porters who were with the expedition during the winter were superior to the Caucasians in physical performance. They repeatedly carried 25-kg loads to the laboratory hut at 5,800 m (19,000 ft) at the same speed as the Caucasians climbing without loads. Only one of these men learned to work satisfactorily on the bicycle ergometer, and a series of blood and respiratory observations was made on this subject.

The study of exercise performance is the study of the integration of all O_2 transport mechanisms. These components include the respiratory system, blood function, cardiac output and its control, and the efficiency of tissue O_2 utilization. Although the interpretation of test results is complex, it is extremely helpful in identifying what physiologic mechanisms may limit the transport of O_2 from air to the tissues. This chapter reviews the available data for Andean, North American, and Himalayan natives and presents new measurements in natives of Cerro de Pasco, Peru.

Many factors, including psychologic ones, determine how much work a person is willing to perform at any given moment. The unpredictability of athletic performance is an example of this fact. Thus, the above descriptions can be regarded only as the subjective impressions of breathless lowland

Table 8.1.   Maximal O_2 uptake in high-altitude natives

Location	Altitude (m)	VO_{2max} (ml/kg/min)	Source
Andes (Nuñoa)	4,200	41	(1)
Andes (Morococha)	4,500	36	(2)
Andes (Morococha)	4,500	39	(3)
Rockies (Leadville)	3,100	38	(4)

Sources: (1) Elsner, Bolstad, Forno 1964; (2) Balke 1964; (3) Hurtado et al. 1956; and (4) Grover et al. 1967.

observers. Pugh's comment illustrates the difficulties in comparing high-altitude natives with sea-level subjects. Cycling is not common in high-altitude communities, and cooperation of natives of remote areas may be difficult to obtain when language is a barrier. In spite of these limitations, there does not appear to be a great difference in the maximal work capacity of natives of different high-altitude regions of the world (table 8.1). Interest in work capacity lies not so much in defining the maximum, but rather in defining what mechanisms must be used to compensate for hypoxia and what physiologic price must be paid for using them.

8.1   Andean High-Altitude Natives

8.1.1   Overall Work Capacity

The definition of work capacity is difficult. At sea level, it is common practice to increase the work load in steps with either a cycle ergometer or a treadmill until the subject reaches exhaustion. Each stage of exercise should be of sufficient duration to allow the subject to come to a "steady state" of O_2 uptake ($\dot{V}O_2$) and CO_2 production ($\dot{V}CO_2$). At sea level, this requires between two and four minutes. If the steady state has been reached at each level, then the $\dot{V}O_2$ at which the external work load can be increased without increasing $\dot{V}O_2$ is taken as $\dot{V}O_{2max}$, the maximal O_2 uptake. Another commonly used measure of work capacity is the endurance time. This is defined as the time to exhaustion when the subject works at some predetermined work level, usually 75–80 percent of $\dot{V}O_{2max}$. These definitions are critically important in the interpretation of studies on the work capacity in high-altitude natives.

High-altitude natives are not accustomed to cycling, because bicycles are not used over the rugged terrain found in the mountains. They may find treadmill exercise slightly less foreign, but it is difficult to transport treadmills to high-altitude laboratories. A treadmill has been available in Morococha, however, since the San Marcos High Altitude Institute was established many years ago, but no similar facility is available in the Himalayas.

Additional difficulties in comparative studies lie in calibration of the equipment, particularly when local power must be relied upon.

Dill (1938) observed that investigation of Andean miners might provide valuable insight into the understanding of high-altitude acclimatization. Many studies followed, but their interpretation was difficult because of a large individual variability in training, motivation, body habitus, age, and possible genetic background. Indians in Morococha have been compared with sailors in Lima and with both athletic and sedentary Caucasian lowlanders acclimatized to altitude. Caucasian natives of intermediate altitudes have been compared with athletic lowlanders at both altitudes, and small numbers of Sherpas have been studied, usually without adequate controls. In all these investigations, different techniques of exercise evaluation have been used by different experimenters.

Hurtado and co-workers studied ten natives of Morococha and compared them with ten sea-level controls (Hurtado et al. 1956). The results, which were summarized in the 1964 *Handbook of Physiology* (Hurtado 1964), are widely quoted as showing evidence of superior exercise performance by high-altitude natives (table 8.2). Details of the selection of subjects are not available, except that the Morococha subjects were "healthy" and the controls were "sailors."

The subjects were well matched in age, but the sea-level subjects were about 4 centimeters taller and 10 kilograms heavier than the Indians. The Morococha subjects had the expected increased vital capacity (see chap. 6), maximal breathing capacity, and hemoglobin concentration. At both locations, subjects were asked to run on a treadmill to exhaustion at an average of 132.4 meters/minute and 11 percent grade.

Under the conditions of this test protocol, the work rate of the Morococha subjects was slightly lower because of their lower weight. Nevertheless, they worked for about twice as long as the lowlanders before they became exhausted, with a higher minute ventilation, lower O_2 uptake, lower heart rate, and, therefore, higher efficiency. The O_2 debt, calculated as the O_2 uptake (over basal requirements) during recovery, was lower for the high-altitude natives, as was their lactic acid production.

Hurtado believed that these studies showed the physical superiority of the high-altitude natives. He felt the superiority resulted from a combination of the training effect of a high degree of physical activity and "adaptive mechanisms" in the subjects. The lower lactic acid accumulation was regarded as protective because it prevented the occurrence of acidosis.

It is striking that the high-altitude natives studied by Hurtado did not exhibit the hypoventilation characteristic of subjects in subsequent studies. Recent work with similar subjects, discussed later in this chapter, also demonstrates a lower blood pH during exercise compared with controls, but the proposed mechanism is reduced ventilation and higher $PaCO_2$. One must

Table 8.2.   Exercise capacity in natives of Lima and Morococha

	Lima	Morococha
	N = 10	*N = 10*
Age (yr)	21.1 ± .3	21.2 ± .5
Hemoglobin (g/dl)	15.8 ± .3	19.5 ± .4
Height (cm)	164.4 ± 1.9	160.6 ± 2.4
Weight (kg)	64.5 ± 2.2	54.5 ± 1.4
VC, (lBTPS)	4.92 ± .22	5.35 ± .36
$\dot{V}_{Emax}$ (l/minBTPS)	175 ± 6	182 ± 9
	Treadmill exercise	
Duration (min)	34.2 ± 4.7	59.4 ± 7.5
Work rate (kgm/min)	935 ± 29	786 ± 21
$\dot{V}_E$ (l/minBTPS)	37.5 ± 1.2	42.4 ± 1.8
$\dot{V}O_2$ (l/minSTPD)	1.333 ± .045	1.167 ± .031
$\dot{V}CO_2$ (l/minSTPD)	1.265 ± .038	1.109 ± .042
RQ	.93 ± .01	.95 ± .01
Calories (min^{-1} m^{-2})	6.699 ± .19	5.809 ± .16
$\dot{V}_E/\dot{V}O_2$	27.8 ± .8	36.1 ± 1.0
Breathing frequency	37.2 ± 1.9	36.4 ± 1.0
Tidal volume (lBTPS)	1.77 ± .11	1.83 ± .10
Heart rate	183 ± 4	160 ± 5
O_2 pulse (ml/min)	12.67 ± .61	11.53 ± .86
	Maximal values	
$\dot{V}_E$ (l/minBTPS)	75.8 ± 2.9	78.2 ± 4.3
$\dot{V}O_2$ (l/minSTPD)	2.56 ± .12	2.11 ± .09
Breathing frequency	44.1 ± 2.6	44.6 ± 1.9
Tidal volume (lBTPS)	2.07 ± .15	2.14 ± .12
Heart rate	202 ± 5	177 ± 3
Lactic acid (mEq/l)	11.89 ± .24	9.94 ± .41
O_2 debt (lSTPD)	5.07 ± .38	3.78 ± .24
O_2 debt/m^2	2.96 ± .18	2.39 ± .11
"Relative" O_2 debt (%)	7.5 ± .83	4.3 ± .43
Net efficiency	19.6 ± .66	22.2 ± .66

Source: Hurtado 1956.
Note: Altitudes are Lima, sea level, and Morococha, 4,500 m.

wonder, therefore, how the subjects were selected for Hurtado's studies and how long they had lived in Morococha before the tests.

At about the same time as Hurtado's work was being performed, Balke (1964) studied five residents of Morococha (table 8.3) and compared their treadmill exercise capacity with that of a single acclimatized Caucasian lowlander on Mt. Evans (altitude 4,300 m). He concluded that both natives and acclimatized lowlanders achieved the same $\dot{V}O_{2max}$. In addition, both achieved a $\dot{V}O_{2max}$ that was comparable with sea-level control values. However, the Morococha subjects did so with a lower pulse rate and O_2 pulse, lower blood pressure, and strikingly lower ventilation. In interpreting

Table 8.3.   Maximal work in high-altitude natives and acclimatized lowlanders

	Minute and/or % grade at 87 m/min					
	10	12	14	16	18	20
$\dot{V}O_2$ (ml/kg/min)						
Normal	23.5	25.8	28.4	31.0	33.6	36.2
A[a]	25.2	28.0	29.6	31.8	34.0	36.0
B[b]	22.6	25.4	28.2	30.4	33.6	36.5
Heart rate (/min)						
A	122	132	140	148	160	167
B	132	140	148	154	160	168
Blood pressure (mm Hg)						
A	136/79	138/80	137/78	142/77	144/77	146/77
B	200/85	200/80	205/75	210/75	215/70	218/70
$\dot{V}_E$ (l/min BTPS)						
A	43.4	47.7	51.8	57.6	63.1	72.5
B	55.6	66.9	77.2	88.5	90.0	139.0
O_2 pulse (ml/min)						
A	12.7	13.4	14.2	14.6	15.5	15.5
B	12.1	12.4	12.4	12.6	12.5	12.9
$\dot{V}_E/\dot{V}O_2$						
A	29.2	29.0	29.8	31.0	31.6	33.7
B	33.2	35.7	37.5	39.4	37.5	52.0

Source: Balke 1964.

[a]A = average of five residents of Morococha, mean weight 59 kg.

[b]B = a single lowland resident after four weeks of acclimatization to 4,500–5,500 m, weight 74 kg.

these results, Balke felt that exercise was limited in the natives by the cardiovascular system and in the acclimatized lowlander by the ventilatory system. These data conflicted with the views of Hurtado and suggested that high-altitude natives are *not* more efficient than lowlanders in work performance.

Further clarification was later provided by Kollias et al. (1968), who studied a group of Peruvian Indians living near the Pennsylvania State field laboratory at Nuñoa, altitude 4,000 meters. They also included athletic sea-level subjects in their control group. Their subjects' ages ranged from twenty-one to forty years, and they were judged typical of the local residents. After repeated familiarization trials on a cycle ergometer, the subjects were asked to follow various exercise protocols. Kollias et al. found that the maximal O_2 uptake ($\dot{V}O_{2max}$) was the same for the Indians and acclimatized lowland athletes, but greater than that of a group of nonathletic acclimatized lowlanders (table 8.4). The Indians could not sustain maximal work as long as the lowlander athletes, and their peak work performance was less. Moreover, after exhaustive work, the Indians' recovery $\dot{V}O_2$ was higher, suggesting an increased O_2 debt. These authors concluded that, while the high-altitude Indians could achieve a $\dot{V}O_{2max}$ as high

Table 8.4. Exercise capacities in high-altitude Indians and in athletic and sedentary lowlanders

	Athletes	Nonathletes	Indians
	$N = 6$	$N = 6$	$N = 8$
$\dot{V}O_{2max}$ (ml/kg/min)	49.2 ± 4.8	37.5 ± 5.6	51.8 ± 3.4
$\dot{V}_{Emax}$ (l/min BTPS)	211.3 ± 17.1	203.6 ± 22.8	153.3 ± 27.2
$\dot{V}_E/\dot{V}O_2$ (STPD)	30.9 ± 3.0	34.9 ± 1.9	26.5 ± 3.4
HR (/min)	165 ± 13	161 ± 22	176 ± 9
Total running time (min)	7.1 ± 1.2	5.4 ± 0.7	4.9 ± 1.0
Peak work (kpm/min)	$1,953 \pm 218$	$1,596 \pm 138$	$1,272 \pm 227$
Recovery $\dot{V}O_2$ (l/10 min)	$5.48 \pm .63$	$5.93 \pm .47$	$6.45 \pm .94$
Gross efficiency[a] (%)	14.5 ± 1.0	14.5 ± 0.7	12.2 ± 1.1

Source: Kollias et al. 1968.
[a]Kcal work in 5 min/(Kcal for 5 min + Kcal in 10 min recovery) $\times$ 100.

as that of well-trained sea-level athletes, their overall efficiency is less, and they cannot sustain maximal work for as long. The results are reminiscent of Barcroft's comments about the spasmodic nature of work patterns of Indians at Cerro de Pasco.

It is probably not possible to determine why these two studies with Peruvian Indians should have arrived at conclusions so different from those of Hurtado, because there are so many differences between the experimental methods used and the subjects selected. However, Hurtado's pioneering work is cited most often, and the idea of a high-altitude "superman" has great emotional appeal. The authors believe these studies show that high-altitude natives are more comparable to sea-level athletes than to sedentary lowlanders. This can be explained by the fact that their lives require more physical activity, not that they need any particular genetic advantage.

8.1.2 The Ventilatory Response to Exercise

The rate of movement of air into and out of the lungs is obviously critical in the uptake of O_2 and is a potentially sensitive point of regulation. For many reasons, exercise generally has not been used to evaluate the regulatory mechanisms that govern ventilation. The main reason for this is that during exercise many variables change in concert as work is increased. The situation at high altitude is even more complex, because hypoxia is superimposed on the other changing conditions, such as $PaCO_2$ and pH. Moreover, it is not easy to standardize exercise test equipment in the field. In recent years, however, equipment has become increasingly reliable and automated, and it is now a relatively simple matter to conduct even complex protocols with naive subjects. Several authors have shown that the relationships between minute ventilation ($\dot{V}_E$) and O_2 consumption and CO_2 production, for example, are quite reproducible for an individual, and the steady state need not be reached to obtain useful information.

In normal sea-level subjects, $\dot{V}_E$ increases linearly with O_2 consumption up to about 70 percent of $\dot{V}O_{2max}$. After that point, the slope of the $\dot{V}_E$ line increases because of the added stimulus of lactic acid accumulation. This point has been called the "anaerobic threshold" by Wasserman and Whipp (1975). The initial $\dot{V}_E/\dot{V}O_2$ slope, which is used to quantitate the ventilatory response to exercise, can be obtained by simple linear regression analysis of data taken several times per minute or even at each breath (fig. 8.1). In practice, the slope of the $\dot{V}_E/\dot{V}O_2$ line is probably more reproducible, in that changes in the respiratory quotient (RQ) caused by diet or other factors will influence the ratio $\dot{V}_E/\dot{V}O_2$ (Jones 1976).

The blunted hypoxic ventilatory drive of high-altitude Andeans may play an important role in maximal exercise efficiency. Kollias et al. (1968) found identical minute ventilation ($\dot{V}_E$) at low work loads, but maximal $\dot{V}_E$ was lower for Indians than for acclimatized lowlanders, whether they were athletic or sedentary. The ventilatory equivalent ($\dot{V}_E/\dot{V}O_2$) was the same in all three groups at rest. However, during exercise, the $\dot{V}_E/\dot{V}O_2$ ratio was 30.9 in the athletic lowlanders and 34.9 in the sedentary lowlanders, but

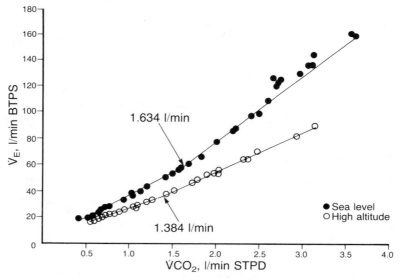

Figure 8.1. A comparison of the ventilatory response to exercise in a resident of Cerro de Pasco with that in an acclimatized lowlander. Note that both curves have two components. The straight line segments are the two best lines that fit the data. The break point between the two lines defines the "ventilatory threshold." This point is more difficult to discern for the high-altitude native because of blunted respiratory drive, but it appears to be about the same as that for the acclimatized lowlander. (Winslow and Monge, unpublished data.)

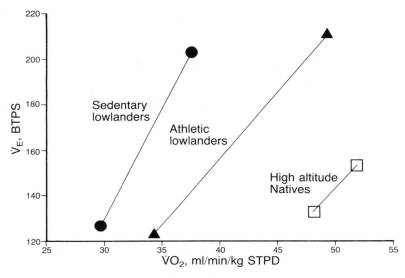

Figure 8.2. A comparison of the ventilatory response to exercise in sedentary and athletic acclimatized lowlanders with that in natives of Morococha at submaximal and maximal exercise. The natives achieve a given $\dot{V}O_2$ with a lower $\dot{V}_E$. (Data from Kollias et al. 1968.)

only 26.5 in the Indians (fig. 8.2). Thus, the Indians exhibited relative hypoventilation during exercise. Some authors have regarded this reduced $\dot{V}_E$ during exercise as an economy of ventilation (Dempsey et al. 1971). However, when $\dot{V}_E$ was related to body size, the $\dot{V}_{Emax}$ of the Indians was about the same as that of the lowlanders.

Hurtado (1964) presented ventilatory measurements from a few subjects in Morococha who had chronic mountain sickness, although he did not give the details of their cases (table 8.5). These studies apparently showed ventilatory rates lower than either "newcomers to altitude" or other high-altitude natives when breathing air or with increased or decreased P_IO_2.

It is tempting to speculate, on the basis of Hurtado's results, that high-altitude polycythemia could be related to hypoventilation. That is, perhaps

Table 8.5. Ventilation with various inspired PO_2 (observations at 4,500 m)

FIO_2	High-Altitude Natives ($N = 18$)	Newcomers ($N = 12$)	CMS Subjects ($N = 5$)
Air	9.50	13.20	7.90
Increased	10.09	11.04	7.32
Decreased	12.78	21.12	9.32

Source: Hurtado 1964.

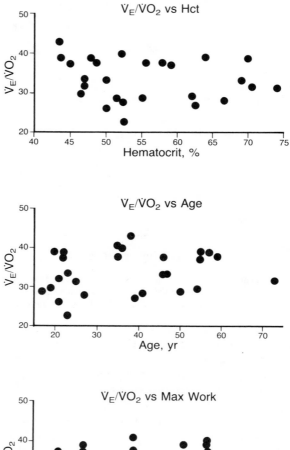

Figure 8.3. The lack of correlation between the ventilatory response to exercise ($\dot{V}_E/\dot{V}O_2$) and the hematocrit, age, or maximal exercise. The control of ventilation during exercise is complex and may not correspond to an individual's "usual" ventilation. (Winslow and Monge, unpublished data.)

subjects whose ventilation is depressed the most might have the lowest PaO_2 and highest erythropoietic drive. As noted earlier, arterial desaturation seems to be a part of chronic mountain sickness, but a cause-and-effect relationship is difficult to establish.

In the authors' own studies, an attempt was made to determine, by measuring the ventilatory response to exercise, whether ventilatory blunting was related to the development of polycythemia in chronic mountain sickness. The subjects, natives of Cerro de Pasco, displayed a large variation in hematocrit, in exercise capacity, and in $\dot{V}_E/\dot{V}O_2$. Figure 8.3 shows the lack of correlation between ventilatory equivalent for O_2 ($\dot{V}_E/\dot{V}O_2$) and hematocrit. Thus, if hypoventilation is the cause of hypoxia in subjects with chronic mountain sickness, the hypoventilation is not manifest as a reduced ventilatory response to exercise. Figure 8.3 also shows that $\dot{V}_E/\dot{V}O_2$ is not correlated with either age or the maximal cycle ergometer work achieved by the subjects in Cerro de Pasco.

8.1.3   The Cardiovascular Response to Exercise

Normal sea-level humans respond to an increased exercise load by increasing their cardiac output. This is achieved mainly by increasing heart rate; the increase in stroke volume is very small. The effect of physical training is to reduce the heart rate at all work loads, reflecting a greater efficiency of O_2 utilization and an increased stroke volume. A useful concept in this regard is the "O_2 pulse," the amount of O_2 delivered to tissue per heartbeat, or simply $\dot{V}O_2/HR$. In other words, with training the O_2 pulse increases. Hypoxia seems to have a direct effect on heart rate, and Åstrand and Åstrand (1958) showed that acclimatized lowlanders cannot raise their heart rate at high altitudes to the same degree as they can at sea level.

Maximal heart rate was found by Kollias et al. (1968) to be about the same for Indians as for both athletic and sedentary lowlanders. At submaximal work loads, the O_2 pulse was about the same for all three groups, but at maximal work the Indians increased their O_2 pulse very little. It may be, therefore, that the Indians could not increase their cardiac output in response to exercise as much as could the lowlanders. A possible explanation could be that increased hematocrit in these subjects led to increased resistance to blood flow (Guyton, Jones, and Coleman 1973). Unfortunately, the hematocrits or hemoglobin concentrations in these subjects were not reported.

The cardiovascular response to exercise was studied in detail by Banchero and co-workers in Morococha (Banchero et al. 1966). They performed right heart catheterization in thirty-five healthy high-altitude residents (mean hematocrit 58.7 ± 6.8 percent) and in twenty-two controls in Lima (mean hematocrit 44.1 ± 2.6 percent). The subjects exercised in the supine position on a cycle ergometer. The results (table 8.6) showed that

Table 8.6. Hemodynamic measurements in natives of Lima and Morococha

	Lima		Morococha	
	20.7 ± 1.3		22.4 ± 3.9	
Age (yr)	20.7 ± 1.3		22.4 ± 3.9	
Hematocrit (%)	44.1 ± 2.6		58.7 ± 6.8	
	rest	*exercise*	*rest*	*exercise*
$\dot{V}_E$ (l/minBTPS)	6.5 ± 1.4	28.1 ± 3.5	8.1 ± 1.4	37.4 ± 7.7
$\dot{V}O_2$ (l/minSTPD)	.153 ± .028	.719 ± .087	.161 ± .019	.779 ± .102
$\dot{V}_E/\dot{V}O_2$	42.5	39.1	50.3	48.0
HR	68 ± 8	128 ± 14	77 ± 13	140 ± 21
SV (ml/min/m^2)	59 ± 13	54 ± 9	52 ± 10	56 ± 8
CI (l/min/m^2)	3.97 ± .98	6.83 ± 1.03	3.97 ± .72	7.70 ± 1.27
PA pressure (mm Hg)	12 ± 2	18 ± 3	29 ± 10	60 ± 17
Arterial pressure (mm Hg)	95 ± 8	112 ± 8	95 ± 8	109 ± 8
Resistance, PA (dynes/sec/cm^{-5})	160 ± 47	125 ± 24	373 ± 147	408 ± 144
Resistance, arterial (dynes/sec/cm^{-5})	1248 ± 304	827 ± 153	1278 ± 271	753 ± 132
Work, RV (kgm/min/m^2)	.55 ± .23	1.73 ± .50	1.49 ± .72	6.60 ± 2.09
Work, LV (kgm/min/m^2)	5.50 ± 1.63	10.27 ± 1.93	5.11 ± 1.04	11.40 ± .37

Source: Banchero et al. 1966.
Note: SV = stroke volume; CI = cardiac index; PA = pulmonary artery; RV = right ventricle; LV = left ventricle.

subjects in both groups increased their cardiac output to about the same extent in response to submaximal exercise, and the increase was due almost exclusively to increased heart rate, with the stroke volume remaining nearly constant. The pulmonary artery pressures doubled in the high-altitude natives, while it increased by only 50 percent in the controls. The resistance to flow in the pulmonary circulation was much higher in the Morococha group, and the resultant work performed by the right ventricle was consequently much higher.

Individual data are not available to judge whether there was a relationship between hematocrit and cardiac output in Banchero's high-altitude group. The ratio $\dot{V}_E/\dot{V}O_2$ for the subjects that were selected in Morococha was quite high (table 8.6). Thus, while the study may characterize healthy subjects in Morococha, they may not be representative of those who have blunted ventilatory response to exercise.

Elsner and co-workers extended the analogy between high-altitude exposure and athletic training by studying leg flow during and after treadmill exercise (Elsner, Bolstad, and Forno 1964). They reported the same pattern for high-altitude natives as for sea-level athletes. Thus, at a given work rate ($\dot{V}O_2$) flow was lower in both groups than in nonathletic sea-level controls.

However, the maximal flow could be forced higher in both athletes and high-altitude residents by increasing the work load. These authors concluded that Indians are like trained sea-level athletes and that tissue blood flow is not limiting to O_2 uptake.

8.1.4   The Acid-Base and Blood Gas Responses to Exercise

An additional striking feature of exercise at high altitudes is that arterial O_2 saturation decreases as work load increases (fig. 8.4). This complex matter, discussed in detail in subsequent chapters, is influenced not only by PAO_2 and ventilation, but also by cardiac output, acid-base balance, and the position of the hemoglobin oxygen equilibrium curve (see chap. 4). The reduced PAO_2 of the high-altitude native falls near the steep descending portion of the OEC. Thus, even small shifts to the right (reduced affinity) will result in decreased saturation at a given PO_2. During exercise, arterial pH decreases because of the accumulation of lactic acid, causing such a right shift. The degree of reduction of PaO_2, however, will be a result of the degree of alveolar ventilation the subject can achieve and of the pulmonary perfusion/ventilation match.

8.1.5   The Production of Lactic Acid

Chronic exposure to high altitudes was observed by Edwards (1936) to reduce the amount of lactic acid that appears in the circulation after exhaustive exercise. Hurtado (1971b) claimed that natives of Morococha had a reduced rate of lactic acid production during exercise as compared with residents at sea level (see table 8.2). This finding is very interesting, because the increase of lactic acid over baseline amounts (the anaerobic threshold) imposes a limit on the duration of exercise that follows (Wasserman 1984). The mechanism of the reduced lactate accumulation in high-altitude natives is not clear, but it could result from decreased production, increased consumption by the heart (Moret 1971), or an increased clearance rate by other tissues. Cerretelli (1983) has studied this problem extensively and views the lower lactic acid concentration as a reduced capacity for accumulation, brought about by reduced plasma bicarbonate that results from decreased $PaCO_2$ and not by any reduction of the maximal rate of phosphocreatine splitting, at least up to an altitude of 4,500 meters.

One study conducted in this area by the authors concerned lactic acid production in subjects with chronic mountain sickness. Tests on excessively polycythemic natives of Cerro de Pasco were based on the hypothesis that polycythemia might lead to a reduced anaerobic threshold. Three subjects were found suitable for the studies; they were able to perform adequately on a cycle ergometer and they consented to hematocrit reduction by phle-

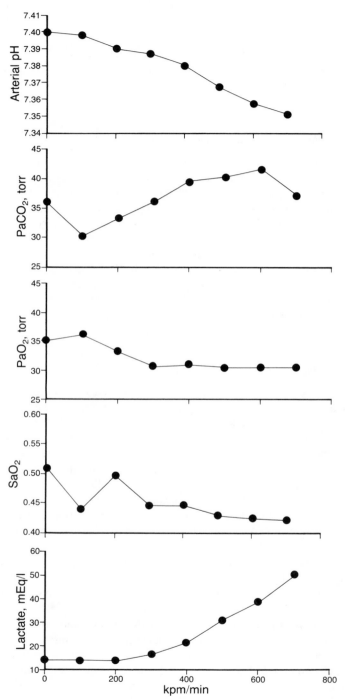

Figure 8.4. Changes in the arterial blood gases during exercise in a native of Cerro de Pasco. The fall in PaO_2 is accompanied by decreasing pH, increasing lactic acid concentration, and increasing $PaCO_2$. The net result is that SaO_2 falls also, a change that is augmented by decreased hemoglobin O_2 affinity attributable to the Bohr effect. (Winslow and Monge, unpublished data.)

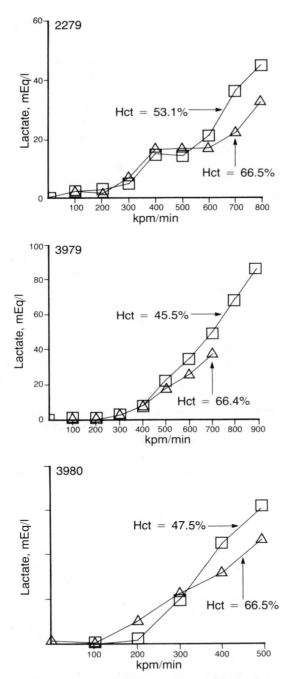

Figure 8.5. The accumulation of lactic acid in three natives of Cerro de Pasco before and after phlebotomy. The hematocrits are indicated. In each case, the maximal lactic acid concentration increased at the highest work rate. Note that the point in exercise at which accumulation begins is approximately the same before and after phlebotomy. (Winslow and Monge, unpublished data.)

botomy. Arterial lactic acid was measured during the last fifteen seconds of each minute of a one-minute exercise test performed in one-minute increments (fig. 8.5). In every case, the maximal lactic acid concentration increased significantly over the prephlebotomy level, indicating a greater "lactactid" capacity (see diPrampero, Mognoni, and Veicsteinas 1981). These results indicate that a part of the reduced lactic acid accumulation seen by various investigators in the past may be due to polycythemia itself. This could result from decreased appearance in the arterial blood because of sluggish flow, decreased clearance from the circulation for the same reason, or from a relatively inadequate supply of O_2 to tissues.

8.2   North American Natives

Exercise capacity in high-altitude natives of Leadville, Colorado, has been studied carefully by the University of Colorado group. At 3,100 meters, Leadville is not as high as other high-altitude sites, but its accessibility makes it very convenient. Grover et al. (1967) carried out studies comparable in design with those by Kollias with Andean natives. In the Leadville study, five young athletes, natives of high altitudes, were compared with similar athletes from a low altitude (300 m). The studies were carried out with both groups at both high and low altitudes. Both groups had very high maximal O_2 uptakes (66–68 ml/kg/min) at low altitude, and both demonstrated a 25 percent reduction at high altitude. In contrast to the studies in the Andes, these high-altitude natives hyperventilated to the same extent at high altitude as did the low-altitude natives. These authors concluded that young athletes of European ancestry who are acclimatized to high altitudes from birth have an O_2 transport system very similar to that of sea-level natives. They went on to speculate that because there are no apparent differences among natives of the Andes, and Leadville, and of athletic sea-level natives, in their maximal O_2 uptake, and because the Andean natives are known to hypoventilate during exercise, the Andeans may have some degree of tissue adaptation that allows a more efficient utilization of O_2.

The Colorado group has provided extensive data on the cardiovascular response to moderate altitude in natives of Leadville (Hartley et al. 1967). They found that when Leadville residents descended to lower altitudes, cardiac output increased by 8 percent and stroke volume, by 15 percent. During exercise the reduced cardiac output was mediated by a reduced stroke volume (Alexander et al. 1967). These changes could not be reproduced by O_2 administration to the same subjects in Leadville, and they could not be explained on the basis of polycythemia or pulmonary artery hypertension. Alexander therefore postulated that the depressed cardiac output at Leadville must be due to a direct depressant effect of hypoxia on the myocardium.

The studies carried out with the Leadville natives, showing a reduced cardiac output at altitude compared with at sea level, do not agree with the Morococha data (Banchero et al. 1966). Unfortunately, no strictly comparable data are available from Morococha, in that the same subjects are not studied at both high and low altitudes. Therefore, it is not possible to determine whether Andeans' cardiac output is unaffected by altitude or whether the subjects selected for study were not well matched. It is unlikely that this issue will be resolved until noninvasive techniques are developed that can be used safely and conveniently in large numbers of subjects at both altitudes.

8.3 Himalayan Natives

In 1964, Pugh et al. reported a limited set of data comparing exercise performances of a single Sherpa porter and two of the members of the 1960–61 Himalayan Scientific and Mountaineering Expedition. In a cycle ergometer exercise test (900 kg-m/min), this Sherpa performed more work than the best of the lowland expedition members, with a higher heart rate and lower $\dot{V}_E$, while his PO_2 was about the same (table 8.7). Pugh, through indirect calculations, estimated that the cardiac output of this subject must have been considerably higher than those of the sojourners. He also estimated a very high pulmonary diffusing capacity for the Sherpa, consistent with his low arterioalveolar O_2 gradient and the fact that he could satisfy his O_2 requirement with less ventilation. He also noted that the Sherpa blood pH dropped more during exercise than did those of the sojourners, because of a lack of hyperventilation. Thus, he argued, the Sherpa's PO_2 remained high at the same saturation as noted in the sojourners.

Table 8.7. Oxygen transport in a Sherpa and in acclimatized lowlanders

	Lowlander 1	Lowlander 2	Sherpa Subject
Age (yr)	32	51	28
Weight (kg)	64	68	63
$\dot{V}O_2$ (l/minSTPD)	2.04	1.61	2.28
$\dot{V}_E$ (l/minBTPS)	115	105	82
Cardiac output (l/min)	17	15	19
Blood pH	7.52	7.55	7.35
D_2O_2 (ml/min/mm Hg)	60	45	97
Oxygen gradient			
$\quad PIO_2$	70	70	70
$\quad PAO_2$	53	55	44
$\quad PaO_2$	29	24	29
$\quad PvO_2$	11	10	10
$\quad (PA - Pa)O_2$	24	31	15

Source: Pugh 1964.

Lahiri and co-workers carried out a systematic study of four Sherpas in 1964, comparing them with acclimatized lowlanders and with sea-level data (Lahiri and Milledge 1965; Lahiri et al. 1967). They found the same relationship between $\dot{V}O_2$ and work rate for the Sherpas and acclimatized lowlanders. At a given work level, Sherpa subjects ventilated less than did the lowlanders, and their rate of increase in ventilation with increasing work was smaller. Breathing 100 percent O_2 during exercise reduced ventilation in the lowlanders but did not in the Sherpas. Heart rates in the Sherpas were lower while at rest, but higher during exercise. Breathing O_2 raised the maximum heart rate in the lowlanders, but lowered it in the Sherpas. The "blunted" hypoxic ventilatory response was manifested by higher $PACO_2$ and lower PAO_2 in the Sherpas. The hemoglobin concentrations in the Sherpas generally were lower than in the lowlanders exposed to the same altitude, and the electrocardiograms were not appreciably different.

The conclusion drawn from these studies was that Sherpas and acclimatized lowlanders do not employ the same physiologic mechanisms to cope with hypoxia. The chief difference is the reduced ventilation of the Sherpas. In addition, however, they also seem to have a different cardiovascular response to inspired O_2 at high altitudes. Lahiri argued, like Pugh, that the resulting lower blood pH should insure a higher PO_2 at a given saturation in the Sherpas compared with similar conditions in the lowlanders.

8.4   The Effect of Polycythemia on Exercise

Many of the above studies show that polycythemia is not essential to performance of muscular exercise at high altitudes, either in natives or in acclimatized lowlanders. Indeed, a number of authors have observed that many healthy high-altitude natives do not show any polycythemic response at all. This fact proved, according to Dill (1938), "that however useful an increased proportion of red cells may be, it is not an indispensable feature of adaptation to low oxygen."

Polycythemia, in fact, may limit the ability of the heart to increase its output during exercise. Thus, Richardson and Guyton (1959) showed that the number of red cells available for O_2 transport is decreased in dogs both by adding to and subtracting from the number of red cells in circulation (fig. 8.6). This striking result was interpreted by the authors as attributable to a fall in cardiac output resulting from increased peripheral resistance.

Extrapolation from experiments with dogs to high-altitude humans could be dangerous. For example, the measurements of Banchero et al. (1966), described earlier, did not show an increased peripheral resistance in Morococha natives, even though their hematocrits were significantly higher than those of the sea-level controls. However, Cerretelli has suggested that

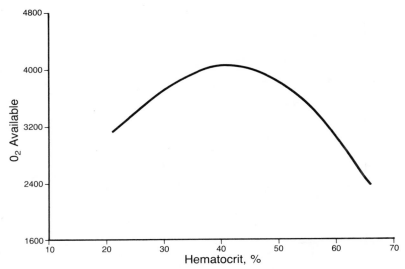

Figure 8.6. The theoretical relationship between the "available" O_2 and the hematocrit. (Modified, with permission from Richardson and Guyton 1959.)

this effect of polycythemia on hemodynamic function could explain reduced $\dot{V}O_{2max}$ in high-altitude natives (Cerretelli and Debijadji 1964) and in acclimatized lowlanders (Ceretelli 1976).

Many of the studies cited in this chapter do not report the hematocrits or hemoglobin concentrations of their subjects, so it is difficult to draw conclusions about what effect, if any, polycythemia has on maximal exercise performance. The authors studied 103 subjects in Cerro de Pasco in 1979–80 and found 49 who could satisfactorily perform cycle ergometer work. Our protocol was not designed to measure steady state $\dot{V}O_{2max}$. Rather, each subject performed work that increased each minute until exhaustion. Each test lasted approximately ten minutes. There is a correlation between hematocrit and maximal work in this protocol ($r = -.6$, $p = .001$) (fig. 8.7). This, of course, does not establish a causal relationship, because the polycythemic subjects tended to be older and more sedentary, and maximal exercise decreases with age (Åstrand et al. 1973). As will be shown in chapter 10, however, the exercise performance of many of the polycythemic subjects improved after their hematocrits were reduced to normal sea-level values, either by phlebotomy or by hemodilution.

8.5 The Economy of Oxygen Uptake during Exercise

For the lowlanders exposed acutely to hypoxia, a brisk hyperventilatory response to exercise seems necessary for sustained heavy exercise (Schoene

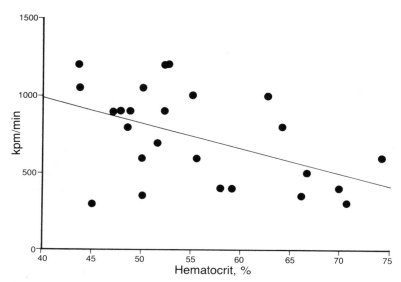

Figure 8.7.   The relationship between the hematocrit and maximal exercise capacity in natives of Cerro de Pasco. The correlation ($r = .49$) is significant ($p = .01$). (Winslow et al. 1985a.)

et al. 1984). However, as has been seen, lifelong natives of high altitudes are not capable of such extreme hyperventilation but they can achieve comparable maximal work rates nevertheless by taking advantage of other physiologic mechanisms. The high-altitude native is able to extract more O_2 per liter of inspired gas than can the acclimatized lowlander, particularly during heavy exercise (fig. 8.1). That is, his diffusing capacity is by definition higher. This observation has been used to support the argument that the high-altitude native is more efficient in gas exchange because the work of breathing is less (Dempsey et al. 1971).

At moderate altitudes (e.g., 3,100 m) it appears that lifelong natives compensate for depressed hypoxic ventilatory drive by means of enhanced alveolar-capillary gas exchange. Several authors have found that this facilitation occurs because of increased lung diffusing capacity, D_LO_2, during vigorous exercise, but that it does not occur at rest (DeGraff et al. 1970; Remmers and Mithoefer 1969; Dempsey et al. 1971). This increased diffusion of O_2 between alveoli and pulmonary capillary blood is probably mediated by an expanded pulmonary blood volume and an increased hemoglobin concentration, as well as by the possible effects of pulmonary arterial hypertension and acidemia in improving the gravity-dependent ventilation/perfusion ratio (Dempsey et al. 1971). Opposing these effects, however, is the possibility that pulmonary blood flow is reduced as a result of increased vascular resistance and decreased cardiac output that accompanies polycythemia (Richardson and Guyton 1959).

In summary, the available data do not seem to bear out the subjective impression that high-altitude natives have increased work capacity, regardless of its definition. Part of the problem is in drawing comparisons: sea-level athletes perform very well at high-altitude, whereas sedentary lowlanders do not. Another problem is that accepted definitions of work capacity have not been used in many of the studies. Additionally, the unique adaptations seen in high-altitude natives (polycythemia, increased pulmonary diffusing capacity, ventilatory blunting, and so on) serve to make such comparisons confusing.

Rather than trying to establish the superiority or inferiority of natives, it is more informative to study their pattern of acclimatization to hypoxia in contrast to the O_2 transport system of lowlanders. The most consistent difference between these two groups is the blunted ventilatory response to exercise that characterizes the high-altitude native, whether he lives in Morococha, Leadville, or the Khumbu Himal. While reduced exercise ventilation may reduce the work of breathing, compensation must occur by a combination of increased lung diffusing capacity for O_2 attributable to polycythemia and, perhaps, increased alveolar surface area and higher right ventricular work resulting from high blood viscosity and pulmonary hypertension.

Whether an individual will develop chronic mountain sickness may depend on how well this balance is struck: inadequate cardiac output will lead to decreased lung perfusion, arterial desaturation, and accelerated erythropoiesis.

CHAPTER NINE
The Comparative Physiology of Hypoxemic Polycythemia

In previous chapters, evidence has been presented to indicate that hypoxemic polycythemia, with its corresponding increase in blood hemoglobin concentration, confers a large burden in the acclimatization process of humans, whether they are sojourners at altitude or high-altitude natives. Although the excessive levels of polycythemia are seen more frequently in the Andes than in the Himalayas, carefully controlled studies by Winslow (unpublished) have shown that Sherpas do also raise their hemoglobin concentrations to the levels of newcomers (see chap. 3). All domestic European animals introduced into South America by the Spaniards also have polycythemia when they acclimatize to the high Andes (Monge C. and Monge M. 1968).

A central question is whether polycythemia is a property that may result from genetic adaptation to high altitudes, or if it is simply a physiologic response to the hypoxic environment. The distinction is important: if it is an adaptation, it must result in improved survival of the species; if not, it may lead only to pathologic consequences. The generation time for human beings is too long and their time of permanent residence at high altitude is too short to draw conclusions. However, the matter can be addressed in the study of other animals whose generation time is shorter and who have been native to high altitudes for very long periods of time. This chapter, therefore, compares the red cell functions and hemoglobin properties of humans at high altitudes with those of animals that have a hypoxic natural habitat and are considered genetically adapted to their environment.

9.1 Polycythemia and Hemoglobin Oxygen Affinity

The South American camelids (llama, alpaca, and vicuña) and rodents (chinchilla and viscacha) do not undergo change in hematocrits when changing altitudes within the ecologic range of their residence (Hall, Dill, and Barron 1936; Hall 1937; Reynafarje et al. 1968). The same is true in burrowing mammals whose habitat is hypoxic (Bullard, Broumand, and Meyer 1966; Bullard 1972). The Himalayan bar-headed goose, born at sea level and acclimatized to 6,100 meters, does not undergo a raised hematocrit. In contrast, the sea-level Pekin duck, acclimatized to the same altitude, undergoes increased hematocrit to about 60 percent above the sea-level values (Black and Tenney 1980).

Schmidt-Nielsen and Larimer (1958) showed that P50, a measure of hemoglobin affinity for oxygen, is correlated with body weight according to the equation

$$P50 = aW^{(-b)} \qquad (9.1)$$

where W is the body weight and a and b are empirical parameters. In figure 9.1, data from sea-level mammals and mammals whose environment is hypoxic have been plotted on a log-log scale. The data were obtained from several publications (Hurtado 1964; Bullard 1972; Schmidt-Nielsen and Larimer 1958; Dhindsa, Hoversland, and Metcalfe 1971; Turek et al. 1980). It can be seen that sea-level mammals present a clearly different correlation from that of species adapted to a hypoxic environment, although the data are not individually shown in the figure. The Andean camelids (llama, vicuña, and alpaca), the rodents (chinchilla and viscacha), and the burrowing squirrels with subterranean hypoxic habitats all fall along the hypoxia correlation

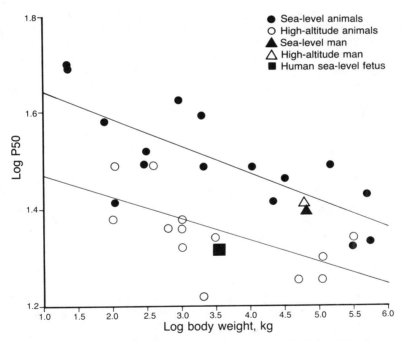

Figure 9.1.   The logarithm of P50 as a function of the logarithm of the body weight of a group of mammals. The upper regression line corresponds to sea-level animals and the lower line corresponds to either high-altitude or burrowing mammals. The points for man, both high-altitude and sea-level natives, fall on the upper line. The plot is based on data of Schmidt-Nielsen and Larimer (1958); Bullard (1972); Dhindsa, Hoversland, and Metcalfe (1971); Hurtado (1964); and Turek et al. (1980.)

line. The gray squirrel, which does not face a hypoxic challenge, has a P50 close to the sea-level group, although it has greater affinity than its sea-level relative, the domestic cow. The guinea pig, although distributed worldwide, has an Andean origin: it was introduced into Europe by Dutch sailors in the sixteenth century (Turek et al. 1980). Its affinity falls inbetween the two lines. High-altitude humans, in contrast to the other mammals whose environment is also hypoxic, have a hemoglobin affinity falling close to the sea-level group. The point for the human fetus falls close to the high-altitude line. The adapted mammals seem to have retained the properties of the fetal hemoglobin.

Reynafarje and Rosenman (1971) studied the concentration of 2,3-DPG in the blood of different mammals. Using a log-log scale, Monge and Whittembury (1976a) showed that the correlation between 2,3-DPG concentration and body weight has a remarkable similarity to that between P50 and body weight (fig. 9.2). Similarly, porpoises that swim faster and dive longer and deeper have a higher hemoglobin oxygen affinity than do the slower-swimming, shallower- and shorter-diving species (Horvath et al. 1968). These authors emphasize the similarity and relationship of the dissociation curves in these sea mammals to those observed in the terrestrial species living in hypoxic conditions.

High-altitude birds also show an increase in hemoglobin affinity (Hall, Dill, and Barron 1936; Black and Tenney 1980). The differences in hemo-

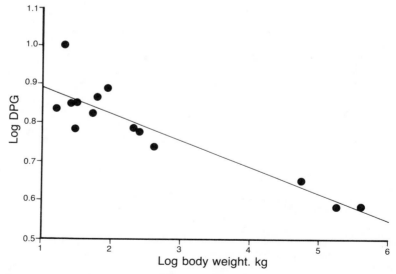

Figure 9.2. The logarithm of 2,3-DPG concentration as a function of the logarithm of body weight. Points represent values obtained in different mammals. (With permission, from Reynafarje and Rosenman 1971.)

globin affinities between mammals and birds from sea level and high altitudes are evident (fig. 9.3).

Ectotherms (poikilothermic animals) have the advantage over endotherms (birds and mammals) of diminishing their oxygen consumption when the ambient temperature falls, such as at high altitudes. To see if this group of animals shared with the birds and mammals the characteristic hemoglobin properties acquired by adaptation to high altitude, a study was undertaken in Peru in toads of the genus *Bufo*, which has subspecies native to sea level, to about 3,000 meters, and to above 4,000 meters. The hemoglobin equilibrium curve is displaced to the left in the maximum-altitude toad (*Bufo spinulosus flavolineatus*). (fig. 9.4). The sea-level toad (*Bufo spinulosus limensis*) and the intermediate-altitude toad (*Bufo spinulosus trifolium*) showed no significant differences in the position of their curves, which were determined at 20° C. In figure 9.4, the oxygen content is also plotted against

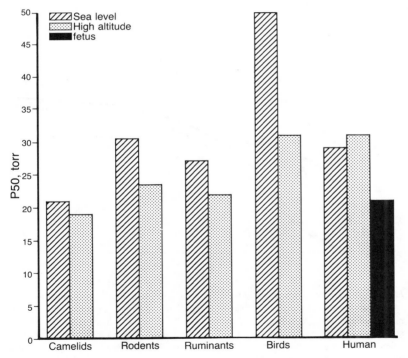

Figure 9.3. P50 values in mammals and birds. The South American (high-altitude) camelids are compared with the African (sea level) camel, the Andean rodents chinchilla and viscacha with the sea-level rabbit, the Himalayan yak with the cow, and the Andean ostrich and goose with sea-level birds (Monge M. and Monge C. 1968). The high-altitude human native is compared with sea-level humans and the human fetus. High-altitude mammals and birds show a lower P50 than that of the corresponding sea-level animals.

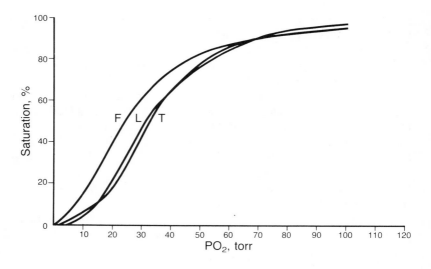

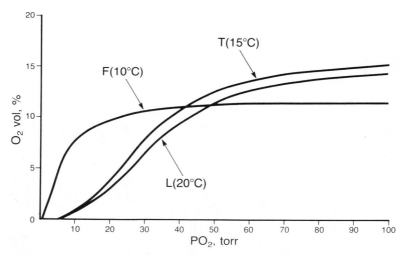

Figure 9.4.   The oxygen affinity and oxygen capacity of toad blood (poikilotherms). *Bufo spinulosus limensis* (*L*) is a sea-level toad. *Bufo spinulosus trifoleum* (*T*) is native to about 3,000 m and *Bufo spinulosus flavolineatus* (*F*) is native to 4,000 m or above. The curves were obtained at 20°C to compare the biochemical properties of the blood. The sea-level and intermediate-altitude curves are similar, but the highest altitude curve is displaced to the left, indicating higher affinity. Oxygen contents were measured at the temperature of the native habitats, 10°C, 15°C, and 20°C for the sea-level, intermediate, and high-altitude toads, respectively. Note that the high-altitude toad has a reduced O_2 capacity but a greatly increased O_2 affinity. (With permission from Ostojic 1979.)

the PO_2 at the ecologic temperatures at which these animals normally live. Because of their lower hemoglobin concentration, the maximum-altitude toad has a lower curve, which is very much displaced to the left. The intermediate-altitude toad has its curve to the left of that of the sea-level subspecies, but close to it. The actual hemoglobin values were 8 grams/deciliter for the maximum-altitude toad and 11 grams/deciliter for the other two. As in the case of the birds and the mammals, this work proved that the high-altitude toads showed no increase in hemoglobin concentration and an increase in hemoglobin affinity (Ostojic 1979). It seems, therefore, that the hypoxic environment selects for these two hemoglobin properties with great pressure, independently of the homeothermic properties of the animals' body fluids.

High-altitude humans, it has been seen, do not employ these properties which, in animals, are an indication of genetic selection to the hypoxic environment. This is not surprising, because in the Andes, at least, humans have not had sufficient time and environmental isolation to allow for sufficient selection pressure in Darwinian terms. The earliest habitation of South America by humans can be dated back about twenty-five thousand years (MacNeish 1971) and there is evidence of early human residence in territories at altitudes above 3,000 meters (Cardich 1960; Lanning 1965). This period of time could have been sufficient for some genetic selection, but the migratory tendencies of Andeans, which Monge M. described (1948), were not favorable. Studies of human population genetics in the steep Andean gradient of Arica in Chile show no evidence of genetic adaptation (Cruz-Coke et al. 1966; Rothammer and Schull 1982). The inhabitants of the Himalayas have not been studied as thoroughly as the Andeans, yet their residence at high altitude is said to date back about five hundred thousand years. Since they do demonstrate a polycythemic response and their hemoglobin affinity is not high (Samaja, Veicsteinas, and Cerretelli 1979), they also seem to lack evidence of genetic adaptation. These statements assume that increased oxygen affinity is an adaptive feature of animals who are selected for high altitudes. Of course, humans may select for other physiologic mechanisms to optimize O_2 transport in a hypoxic environment.

Previous chapters have shown that hypoxemic polycythemia leads to a reduced plasma volume and to high blood viscosity. In this regard certain rodents (the golden mantle ground squirrel and the yellow-bellied marmot), although native to a region of approximately 3,800 meters, do not display marked polycythemia, but they have high red cell and plasma volumes relative to body weight (Bullard et al. 1966). Thus, the red-cell volume increase may be an initial response and an expansion of plasma volume may represent a secondary adaptation. The adverse effects of an increased hematocrit thus would be reduced at the expense of an increase in total volume. It is evident that more integral hemodynamic studies such as the one done by

Monge C. in humans are needed in animals genetically adapted to sea level and to high altitudes (Monge et al. 1955).

European animals were introduced into South America only five hundred years ago at the time when the Inca dynasty was conquered by the Spaniards. All these animals develop polycythemia when living in the mountains and are susceptible to chronic mountain sickness, as are humans (Monge M. and Monge C. 1966).

The above considerations are applicable to a biologic interpretation of chronic mountain sickness. Humans and domestic European animals use their phenotypic capacities to acclimatize to the hypoxic environment and therefore have narrow limits of tolerance to high altitudes. Their use of polycythemia with normal or reduced hemoglobin oxygen affinity as adaptive mechanisms puts the burden of acclimatization on the circulation, with increasing demands of energy used in the transport of viscous blood and probably with a diminished efficiency of capillary function. The high-altitude, genetically selected animals do not need these intravascular transport adaptations and are able to live with low tissue PO_2. Chronic mountain sickness has not been described in them.

9.2   Tissue PO_2 and Adaptation to High Altitudes

A lack of polycythemic response to hypoxia, accompanied by high hemoglobin oxygen affinity, should result in a marked drop in tissue PO_2. In fact, animals having these blood properties have a low $P\bar{v}O_2$ even at sea level. Tenney (1974), using a mathematical model, has shown that $P\bar{v}O_2$ is a good approximation of tissue PO_2. The $P\bar{v}O_2$ values at sea level and at high altitudes were compared for humans, llamas, Pekin ducks, the Himalayan bird, and the bar-headed goose (fig. 9.5). In the case of the llama, although the experimental altitude selected for the comparative study was moderate (3,400 m), its $P\bar{v}O_2$ suffers a very small drop in the hypoxic environment. The comparison between sea-level and high-altitude birds leaves no doubt that the higher the sea-level PO_2, the larger the $P\bar{v}O_2$ drop at high altitude. The $P\bar{v}O_2$ of the Himalayan bird is low at sea level, and it drops moderately at very high altitude (6,100 m). In the case of the Pekin duck, a rise in hematocrit of 60 percent greater than the sea-level value did not prevent a marked drop in the $P\bar{v}O_2$ at the same elevation. As Rahn (1966) pointed out, the oxygen conductance depends more on the shape of the oxygen equilibrium curve than on any other extracellular adaptive parameter, such as ventilation or polycythemia. When the $P\bar{v}O_2$ is low, the curve operates on its steep slope and favors oxygen release with a reduced oxygen pressure drop (see chap. 4). Chapter 7 noted how the kidney, an organ with high PvO_2, is more sensitive to hypoxia than is the systemic circulation, which has a lower $P\bar{v}O_2$.

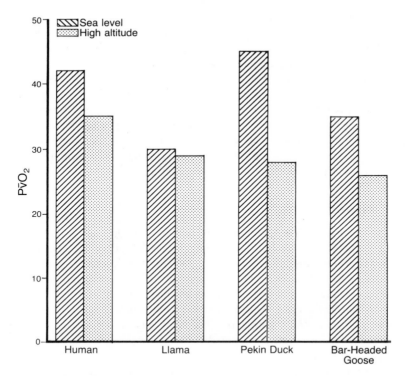

Figure 9.5.   Mixed venous PO_2 for various animals at sea level and at high altitude. The native high-altitude animals (llamas and bar-headed geese) have a lower $P\bar{v}O_2$ at sea level and a smaller $P\bar{v}O_2$ drop at high altitude than do the native sea-level animals (human and Pekin duck). Data for humans are from Hurtado (1964); for llamas, from Banchero, Grover, and Will (1971); and for Pekin ducks and bar-headed geese, from Black and Tenney (1980).

An example taken from the work of Banchero (Banchero, Grover, and Will 1971) shows this concept applied to the llama blood O_2 conductance. This value (G) can be obtained by:

$$G = \dot{V}O_2/(PaO_2 - P\bar{v}O_2) \qquad (9.2)$$

In llamas taken from sea level to an altitude of 3,420 m for ten weeks, $\dot{V}O_2$, blood flow, and hematocrit showed slight variations, yet the blood conductance increased markedly at high altitude. The relation between high-altitude (G') and sea-level (G) conductance can be obtained as (PO_2 in torr):

$$\frac{G'}{G} = \frac{PaO_2 - P\bar{v}O_2}{P'aO_2 - P'\bar{v}O_2} = \frac{90 - 30}{53 - 29} = 2.5 \qquad (9.3)$$

These animals increased their hematocrits and blood flow by only about 10 percent. Therefore, the appropriate shape and position of the oxygen equilibrium curve reduced the $P\bar{v}O_2$ drop at high altitude by only one torr, with minimal additional conductance contributions.

Barbashova (1964) differentiated the "struggle for oxygen" from true adaptation. She believed that true adaptation depended mainly on the capacity of the tissues to tolerate hypoxia and that efforts directed mainly to transporting oxygen to them were of limited adaptive value. From the authors' review, this point of view is judged to be correct; her analysis came from in vitro experiments with tissue sections, but the in vivo work reviewed here serves to confirm these in vitro observations.

9.3 Properties of Red Cells

The PO_2 is the driving force that mobilizes O_2 from the capillaries into the tissue fluids, into the cells, and into the respiring mitochondria. The hemoglobin concentration in the blood and its affinity for oxygen are parameters directly related to the blood PO_2. Because of this, other red cell properties have received less attention in studies related to high altitudes. If one keeps in mind that, at the level of the microcirculation, conditions like the red cell shape, diameter, and osmotic fragility play very important roles in the efficiency of oxygen transport, then those properties should also be assessed from a comparative point of view.

Microcytosis is of definite importance in increasing the red cell oxygenation rate. Figure 9.6 shows the correlation between the reaction velocity constant ($k'c$) and the reciprocal of the red cell radius ($1/r$) when the red cell is assumed to be spherical (Monge C. and Whittembury 1976a). The values predicted for llamas and vicuñas are indicated. Camelids, which share with sheep and goats a high oxygenation rate, thrive at high altitudes. Humans occupy the lower end of the mammal scale.

The viscosity of blood is a logarithmic function of the hematocrit (Pirofsky 1953). The nature of the curve is such that the viscosity shows a modest increase when hematocrit values are moderately high, but the viscosity reaches very high levels at higher hematocrits. The viscosity value for the alpaca falls very close to the human line at the alpaca's normal hematocrit, but the slope differs from that in humans (fig. 7.3) (Whittembury et al. 1968). Calculations of optimal hematocrit, according to Crowell and Smith (1966), give a value of 25 percent for the alpaca, which corresponds to its normal value of 27 percent. For humans, this value is 34 percent, lower than the normal figure (Monge C. and Whittembury 1982). Monge C. has considered that this may be the hematocrit of primitive humans. Like the blood pressure, it is possible that hematocrit increases with modern habits of life, such as overnutrition, sedentarism, and ambient contamination. The max-

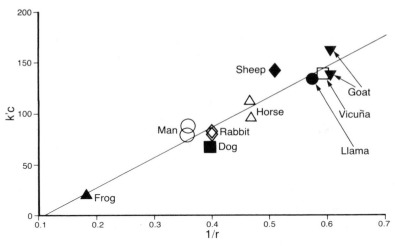

Figure 9.6.   The velocity constant of red-cell oxygenation ($k'c$) as a function of the reciprocal of the red-cell radius ($1/r$). The red cell is assumed to be spherical (Holland and Forster 1966). Values for llama and vicuña are from Banchero, Grover, and Will (1971) and Hall, Dill, and Barron (1936).

imal normal male sea-level hematocrit is about 54 percent (Wintrobe 1981), a figure already showing a significant increase in blood viscosity.

In contrast with this high figure found in humans, the South American camelids have hematocrits on the order of 27 percent, the lowest figure found in mammals. Nature has selected a lower viscosity and a higher hemoglobin concentration in the red cells of camels in general (Bartels et al. 1963). Camel red cells are also remarkably resistant to hypotonic lysis (Perk 1963; Yagil, Sod-Moriah, and Meyerstein 1974). These properties are ideal for desert life and are adequate for high-altitude adaptation in the Andes, where hypoxia and atmospheric dryness are climatologic challenges that act in combination. Therefore, one cannot attribute these red cell properties to selection for the hypoxic environment in the case of the South American camelids. Most probably the selection occurred before their introduction into the South American continental mass about 3.5 million years ago.

The Asian camels tolerate high altitudes well both in Tibet and in Afghanistan, but their anatomy and some metabolic functions seem to be better selected for sea-level deserts. These are typical examples of the so-called preadaptation in the language of evolutionary biology. What makes the difference between the South American camelids and their relatives in Asia and Africa is that in the former the hemoglobin affinity, when corrected for body weight by the appropriate equation, is significantly higher. Chiodi (1970) has given direct experimental evidence that, despite their lighter weight, the four South American camelids have hemoglobin concentrations with higher affinity than those of the sea-level camels.

Isaacks and Harkness (1983), in an extensive review of the role of erythrocyte organic phosphates and hemoglobin function in domestic animals, classify their subject matter broadly into two groups: those with an intrinsically high oxygen affinity, which is lowered in the red cell by high concentrations of 2,3-DPG (camel, llama, pig, dog, rabbit, horse, and elephant) and those with an intrinsically low oxygen affinity, which respond little if at all to 2,3-DPG and whose erythrocytes contain only small amounts of this compound (cow, goat, sheep, and cat). In the case of birds, inositol pentaphosphate apparently regulates hemoglobin affinity (Isaacks and Harkness 1980). Despite the diversity and intricacies of the biochemical mechanisms regulating hemoglobin affinity in different species, there is a clear correlation between P50 and body weight (fig. 9.1), and hypoxia-selected animals significantly deviate from the sea-level regression equation. The correlation with body weight seems also to hold in the case of birds (Lutz, Longmuir, and Schmidt-Nielsen 1974), but correlation studies with high-altitude birds, taking into consideration their body weights, have not been done.

9.4   Chronic Mountain Sickness in Animals

All the European domestic animals introduced into South America during the Spanish conquest develop polycythemia in response to the high-altitude environment (Monge M. and Monge C. 1968). Chronic mountain sickness has been observed in cattle, sheep, horses, dogs, and chickens. Brisket disease, or chronic mountain sickness of cattle, was described first in Colorado. The ventilatory response of cattle when taken to high altitudes may be inadequate, according to Grover et al. (1963), and these animals show marked elevation of their pulmonary arterial pressure. This tendency to high pulmonary artery pressure may lead to heart failure. The clinical picture has been described by Hecht et al. (1962), and a similar picture has been described in sheep by Cuba-Caparó (1950) in the Peruvian Andes. Its occurrence is more of academic than of practical importance, however, for these animals thrive at high altitudes in the Andes of Peru, and their population reaches approximately twenty million.

Chickens are very sensitive to chronic mountain sickness. The incidence is high, and the clinical picture of right heart failure is severe in some breeds (Cueva et al. 1970).

Chronic mountain sickness in nonhuman animals is mainly diagnosed by the symptoms of right heart failure. Right heart failure can be observed in humans, but it is rare. Perhaps most patients with this condition seek lower places of residence before the disease advances; alternatively, humans may have less tendency to severe pulmonary hypertension. In the case of cattle, a possible explanation for the high pulmonary pressure was offered by Grover et al. (1963), who suggested that increased pressure may serve to better perfuse the upper poles of the lungs, which are well above the heart in the animal's deep chest. The fact that chickens and pigeons, with a very different anatomy (McGrath 1971), develop pulmonary hypertension at high altitudes demands a more general explanation; hypertension is an intriguing response with adaptation benefits that are difficult to understand.

9.5   Animal Models

Although the rat has been extensively and productively used as an animal model in chronic hypoxia experiments, it reacts more intensively than do other animals to the low PO_2 of moderate altitudes (Turek, Grandtner, and Kreuzer 1972; Turek et al. 1972; Turek et al. 1973). In addition, rats do not thrive at very high altitudes in the Peruvian Andes. An interesting strain of rats described by Ou and co-workers seems to be exquisitely sensitive to high altitudes. They develop severe polycythemia and right ventricular pressure and hypertrophy, in association with increased mortality. In careful studies, the researchers have not been able to attribute these genetic differences to altered ventilatory or pulmonary vascular response to hypoxia (Ou and Smith 1984; Hill 1984).

Because of the difficulties with the rat model, the mouse was selected as a convenient animal model in the studies carried out in the Biophysical Laboratory of the Cayetano Heredia University, Lima. Preliminary reports on feral mice, native to the Peruvian mountains above 4,000 meters, indicated that polycythemia may be a genetic adaptation, since the hematocrits in these animals remained high even after several generations at sea level (Morrison and Elsner 1962; Morrison et al. 1963). These native high-altitude rodents could be cross-bred with white laboratory mice, making possible the investigation of the genetic control of red cell production (Whittembury 1983).

White laboratory mice were exposed to intermittent hypobaric hypoxia, and their litters were divided into two groups. The first group was kept at sea level as controls, and the second was exposed after twenty-one days to a simulated altitude of 4,500 meters for twenty hours a day. The hypoxic exposure of this group continued until the animals died spontaneously or were removed for experimental purposes. Their hematologic parameters were compared with body weight and brain weight (fig. 9.7). Although body weight diminished significantly in the hypoxic mice, brain weight remained unchanged. Hematocrit, total blood volume, and cerebral blood volume were higher in the hypoxic animals.

Brain hematocrit was determined in the mice by injection of Evans blue

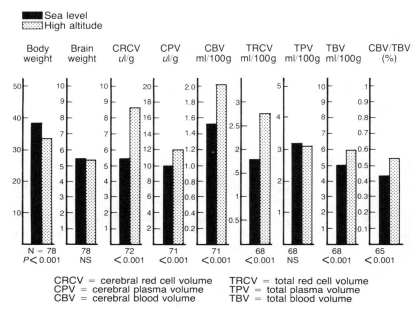

Figure 9.7. A comparison of the body-weight, brain-weight, and blood volume fractions in mice at sea level and at high altitude. (With permission, from Whittembury 1983.)

dye to determine plasma volume and by extraction of hemoglobin from the brain to determine red cell volume (Correa 1978). The results showed that the brain hematocrit was higher in the hypoxic mice than in the controls. Cerebral hematocrits and large vessel hematocrits were compared in these animals (fig. 9.8). The linear regression line with positive slope falls close to a similar one obtained in humans by Larsen and Lassen (1964). These hematologic studies show great similarities between mice and humans, despite the enormous difference in metabolic rates between the two species.

Lahiri (1971) pointed out that humans seem to be the only animals to show a blunted hypoxic ventilatory response after chronic exposure. White mice acclimatized to intermittent chronic hypoxia also show functional chemodenervation like that described in humans. These mice also showed very little difference in ventilation in response to augmented inspired O_2 and a slight increase in ventilation in response to hypercapnia (Barclay-Piazza 1982, 1983). Blood gas studies done after exposure to acute hypoxia confirmed the functional measurements (Muños 1983).

These animal studies indicate that mice, from ecologic, genetic, and physiologic points of view, make an ideal model for high-altitude studies, and that an intelligent combination of these biologic conditions can be extremely useful in future hypoxia research.

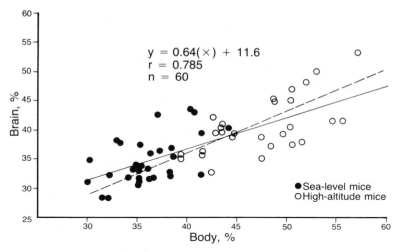

Figure 9.8. The brain hematocrit as a function of the body hematocrit in mice at sea level and at high altitude. The continuous line fits the experimental points (Correa, Monge C., and Whittembury 1979). The broken line corresponds to values calculated from in vivo determinations in humans. (Larsen and Lassen 1964.)

9.6 Comparisons of Animals with Humans

Hemoglobin synthesis in response to hypoxia appears early in evolutionary history. For example, crustaceans such as *Artemia salina* (Farley 1968) turn red when the concentration of sodium chloride in their salt-water habitat increases, diminishing, in turn, the oxygen concentration in the water (the solubility of O_2 in saline is less than it is in distilled water). For reasons that are difficult to explain, whole groups of animals, such as amphibians and reptiles, do not respond with hemoglobin synthesis to the lack of oxygen.

With the exception of those adapted to a hypoxic environment who also have a high hemoglobin affinity, mammals do respond with polycythemia and hemoglobin synthesis to the hypoxemic condition. That hypoxia is the acting selection force seems to be proved in high-altitude, fossorial, and deep-diving mammals and in high-altitude birds. In contrast with high-altitude humans, who develop polycythemia without changing hemoglobin affinity when acclimatized to high altitudes (Winslow et al. 1981), humans with mutant high-affinity hemoglobins develop polycythemia at sea level. Also of interest are hypoxia-selected mammals that have a high-affinity hemoglobin and are not polycythemic in the hypoxic environment.

A high hemoglobin-oxygen affinity without polycythemic response to the ecologic altitude level seems to be a genetic mark of high-altitude adaptation in amphibians, birds, and mammals. These characteristics do not necessarily mean that the habitat has to be hypoxic for the success of the species so adapted. In fact, the deep divers and the fossorial mammals experience intermittent, rather than continuous, hypoxia, and most so-called high-altitude animals thrive and reproduce at sea level. This characteristic is an indication of the sensitivity of the hemoglobin molecule to being selected for high affinity and diminished synthesizing response to hypoxia, as well as of how fixed this characteristic remains after generations at sea level. It seems that this selection expands the phenotypic capacity to acclimatize, without selecting exclusively for the hypoxic environment.

Chronic mountain sickness can be better understood in the context of comparative physiology when humans are compared with mammal relatives genetically selected for the hypoxic environment. Humans, whether they be sea-level or high-altitude natives, show no obvious indication of genetic selection. We seem to use limited phenotypic capacity to acclimatize, and we have diminished reserves at high altitudes. Our polycythemic response is more a maladaptation than an advantage, and although we are able to thrive, reproduce, and develop at high altitude, humans pay tribute to the hostile environment.

By integrating such broad fields as paleontology, archeology, evolution-ary biology, and comparative physiology with studies of the clinical and public health problems of the mountainous communities of the world, there will come eventually a better understanding of the capacities of humans and animals in the hypoxic environment.

CHAPTER TEN
Bloodletting

A distinction needs to be made between normal and excessive high-altitude polycythemia. A mild elevation of hematocrit seems to be the normal response to the altitude of Cerro de Pasco (see fig. 3.6), but a subset of the population develops hematocrits that are significantly higher than this and often shows symptoms of chronic mountain sickness. It is well known in Andean villages that descent to sea level or phlebotomy relieves these symptoms. In addition, it is common practice to remove blood from high-altitude surgical candidates to reduce the risk of excessive bleeding (Monge M. and Monge C. 1966). These subjective observations indicate that excessive polycythemia is detrimental to oxygen transport to tissues. Previous chapters have also indicated that an additional mechanical burden is placed on the circulatory system such that heart failure can occur.

Although mild polycythemia may be a *normal* response to hypoxia, does it necessarily follow that it is *good?* As chapter 1 showed, the connection between normality and advantage probably began with the work of Paul Bert; it was fostered by governments eager to attract workers and soldiers to the high mountains. It is now known that polycythemia, when excessive, may have a number of detrimental consequences. Therefore, perhaps the advantages of normal high-altitude polycythemia also should be considered.

Two questions need to be examined. The first is: Is *excessive* polycythemia more detrimental than it is beneficial? Clinical observations suggest that the problems caused by a tremendous increase in red cell mass are not outweighed by the advantages of increased O_2 carrying capacity. The second is more difficult: Is *normal* high-altitude polycythemia beneficial to oxygen transport? Here there is less to go on. Because it is a normal response, mild polycythemia can be considered beneficial. To be objective, however, one must not use an extension of the argument that it is better to have a normal hematocrit than it is to be anemic. One way to approach these questions is to observe the physiologic responses to hematocrit reduction in high-altitude natives. This chapter examines the available data from phlebotomy and hemodilution studies.

10.1 The Effect of Polycythemia on Gas Exchange

The idea that polycythemia itself could aggravate hypoxia is not new. Newman and co-workers reviewed the existing literature on this point (see table 10.1) and suggested that in polycythema vera, vital capacity and total lung volume are reduced and that residual air is decreased, presumably because

Table 10.1. Pulmonary functions in polycythemia vera

	N	Observation	Source
Vital capacity	1	Decreased to 45% predicted	(1)
	1	Decreased, improved with phenylhydrazine[a]	(2)
	3	Normal in 2, decreased in 1; no change after phlebotomy	(3)
	3	Reduced in all 3; increased in one after phlebotomy	(4)
Residual air	7	Increased	(5)
	1	Increased; reduced after phlebotomy	(2)
Total lung capacity	7	Normal	(5)
	1	Decreased in 1 case; improved after phlebotomy	(2)
SaO$_2$ at rest	—	Decreased	(5)
	17	9 cases significantly low	(6)
SaO$_2$, exercise	3	Decreased in all 3	(5)

Sources: (1) Isaaks 1923; (2) Brooks 1936; (3) Altschule, Volk, Henstell 1940; (4) Stewart 1941; (5) Harrop 1927; and (6) Wasserman 1949.
[a]Phenylhydrazine reduces hematocrit by inducing hemolysis.

of the increased volume of blood in the chest (Newman, Feltman, and Devlin 1951). They noted that in most cases these effects could be reversed by phlebotomy.

Newman added studies in five additional cases of polycythemia vera in which a mean hematocrit reduction of 67.6 percent to 46 percent was achieved by repeated venesection. All five of these subjects increased their maximal breathing capacity, and it was suggested this was due to decreased resistance, less anoxia, and decreased blood volume. In two of the cases, $\dot{V}_E$ did not change during exercise despite decreasing pH, increasing PCO$_2$, and decreasing PaO$_2$. It was suggested that these subjects had respiratory center damage that was only partially reversed by phlebotomy. The argument was made that polycythemia leads to a ventilation/perfusion mismatch[1] that can be reversed by phlebotomy.

These studies in polycythemia vera suggested to Newman that the increased volume of blood in the chest decreases elasticity of the lung, decreases the volume of the chest available for gas exchange, and decreases the vital capacity and alveolar ventilation. The increased viscosity of the blood also leads to underperfusion of some lung regions. Furthermore, when these changes are of long duration, respiratory center depression can occur. All of these changes can lead to compromised oxygenation of the blood and, when superimposed upon high-altitude hypoxia, could have even more severe effects.

10.2　Bloodletting in High-Altitude Natives

Studies in high-altitude natives have been less extensive. Remarkably few data in the scientific literature document the known physiologic benefits of bloodletting in high-altitude natives with chronic mountain sickness. Monge C., Lozano, and Whittembury (1965) reported studies on three subjects in Cerro de Pasco (4,300 m) from whom small amounts of blood were removed (600 ml, 750 ml, and 1,350 ml). They found no changes in symptoms, slight reductions in $PaCO_2$, increases in plasma pH, and no regular pattern of change in SaO_2. They concluded that the studies were not representative because clinical improvement was generally well known, and they suggested that larger amounts of blood should have been taken.

In the discussion of a paper presented at the 1971 Ciba Foundation symposium, Peñaloza described studies in six subjects with a mean hematocrit of 72 percent, SaO_2 of 63.8 percent, and a mean pulmonary artery pressure of 39 millimeters Hg.[2] Five days after the hematocrit was reduced to 66 percent by phlebotomy, the SaO_2 had increased to 73.4 percent, mean pulmonary artery pressure had decreased to 30 millimeters Hg, and there was no change in the cardiac output (Peñaloza, Sime, and Ruiz 1971). These results are consistent with the polycythemia vera data suggesting that decreased viscosity after phlebotomy led to improved lung perfusion in spite of the drop in pulmonary artery pressure.

Cruz et al. (1979) reported phlebotomy studies in four subjects with chronic mountain sickness at La Oroya (3,700 m). One had atrial fibrillation; another had right bundle branch block and signs of heart failure. Before phlebotomy, two of the patients had abnormal spirometry and gas exchange. These studies demonstrated a small but significant improvement in static pulmonary function in all four after phlebotomy. In addition, they found increased PaO_2, decreased $PaCO_2$, and a reduced $(A - a)O_2$ gradient. They could not attribute improved gas exchange to changes in alveolar ventilation, but they postulated a more even $\dot{V}_A/\dot{Q}_c$ ratio because physiological dead space decreased. The literature on phlebotomy in other polycythemic patients was reviewed, with the conclusion that when gas exchange is already impaired, as, for example, in chronic lung disease, polycythemia worsened hypoxia and that the most improvement could be expected after phlebotomy in the subjects who are most hypoxic.

10.3　Studies of Bloodletting in Cerro de Pasco

The authors' own phlebotomy studies at Cerro de Pasco were undertaken to extend the data on high-altitude natives by performing even more drastic hematocrit reductions. Exercise testing was used to evaluate the results of reduction of hematocrits either by simple phlebotomy or by hemodilution.[3]

The physiological changes that follow these procedures were expected to be complex, but overall exercise performance should be an indicator of the efficiency of O_2 transport, regardless of the specific alteration in the pathway of O_2 utilization.

In all, 103 potential candidates for the studies were interviewed, examined, and given trial runs on the cycle ergometer. Some were unable to operate the ergometer and were therefore rejected. Eight of these candidates were selected for phlebotomy or hemodilution; six high-altitude natives who had "normal" polycythemia served as exercise test controls; and three members of the expedition team served as acclimatized lowlander controls. These subjects are described in table 10.2. The criteria for selection were a hematocrit significantly above the mean for the population (see fig. 3.6), ability to cooperate in the exercise tests, and reliability in returning to the laboratory for the necessary follow-up studies. Three of the subjects underwent repeated phlebotomy, and five underwent hemodilution with a Haemonetics cell separator. These two groups were well matched in regard to age, height, weight, hematocrit, hemoglobin concentration, and spirometry.

The exercise test protocol was adapted from the methods of Wasserman and Whipp (1975), in which the work level is increased each minute until the subject reaches exhaustion. The maximal level was taken as the last one at which a full minute of work was performed.[4] The subject always pedaled at a rate of 60 rpm.

Large amounts of blood were removed from subject 3979, a phlebotomy subject, over a period of eight days (fig. 10.1). Nevertheless, the hematocrit

Table 10.2.   Effects of familiarity on exercise test results

Subject	Hct (%)		Max Work (kpm/min)		Max HR (/min)		Max $\dot{V}_E$ (l/min BTPS)	
Test	1	2	1	2	1	2	1	2
1979	53.0	53.0	1,000	1,000	134	137	73.3	66.6
2279	68.0	66.5	600	800	114	139	69.1	70.4
3779	54.9	54.9	900	800	158	156	90.5	64.4
3979	66.4	67.1	600	700	145	143	48.5	66.7
4279	53.0	53.0	1,000	1,350	145	155	99.3	84.3
5079	49.5	49.5	1,000	1,050	157	169	180.8	144.1
5779	57.0	57.0	700	700	144	150	60.5	60.5
680	47.9	47.9	900	900	179	172	—	—
N	8.0	8.0	8	8	8	8	7.0	7.0
Mean	56.2	56.1	837	912	147	153	88.9	79.6
SD	±7.4	±7.2	±177	±218	±19	±13	±44.0	±29.4
Change	−0.1		+75		+6		−9.3	
p	ns		ns		ns		ns	

Source: Winslow and Monge C., unpublished data.

and the bulk viscosity[5] continued to change over the entire seventeen-day period of study. The striking improvement in symptoms seemed to be concurrent with the abrupt decrease in viscosity.

Red cell 2,3-DPG decreased over the period of study; this result was not

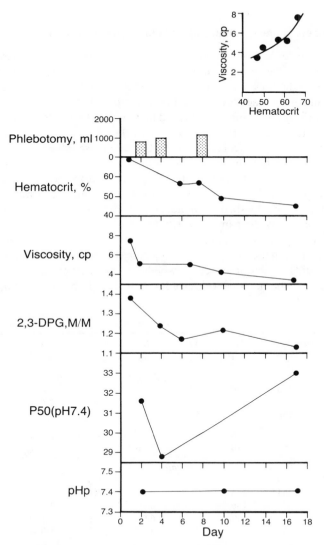

Figure 10.1.   The time course of the change in hematologic parameters during phlebotomy in a polycythemic subject. The amounts of blood removed are shown in the top panel. Viscosity and 2,3-DPG closely follow the hematocrit changes. (Winslow and Monge, unpublished data.)

expected—one usually expects 2,3-DPG to increase in anemia or in situations of oxygen lack (see chap. 4). This matter, which was a consistent finding among the phlebotomy subjects, remains unexplained. In the hemodilution subjects, little change in 2,3-DPG was observed, possibly because the period of observation was too short.

10.4   Exercise Performance after Hematocrit Reduction

In all the Cerro de Pasco studies, the authors attempted to familiarize the subjects with the experimental procedures by repeated exercise runs before hematocrit reduction. This was not possible in all cases because of the short time permitted for the studies and because most of the subjects were employed by the mining company and had limited time to devote to the project.

Control tests were performed to estimate the effect on exercise of familiarization with the protocol (table 10.3). Some of these subjects later participated in the phlebotomy or hemodilution studies. In three of them the maximal work level increased slightly; it dropped in one, but the mean increased by only 76 kpm/minute. The mean maximal heart rate in these tests increased only by six per minute. None of these changes was significant when evaluated by the paired t-test.

Table 10.4 gives the overall exercise performance before and after hematocrit reduction in the experimental subjects. The most striking result is that in no case did hematocrit reduction, whether by phlebotomy or by hemodilution, decrease the maximal exercise level. Although the changes in hema-

Table 10.3.   Exercise results in subjects chosen for phlebotomy or hemodilution

Subject	Age (yr)	Ht (cm)	Wt (kg)	Hct (%)	Hb (g/dl)	VC (l BTPS)	FE$_1$ (% VC)
Phlebotomy Subjects							
2279	55	160	70	68.0	24.5	4.423	72
3979	46	178	64	66.4	20.7	2.601	52
4579	58	160	60	75.0	27.5	3.279	87
Mean	53	166	65	69.8	24.2	3.434	70
SD	±6	±10	±5	±4.6	±3.4	±.921	±18
Hemodilution Subjects							
3280	59	151	61.5	66.0	21.8	3.587	73
3680	54	148	50.0	62.0	22.4	3.615	78
3780	73	156	59.0	69.0	24.6	2.966	97
3880	57	149	69.0	69.9	22.8	3.530	81
3980	41	164	61.0	66.5	22.7	5.074	79
Mean	57	154	60.1	66.7	22.9	3.754	82
SD	±11	±7	±6.8	±3.1	±1.0	±.784	±9

Source: Winslow and Monge C., unpublished data.

Table 10.4. The ventilatory response to exercise

	Hematocrit (%)			Age (yr)			AT (ml/min/kg)			$\dot{V}_E$ at AT (l/min)		
	N	Mean	SD	N	Mean	SD	N	Mean	SD	N	Mean	SD
Type A[a]	19	56.7	± 8.7	18	39.0	± 17	18	18.1	± 6.2	20	37.0	± 11.5
Type B	6	51.5	± 9.3	5	42.4	± 15.5						
Prebleed	5	60.0	± 3.4	5	56.8	± 11.5	4	17.4	± 5.4	4	30.1	± 9.5
Postbleed	5	47.7	± 3.9	5	56.8	± 11.5	3	18.1	± 2.0	2	31.8	± 3.1
Controls	3	44.5	± 5.9	3	41.5	± 16.9	3	23.6	± 5.6	3	59.8	± 12.0

	$\dot{V}CO_2$max (l/min)			$\dot{V}_E$max (l/min)			Init Slope (l/min/kg)			$\dot{V}E/\dot{V}CO_2$		
	N	Mean	SD	N	Mean	SD	N	Mean	SD	N	Mean	SD
Type A[a]	18	29.7	± 10.8	19	60.6	± 23.7	18	1.721	± 0.351	18	2.004	± 0.304
Type B	5	24.8	± 7.5	5	51.6	± 11.5	5	2.200	± 0.523	5	2.137	± 0.424
Prebleed	5	25.5	± 6.7	5	51.3	± 11.6	5	1.847	± 0.421	5	2.046	± 0.451
Postbleed	5	23.9	± 6.1	5	46.8	± 9.2	5	2.015	± 0.688	5	2.006	± 0.425
Controls	3	43.7	± 9.6	3	129.4	± 34.4	3	2.394	± 0.094	3	2.942	± 0.154

Source: Winslow and Monge C., unpublished data.
[a] In Type A (but not Type B) tests, a definite "breakpoint" could be identified.

tocrit was approximately the same in the two groups (-17.6 percent for phlebotomy vs. -20.8 percent for hemodilution), the former demonstrated a more definite increase in overall maximal work level ($+167$ kpm/min vs. $+50$ kpm/min). Although the increased maximal work level in certain individuals was striking, the statistical significance for the two groups together could not be established.

In persons whose maximal work level increased, the degree of increase did not correlate with original hematocrit, the degree of reduction, or the initial maximal work level. The most dramatic increase was in subjects 4579 and 3780, who had the most severe symptoms of chronic mountain sickness. Subject 4579 reported that after hematocrit reduction he slept well and could concentrate on his work for the first time in many years. In both, the maximal work level doubled.

The maximal heart rate increased after hematocrit reduction. Despite the difference in maximal work level, the phlebotomy and hemodilution groups were very similar in their mean changes in maximal heart rate ($+28$/min, phlebotomy; $+22$, hemodilution; $+6$, controls). In these studies, maximal heart rate refers to the heart rate at the maximal work level. The actual change in individuals was not predictable from initial hematocrit, maximal work level, or any other measured value. The largest change ($+35$/min) occurred in two of the hemodiluted subjects (3880 and 3980), but one of the phlebotomy subjects (3979) increased his maximal heart rate by twenty-four per minute. The increased maximal heart rate for the entire group was significant ($p = .001$).

Maximal $\dot{V}CO_2$ (the $\dot{V}CO_2$ at maximal work level) was calculated only in the hemodiluted subjects, because detailed analysis of expired gas was not done in the phlebotomy studies. A very small mean increase was noted, but because the maximal work level also increased slightly in this group, the overall work efficiency did not appear to change. The increased $\dot{V}CO_2$ was not statistically significant.

10.4.1   The Ventilatory Response to Exercise

The ventilatory response to exercise was estimated by breath-by-breath analysis of expired gas during incremental exercise tests. Examples of tests in a sea-level control and a high-altitude native are shown in figure 8.1. The high-altitude native was a twenty-seven-year-old man (subject 2680) in good health who played soccer regularly. His hematocrit was 52.4 percent, close to the average for Cerro de Pasco. The sea level subject was a thirty-nine-year-old member of the research team who was also in good health, moderately athletic, and had a hematocrit of 43.5 percent. The exercise test on this subject was carried out in the Cerro de Pasco laboratory after three weeks of acclimatization. These data were subjected to a linear regression analysis that selected the best two lines to pass through the points. The ventilatory thresholds[6] are indicated, and they suggest that the anaerobic threshold (Wasserman 1984) may have occurred at a slightly lower $\dot{V}CO_2$ in the high-altitude native (1.384 ± .086, SE) as compared to the acclimatized lowlander (1.634 ± .146, SE). In addition to the ventilatory threshold, this analysis provides other useful data to characterize the exercise test results; $\dot{V}_E$ at the ventilatory threshold, maximal ventilation (the $\dot{V}_E$ at the maximal work level), and the initial slope of the $\dot{V}_E/\dot{V}CO_2$ line.

The results of the twenty-six exercise tests in which breath-by-breath gas analysis was carried out are summarized in table 10.5. In six of the tests, no ventilatory threshold could be identified. These are designated "type B" tests, in contrast to "type A" tests, in which a threshold was clearly present. The type B subset was not different from the group as a whole in regard to hematocrit or age. These subjects did not achieve as high a maximal $\dot{V}CO_2$ as those who showed a definite threshold, but because of the wide variation in individual responses to exercise, and the disparity in the numbers of individuals in the two groups, statistical significance in regard to maximal $\dot{V}CO_2$ could not be established. All high-altitude subjects ventilated significantly less than did the sea-level controls ($p = .001$) at the ventilatory threshold.

Both type A and type B subjects demonstrated significantly lower maximal $\dot{V}CO_2$ as compared to the three sea-level controls ($p = .001$). No distinction could be made, however, among type A, type B, and the poly-

Table 10.5. The effect of hematocrit reduction on exercise performance

Subject	Hct (%)		Max Work (kpm/min)		Max HR (/min)		Max $\dot{V}CO_2$ (ml/min/kg)		Max $\dot{V}_E$ (l/min BTPS)	
Test	1	2	1	2	1	2	1	2	1	2
2279	68.5	53.0	600	800	114	146	—	—	70.4	63.2
3979	66.4	45.5	600	900	145	167	—	—	64.1	68.1
4579	75.0	58.0	300	600	117	147	—	—	33.6	51.7
3280	66.0	52.8	400	600	167	182	27.6	21.5	62.0	46.3
3680	62.0	42.2	600	600	169	184	36.2	34.1	56.4	57.4
3780	70.5	49.5	300	600	128	134	19.2	19.3	37.7	33.6
3880	66.5	47.0	500	500	133	168	22.0	19.8	59.8	53.3
3980	66.5	47.0	500	500	133	168	22.6	24.7	39.6	43.5
N	8.0	8.0	8	8	8	8	5.0	5.0	8.0	8.0
Mean	67.0	49.4	475	638	138	162	25.5	23.9	53.0	52.1
SD	±3.8	±5.0	±128	±141	±21	±18	±6.7	±6.1	±13.9	±11.1
Change	−18.3		+163		+24		−1.6		−0.9	
p	.0001		ns		.001		ns		ns	

Source: Winslow and Monge C., unpublished data.
Note: Hematocrits were reduced by phlebotomy in subjects whose numbers end in 79, and by hemodilution in those whose numbers end in 80.

cythemic subset chosen for hematocrit reduction. Moreover, the maximal ventilation or the $\dot{V}_E/\dot{V}CO_2$ at the maximal exercise level was not different among these three groups.

Respiratory chemosensitivity, as measured by the initial $\dot{V}_E/\dot{V}CO_2$ slope, was the same in type A, type B, and polycythemic groups. All three, however, had significantly lower slopes than did the sea-level controls (p = .001). Finally, even though the reduction in the hematocrit in the subjects shown in table 10.4 was marked (60.0 percent to 47.7 percent), no statistically significant differences were observed in ventilatory threshold, $\dot{V}_E$ at the ventilatory threshold, maximal $\dot{V}CO_2$, or the initial $\dot{V}_E/\dot{V}CO_2$ slope. These results suggest that blunted chemosensitivity of the respiratory center is not reversed by hematocrit reduction, at least over the short time period of the studies.

10.4.2   Analysis of Arterial Blood during Exercise

Arterial blood was sampled in three subjects at each exercise level before and after hematocrit reduction (fig. 10.2). In two of these subjects (2279 and 3979) reduction was by phlebotomy, and in the third (3980) it was by hemodilution. All the subjects demonstrated reduced $PaCO_2$, suggesting increased alveolar ventilation, since as $\dot{V}CO_2$ did not change appreciably in any of them (see table 10.5). In two of the subjects, PaO_2 increased correspondingly. The third subject may have had an additional block to pulmonary O_2 uptake that could not be overcome by increased alveolar ventilation. The changes in arterial pH were irregular: in subject 2279 pH was higher at all exercise levels after hematocrit reduction, whereas in the other two it was lower. In all tests, regardless of the hematocrit, pH decreased as work rate increased.

The work level at which lactic acid began to accumulate (the anaerobic threshold) was nearly unaffected by the hematocrit reduction. This is in agreement with the ventilatory threshold estimates from $\dot{V}_E/\dot{V}CO_2$ analysis (see table 10.4). However, the maximal concentration of lactic acid was higher in all three subjects after hematocrit reduction.

10.5   Invasive Gas Transport Measurements

A complete set of O_2 transport data was obtained in a single individual (subject 3680) whose hematocrit was close to that considered "normal" for Cerro de Pasco (Winslow, Monge, Brown, et al. 1985,). This study was possible because of the availability of specially constructed catheters (Brown et al. 1985), instrumentation to carry out the hemodilution procedures in the Cerro de Pasco laboratory (Klein 1983), and on-line computer analysis of exercise test data (Winslow and Mckneally 1986).

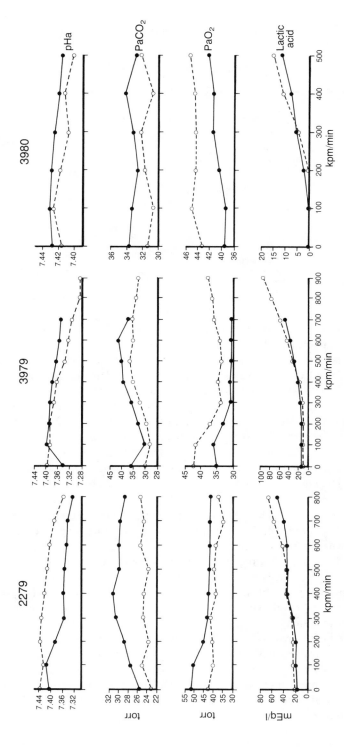

Figure 10.2. An analysis of arterial blood during exercise in three subjects in Cerro de Pasco. Tests done before hematocrit reduction are represented by closed symbols and solid lines; those after reduction, by open symbols and dashed lines. Reduced $PaCO_2$ in all three and increased PaO_2 in two suggest a higher alveolar ventilation after the hemodilution. (Winslow and Monge, unpublished data.).

Table 10.6.   Changes with hemodilution
in subject 3680

	Before	After
Hct (%)	62	42
2,3-DPG (mol/mol)	.80	.87
Hb (g/dl)	22.4	16.0
Red cell mass (ml/kg)	48	
Vital capacity (lBTPS)	3.615	3.630
Percent predicted	113	114
FEV_1 (% VC)	78	84
Resting heart rate (/min)	82	92
R (mV)	0.41	0.59[a]
S (mV)	−0.27	−0.21[a]
QRS (s)	0.07	0.05[a]
Q − T/R − R (s)	0.37	0.34[a]

Source: Winslow et al. 1985a.
[a]$p < .05$.

The subject was of Quechua ancestry, was born in Cerro de Pasco, and had lived there all his life (table 10.6). He had never visited sea level, and his symptoms were typical of those suffering from chronic mountain sickness: fatigue, headache, sleeplessness, and confusion. His hematocrit, 62 percent, was within one standard deviation of the mean observed by the authors in Cerro de Pasco (see fig. 3.6). His red cell volume, 48 milliliters/kilogram, was clearly elevated above sea-level normal, and it agreed well with measurements reported by Sánchez (Sánchez, Merino, and Figallo 1970) in subjects at similar altitudes with similar hematocrits (see chap. 3).

His vital capacity was elevated by about 10 percent over predicted values for sea-level residents. He had no symptoms of lung disease and did not use tobacco. His one-second forced expiratory volume (FEV_1) was within the normal range, and a chest X ray taken at the Cerro de Pasco Mining Center Hospital was normal. Thus, there is no evidence that lung disease could account for his polycythemia.

The hemodilution procedure required about two hours, resulting in a reduction of venous hematocrit from 62 percent to 42 percent (table 10.5). The subject's symptoms improved immediately and continued to do so over the several days following the procedure. His weight did not change.

After pulmonary and radial artery catheters were inserted, exercise testing with breath-by-breath monitoring of gas exchange was performed. Hemodilution was carried out, and four days later the catheters were reinserted and the tests were repeated. The catheters were equipped with fiber optics for measurement of O_2 saturation, and the arterial catheter also contained a PO_2 electrode (Brown et al. 1985). Thus, $(a - \bar{v})O_2$ difference could be monitored continuously, and cardiac output could be measured both by the thermodilution and the O_2 Fick techniques.[7] The data obtained allow a complete characterization of the physiologic changes that follow acute reduction in hematocrit in this subject.

10.5.1   Electrocardiographic Changes

Mean QRS complexes were calculated at several levels of work during an incremental exercise test, before and after hemodilution (fig. 10.3). The figures represent averages of at least ten successive individual complexes. Measured amplitudes and durations from the resting ECG also were taken before and after the hemodilution (table 10.6). Significant changes included increased heart rate, R wave amplitude, decreased S wave amplitude, and decreased QRS and QT intervals. Results similar to these have been associated with improved cardiac filling (Brody 1956), and suggest increased venous return to the heart.

10.5.2   Pulmonary Hemodynamics

Pulmonary artery pressure was measured during hemodilution (fig. 10.4) with the subject supine. Cardiac output, measured by the thermodilution technique, changed from 6.06 ± 0.03 liters/minute to 6.66 ± 0.46 liters/minute after the two hours required for the procedure, but it increased to 6.99 ± 0.46 liters/minute two days after hemodilution. The pulmonary arterial ejection slope, dP/dt, followed a similar pattern: there was very little change during the hemodilution itself, but it was markedly reduced two days later.

In contrast, pulmonary artery pressure decreased immediately and dramatically. Before the procedure, the pressure was 40/30 millimeters Hg, and after it, 23/15 millimeters Hg, a value in the range of sea-level normal (Altman and Dittmer 1971).[8] Measurements made at the second exercise test show that the pulmonary artery pressure remained low.

10.5.3   Alveolar Gas Exchange

Measurement of true alveolar gas exchange is difficult because of breath-to-breath variation in O_2 uptake and CO_2 production. This is particularly true in subjects who are untrained. Auchincloss (Auchincloss, Gilbert, and Baule 1966) suggested that this is caused by a variable residual gas volume in the lung after expiration, and several authors have used approximate numerical procedures to estimate the true alveolar gas exchange (Swanson 1980; Giezendanner, Cerretelli, and DiPrampero 1983; Beaver, Lamarra, and Wasserman 1981). These require that the initial functional residual capacity (FRC at rest) is known or can be estimated.

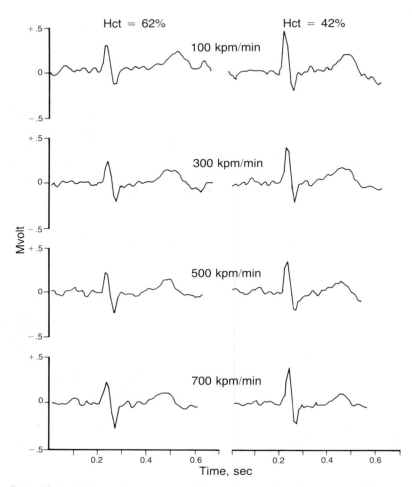

Figure 10.3. QRS complexes recorded during exercise cycling. Each curve represents the average of ten successive QRS complexes. At all work levels, the QRS amplitude is higher following hematocrit reduction. (Winslow and Monge, unpublished data.)

The Cerro de Pasco studies used a curve-fitting technique to estimate the FRC during two minutes of unloaded pedaling before and after hemodilution. The estimated FRC for O_2 decreased from 2.6 liters to 1.6 liters (BTPS) and for CO_2, from 2.8 liters to 1.8 liters (BTPS). Note that this is in opposition to the results of Newman in polycythemia vera patients. These studies need to be extended to include conventional measurements of FRC by inert gas techniques. They raise the interesting possibility that the large quantity of blood in the chest could serve as a substantial reservoir of O_2 and

CO_2 that could damp the dynamics of gas exchange, particularly during exercise.

10.5.4   Exercise Tests

Figure 10.5 shows the results of incremental exercise tests carried out before and two days after the hemodilution. The hematocrit at the time of the

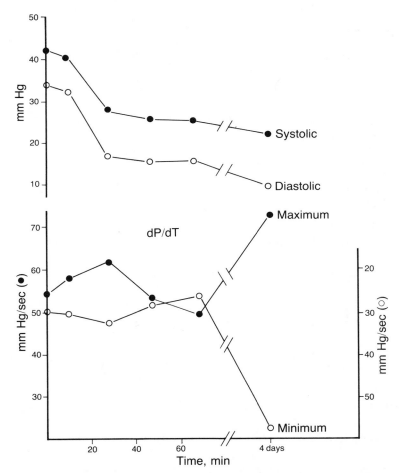

Figure 10.4.   The effect of hemodilution on pulmonary circulation. Pulmonary artery pressure and maximum (systolic) and minimum (diastolic) slopes are shown during the procedure and again four days later. Note that changes in cardiac output and pulmonary artery pressure are immediate, whereas the increase in ejection slope (*dP/Dt*) is gradual. (Winslow, Monge, Brown, et al. 1985.)

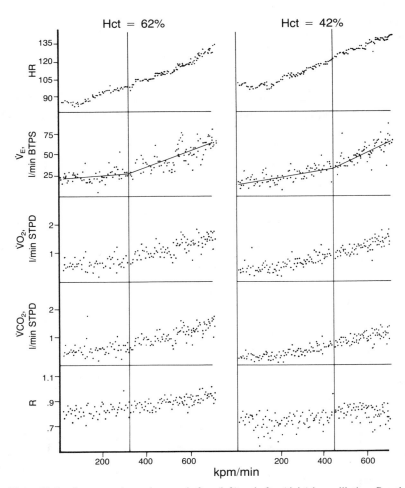

Figure 10.5. Incremental exercise tests before (left) and after (right) hemodilution. Breath-by-breath analysis of $\dot{V}_E$, $\dot{V}O_2$, and $\dot{V}CO_2$ are shown. The heart rate (top panel) is given for each breath. The vertical line was drawn at the best estimate for the anaerobic threshold. R is the gas exchange ratio. (Winslow, Monge, Brown, et al. 1985.)

second test was 42 percent. There was a clear increase in the heart rate throughout the test, with the maximum reaching 142 per minute. The age-adjusted maximal heart rate predicted from sea-level normal values for this subject is 175 per minute (Altman and Dittmer 1971). Thus, he more nearly achieved his maximal rate after the hemodilution. Nevertheless, the maximal work level attained was the same for the two tests.

The ventilatory threshold analysis (fig. 10.6) suggests that the threshold is increased after hemodilution from 316 kpm to 438 kpm/minute, corre-

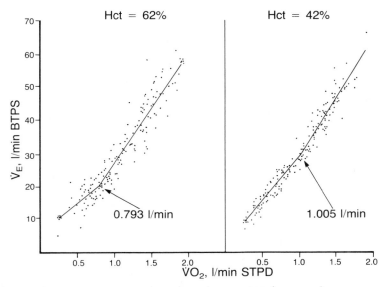

Figure 10.6. The ventilatory threshold, determined by plotting $\dot{V}_E$ against $\dot{V}O_2$. This subject shows a shift of the ventilatory threshold to higher work. (Winslow and Monge, unpublished data.)

sponding to $\dot{V}CO_2$ of 0.793 liter/minute and 1.005 liter/minute, respectively.

After an assessment of overall exercise capacity in the incremental test, steady-state tests were performed with the catheters in place (figs. 10.7 and 10.8). The design was to establish the steady state at no load, then to increase the work abruptly to a level less than the ventilatory threshold. In the first test the subject developed several premature ventricular contractions after the increase, and the test was terminated before a steady state was reached at the higher level.

Nevertheless, the results do provide useful information. First, the $\dot{V}O_2$ and $\dot{V}CO_2$ changed very little in the first test after the work increase; they changed a little more in the second. This indicates an O_2 debt that does not seem to be repaid during the higher exercise. The mixed venous PO_2 and SO_2 dropped dramatically in both tests. Heart rate is much higher in the second test, in agreement with the observations in the incremental test. The $\dot{V}_E$ increased somewhat, providing an increased PAO_2 and PaO_2.

Table 10.7 presents a summary of the blood gas measurements and table 10.8 gives the gas exchange data in the two steady-state exercise tests. The data are from the last fifteen seconds at the specified work levels. Arterial and mixed venous O_2 saturations are taken from the catheter studies. The PaO_2 values were as measured with blood gas samples withdrawn at the

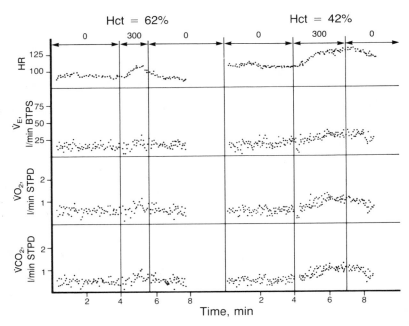

Figure 10.7. Steady-state exercise tests before (left) and after (right) hemodilution. Breath-by-breath analysis of $\dot{V}_E$, $\dot{V}O_2$, and $\dot{V}CO_2$ are shown. Heart rate is given for each breath. The subject was able to sustain a longer period of work at 300 kpm after hemodilution. (Winslow, Monge, Brown, et al. 1985.)

Table 10.7.   Blood-gas measurements during constant work-rate exercise in subject 3680

	Prehemodilution Rate (kpm/min)		Posthemodilution Rate (kpm/min)	
	0	300	0	300
PaO_2 (torr)	42.3	39.8	46.2	39.7
SaO_2 (%)	80.0	71.0	85.0	70.2
$P\bar{v}O_2$ (torr)	19.2	11.0	25.9	15.1
$S\bar{v}O_2$ (%)	30.0	11.4	43.0	17.1
$P(A - a)O_2$ (torr)	4.5	6.8	4.4	12.3
$C(a - \bar{v})O_2$ (ml/dl)	15.0	17.9	9.0	11.3
$PaCO_2$ (torr)	30.8	31.6	31.0	31.4
pHa	7.451	7.435	7.427	7.413
BE (mEq/L)	−1.7	−2.7	−3.3	−4.9

Source: Winslow et al. 1985a.
Note: Hematocrit readings were 62% before and 42% after hemodilution.

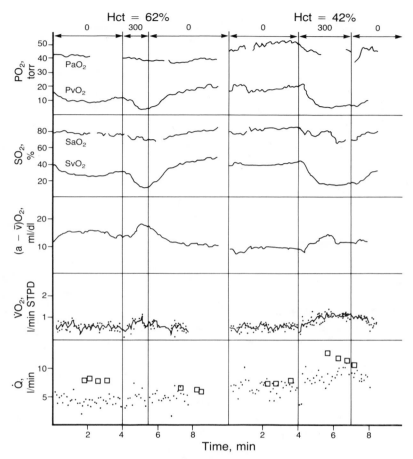

Figure 10.8. Parameters of oxygen transport during exercise. Arterial and venous PO_2 and SO_2 before (left) and after (right) hemodilution were used to calculate the $(a - \bar{v})O_2$ difference. The breath-by-breath O_2 uptake allows calculation of the Fick cardiac output for each breath. The results are compared with thermodilution measurements in the bottom panel. (Winslow, Monge, Brown, et al. 1985.)

appropriate times; they correspond to those measured continuously with the arterial catheter.

The effect of hemodilution on exercise breathing patterns was primarily to increase breathing frequency, while tidal volume remained almost unchanged. The minute ventilation increased at both zero and 300 kpm/minute. This pattern of change resulted in an increased VD/VT ratio[9] at 0 kpm/minute, which decreased at the highest work rate.

Both $\dot{V}CO_2$ and $\dot{V}O_2$ increased slightly, as did their ratio, R. These measurements increase $\dot{V}_A$, since $\dot{V}_A$ is proportional to $(\dot{V}CO_2/PaCO_2)$.[10]

Table 10.8. Pulmonary gas exchange during constant work-rate exercise in subject 3680

	Prehemodilution Rate (kpm/min)		Posthemodilution Rate (kpm/min)	
	0	300	0	300
FB (min^{-1})	16.7	18.2	26.5	25.2
TV (l) BTPS	.847	1.167	.852	1.297
$\dot{V}_E$ (l/minBTPS)	14.6	21.1	22.2	32.31
VD/VT	.185	.095	.490	.132
$\dot{V}_A$ (l/minBTPS)	11.7	18.8	14.8	22.9
PECO$_2$ (torr)	25.1	28.6	20.4	26.4
PAO$_2$ (torr)	46.8	46.6	50.6	52.0
$\dot{V}CO_2$ (l/minSTPD)	.418	.689	.553	.983
$\dot{V}O_2$ (l/minSTPD)	.524	.847	.613	1.081
R	.798	.814	.862	.909
$\dot{V}A/\dot{Q}$ (Fick)	2.83	4.05	2.72	2.90
$\dot{V}A/\dot{Q}$ (thermodilution)	1.56	—	2.00	2.45

Source: Winslow et al. 1985a.

This increase is particularly impressive at 300 kpm/minute. Concomitant with this result is an increase in PAO$_2$.

The pulmonary alveolar ventilation to blood-flow ratio ($\dot{V}_A/\dot{Q}_c$) is better matched after the hemodilution. Because the ratio is proportional to the ($a - \bar{v}$)O$_2$/PaCO$_2$ ratio, its calculated reduction is due primarily to decreased ($a - \bar{v}$)O$_2$ content.

Resting PaO$_2$ and SaO$_2$ increased after hemodilution as a result of increased PAO$_2$. The alveolar-to-arterial O$_2$ gradient ($A - a$)O$_2$ changed insignificantly after the 0–300 kpm/minute transition in the first test, but after hemodilution the increase was striking (from 4.4 to 12.3 torr). Thus, in the second test, O$_2$ transfer from the alveolus to capillary blood may have been limited by the diffusion gradient, while in the first test some other barrier (e.g., blood flow) was limiting.

A very important result is that both P$\bar{v}$O$_2$ and S$\bar{v}$O$_2$ increased at both exercise levels after hemodilution, despite reduced O$_2$ content. This obviously reflects favorable tissue O$_2$ supply and could occur only if blood flow in tissue capillary beds improved.

The pH values at a constant work rate diminished somewhat during both exercise levels after hemodilution. The base excess values were slightly lower, however, during the second test. Unchanged PaCO$_2$ and lower base excess probably reflect a difference in blood buffering after hemodilution. The significance of these changes remains to be explored.

10.5.5 Cardiac Output

Cardiac output was estimated from the O_2 Fick equation and compared with direct thermodilution measurements. The thermodilution values are shown as the boxes in the lower panel of figure 10.8. Unfortunately, no injections were made during the period of increased work in the first test because of the development of cardiac irritability. However, in the second test, thermodilution cardiac output clearly increased in response to increased work. The O_2 Fick cardiac output, calculated for each breath of the test, showed little response in the first test when the work increased. In the second test, the initial (0 kpm/min) Fick cardiac output is greater than in the first test and appears to increase as the work increases, but it remains somewhat below the thermodilution values throughout the test. The heart rate increased at both work levels.

10.5.6 Stroke Volume

Stroke volume was calculated from the Fick cardiac output and the heart rate (table 10.9). From normal data (Altman and Dittmer 1971), subject 3680 (estimated body surface area 1.421 m^2) would be expected to have a left ventricular volume of about 50 milliliters and an ejection fraction of 0.67.[11] These theoretical figures give an estimated end-diastolic volume of 33 milliliters, a value close to that observed.

In the first exercise test, the stroke volume does not increase with increased work load. In contrast, stroke volume increased when the hematocrit was lowered to sea-level normal and increased further at higher work load. These findings support the interpretation of the electrocardiographic changes with hemodilution (see fig. 10.3) that increased R wave slope and amplitude correlate with stroke volume.

Table 10.9. Hemodynamics during constant work-rate exercise in subject 3680

	Prehemodilution Rate (kpm/min)		Posthemodilution Rate (kpm/min)	
	0	300	0	300
CQ̇ (l/min) Fick	4.12	4.64	5.43	9.624
CQ̇ (l/min) thermodilution	7.5	—	7.4	11.4
HR (min^{-1})	93	106	109	132
SV, Fick (ml)	42	42	61	79
SV, thermodilution (ml)	81	—	68	86

Source: Winslow et al. 1985a.
Note: SV = stroke volume.

10.5.7   The Ventilation/Perfusion Ratio

Alveolar ventilation can be calculated from the measured $PaCO_2$ and $\dot{V}CO_2$. Pulmonary blood flow, $\dot{Q}_c$, is then calculated from $PaCO_2$, $\dot{V}_A$, $(a - \bar{v})O_2$, and the RQ. The ratios, $\dot{V}_A/\dot{Q}_c$, are 2.83, which increases to 4.05 in the first test, and 2.72, which increases to 2.90 on exercise in the second test.

It is difficult to find studies comparable with the authors' Cerro de Pasco ones in the literature, and the available data are somewhat contradictory. The results of O_2 Fick studies of four natives of Leadville, Colorado (3,100 m), showed a slightly decreased cardiac output but an increased $(a - \bar{v})O_2$, at a given $\dot{V}O_2$ compared with sea-level controls (Hartley et al. 1967). The decrease in cardiac output was mediated by decreased stroke volume and was not reversed by administration of O_2 at altitude; cardiac output increased after descent to sea level. These subjects were born at a high altitude, but their parents were lowlanders. Their mean hematocrit was 48.5 percent, body weight was 71.2 kilograms, and surface area was 1.87 square meters.

Banchero et al. (1966) studied thirty-five male natives of Cerro de Pasco, also using the O_2 Fick technique. Although individual data are not given in their report, they found mean cardiac output and the $(a - \bar{v})O_2$ difference was not different from those of a sea-level control group of twenty-two subjects. In Banchero's high-altitude group, mean body surface area was 1.55 square meters (1.63 m^2 for the sea-level group), and mean hematocrit was 58.7 percent. They noted that the increase in cardiac output with exercise was mediated almost exclusively by an increase in heart rate, the stroke volume being essentially fixed.

The authors' O_2 Fick data are compared with these two data sets in figure 10.9. The caridac output has been adjusted for body surface area (cardiac index) in an attempt to correct for differences in body size. Although the number of subjects is small, there does appear to be a difference between the Morococha and the Leadville data in regard to cardiac index, while the $(a - \bar{v})O_2$ differences are not distinguishable. This may reflect the differences in body habitus and surface area, or it may be due to these subjects' different genetic backgrounds or levels of adaptation. Our subject had a strikingly low cardiac index and a high $(a - \bar{v})O_2$ difference before hemodilution. After his hematocrit returned to 42 percent, however, both values fell into the range reported in the previous studies.

The contradictory cardiac output measurements by the two methods, thermodilution and O_2 Fick, could be resolved in at least two ways: error in the thermodilution measurements due to excessive polycythemia or lack of steady-state conditions in the measurement of $\dot{V}O_2$ for the O_2 Fick calculations. Although rejection of the thermodilution data would reconcile the authors' data with those of previous studies, the technique has been evalu-

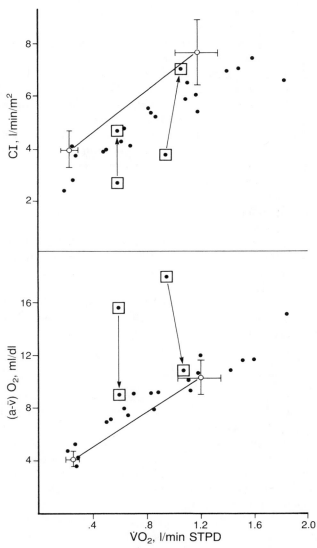

Figure 10.9. A comparison of the cardiac index *(CI)* and $(a - \bar{v})O_2$ with previous studies. Means for thirty-five male Andean natives of 4,500 m are shown with 1 SD range *(open circles)*. Measurements in four male North American residents of 3,100 m at various work rates are also shown *(closed circles)*; studies in the authors' subject 3680 are given *(boxed)* for comparison. Changes following hemodilution are indicated by arrows. Note that this procedure moves the values into the range observed for the other groups. The Andean data are from Banchero et al. (1966), and the North American data are from Hartley et al. (1967).

ated extensively and has even been shown to be accurate in subjects with shock (Levine and Sirinik 1981) when blood flow is minimal. Moreover, the authors are not aware of comparable cardiac output measurements with indicator dilution techniques in high-altitude natives.

The older literature extensively discusses the necessity of steady-state conditions to calculate cardiac output by the O_2 Fick technique. For example, in a study by Fishman et al. (1952) of subjects with hypoxic lung disease, definition of the steady state required: (1) emotional stability, (2) constant $\dot{V}O_2$, and (3) constant RQ. They rejected any measurements when the RQ was greater than one or the variation from basal conditions was greater than 0.11, noting that cardiac output under non–steady-state conditions will severely underestimate the actual value, particularly in the hypoxic state.

The explanation for this underestimation of cardiac output may lie in the mobilization of tissue O_2 stores in hypoxia or exercise. Whem pulmonary O_2 uptake of the blood is limited by diffusion, as it is at high altitude (West and Wagner 1981), increased demand for O_2 may be satisfied by some combination of widened $(a - \bar{v})O_2$ and cardiac output. When $S\bar{v}O_2$ decreases, as it clearly did in the authors' subject during exercise, there will be a net flux of O_2 out of tissue reservoirs. Very large stores of O_2 may be found in stagnant blood in the lung (Hamilton 1964) and myoglobin-bound O_2 in muscle (see chap. 5).

10.5.8 Oxygen Debt

No direct estimation of the size of the stagnant pulmonary blood pool can be made from the authors' Cerro de Pasco data, but our estimation of FRC may provide a clue. The estimated residual volume for gas distribution before hemodilution (2.6 liters for O_2) is much larger than after hemodilution (1.6 liters). Vital capacity did not change after hemodilution (see table 10.3), so these observations could also be explained by a decreased pulmonary blood volume, in that blood contents of both gases will be much larger than gas-phase contents, particularly at low partial pressures.

The second major source of tissue O_2 is muscle. Normally, very little O_2 is supplied to the blood from this reservoir, since the P50 of myoglobin, under physiologic conditions, is about 2.5 torr (Rossi-Fanelli and Antonini 1958). However, in the Cerro de Pasco subject, mixed venous SO_2 decreases to 12.7 percent in the first test and to 20.9 percent in the second, corresponding to PO_2s of 13.7 torr and 16.9 torr, respectively. The venous PO_2 in the leg during exercise in our subject could not be estimated, but in experiments of Jorfeldt and Wahren (1971) it was found that about two-thirds of the cardiac output went to the legs during bicycle ergometer exercise, and the actual leg blood flow was directly proportional to $\dot{V}O_2$. Thus, a simple calculation suggests that femoral vein blood in the subject during exercise could have had a PO_2 of very nearly zero; if true, large quantities of O_2 could have been made available from myoglobin stores.

10.6   Conclusions from Hematocrit-Reduction Studies

Some variation among individuals precludes a strict characterization of the physiologic response to phlebotomy or to hemodilution in the authors' studies or from the literature. However, reduction of blood viscosity and improved circulation must be an overriding feature of the adjustment. Certainly symptomatic improvement is a universal finding, regardless of subsequent exercise performance. Increased PaO_2 in the authors' subjects was not always accompanied by increased minute ventilation, but decreased $PaCO_2$, in most cases, suggests increased alveolar ventilation.

The stimulation of ventilation, regardless of whether hematocrit reduction was effected by phlebotomy or hemodilution, was one of the most consistent findings. It is well known that high-altitude natives have "blunted" hypoxic respiratory drives (see chap. 6), and the results suggest the possibility that at least some of this reduced chemoreceptor sensitivity may be reversible and that it may be attributable to excessive polycythemia. This interpretation would seem to be at odds with the traditional view that hypoventilation is the essential cause of excessive polycythemia, but a similar argument has been used to explain improvement of sleep apnea in polycythemia vera patients after phlebotomy.

It is perhaps of greatest significance that in no case, either in the literature or in the authors' own experience, was exercise capacity impaired after a reduction of the red cell mass. This is, in itself, strongly suggestive that the increased O_2 capacity resulting from excessive polycythemia in these high-altitude natives serves no useful purpose.

The Cerro de Pasco studies were intended to determine to what extent polycythemia may limit exercise performance because of increased viscosity of the blood and consequent fall in cardiac output. The increase in maximal lactic acid concentration indicates a greater "lactacid" capacity (diPrampero, Mognoni, and Veicsteinas 1981). Thus, a part of the reduced lactic acid accumulation seen by various investigators in the past may be due to polycythemia. Why polycythemia should lead to decreased lactic acid production is not clear, but it may be a reflection of reduced tissue O_2 supply.

A decreased ratio of red cell 2,3-DPG to hemoglobin was an unexpected finding. Hypoxia (Lenfant, Torrance, and Reynafarje 1971) and alkalosis (Espinos, Alvarez-Sala, and Vellegas 1982) are both associated with increased 2,3-DPG/hemoglobin ratios. However, 2,3-DPG/hemoglobin decreased in the authors' subjects even though arterial O_2 content decreased and hyperventilation followed. Perhaps the explanation is that the respiratory alkalosis was compensated, and that PaO_2 actually increased after hematocrit reduction. If so, it suggests that O_2 pressure, not content, is more important in regulating 2,3-DPG concentration.

The authors' experience does not allow a clear definition of what hematocrit is "excessive," nor does it enable a distinction to be made between gradual phlebotomy and hemodilution. The latter procedure is attractive because it is rapid, simple, and safe, and it requires only one visit by the subject to the clinic. However, the former procedure probably allows reduction in blood volume to parallel reduction in O_2 capacity and viscosity.

Increased work capacity seems to be more pronounced after phlebotomy than of the hemodilution, but the response to either procedure was too variable to be certain of the validity of this generalization. However, it is possible that fluid shifts after the phlebotomy could result in increased blood volume, and, therefore, increased cardiac output. It would be of interest to measure plasma volume after such therapy. More studies of the specific physiologic responses to a hematocrit reduction would be of use.

CHAPTER ELEVEN
Summary and Conclusions

It can be said that chronic mountain sickness is the sum of a number of physiological responses to hypoxia, superimposed on other normal mechanisms. Two such mechanisms are the decreased ventilation with age and the lower hypoxic ventilatory drives found in many normal persons, regardless of altitude of residence. This does not mean, however, that much important information cannot be gained from studies of high-altitude natives. This chapter summarizes each of the foregoing chapters and points out where additional work most urgently needs to be done.

In the absence of data to establish that high-altitude natives are genetically different from lowlanders, one cannot regard high-altitude natives as representing a special breed of the human race. Rather, they must be viewed as individuals who demonstrate a logical extreme of lifelong physiologic reaction to a hostile environment. Because modern definitions of chronic mountain sickness are diffuse and confusing, this book has tried to observe the differences between sea-level and high-altitude physiologic responses and to interpret them in reference to their advantages and disadvantages for the high-altitude resident native.

The authors believe, like those who have gone before them, that polycythemia is a normal response to altitude hypoxia; however, sufferers of chronic mountain sickness have an excessive response. To test polycythemia as an adaptive mechanism, we have studied exercise and the response to bloodletting. We have also extensively reviewed the literature to obtain relevant data and opinions, thereby resisting the development of a rigid theory based on our studies alone. On the contrary, we have enlisted the aid of many foreign scientific and methodologic fields in order to interpret our findings. The conclusion is that excessive polycythemia in high-altitude natives serves no useful purpose. Indeed, it is doubtful whether there is any physiologic value in "normal" polycythemia.

11.1 The History of Chronic Mountain Sickness

The study of high-altitude polycythemia began in the small mining town of Morococha, Peru, altitude 4,500 meters. This town is only three hours by car from Lima, but when Viault went there in 1894 and when Barcroft went in 1921, it was an extremely arduous trip by rail up endless switchbacks on the steep slopes of the Andes.

The first description of chronic mountain sickness, or excessive polycythemia, was made by Carlos Monge M. in 1925 of a native of another small Peruvian town, Cerro de Pasco (4,300 m). Soon after, the Chilean, Argentinean, and Bolivian Cordilleras became hosts to fundamental studies defining the effects of chronic exposure to high altitudes. Alberto Hurtado was perhaps the most prolific of a large number of young Peruvian scientists who were influenced by Monge M., and under his guidance many of the fundamental discoveries of chronic acclimatization to high altitudes were made. As the high-altitude story unfolded, numerous North American scientists visited Peru to study aspects of acclimatization that touched their particular fields of expertise. All of the investigators were deeply influenced by Monge M. and Hurtado, and the collaborative studies not only furthered understanding of high-altitude humans but also contributed to the modern understanding of the physiologic effects of hypoxia in general.

High-altitude research now has extended to the North American Rockies, to Tibet, Nepal, and India, to China, to the Soviet Union, and to other mountainous areas of the world. Three significant populations have been studied: the Andeans, the Nepali Sherpas, and the Tibetans. Some authors have suggested genetic differences among these groups that might account for differences in apparent abilities to acclimatize. Comparative studies are needed to establish whether such differences exist. Modern electronic technology, rapid travel, and the development of noninvasive instrumentation make such studies possible for the first time, and genetic studies will contribute yet another chapter to this story.

11.2   High-Altitude Natives and Chronic Mountain Sickness

Chronic mountain sickness is an elusive clinical syndrome. There is no doubt that at higher altitudes the "normal" hemoglobin concentration increases and that some high-altitude natives develop excessive, symptomatic polycythemia. Most high-altitude clinicians have agreed upon a definition of *chronic mountain sickness:* a hypoventilatory disorder affecting the high-altitude native or long-term resident, which, by aggravating hypoxemia, leads to excessive polycythemia. The degree of polycythemia is defined as a hematocrit above the statistical maximum for the altitude in question.

The detailed clinical description by Monge M. of the first case of chronic mountain sickness emphasized the limitations imposed on the individual by a high hematocrit, particularly in regard to the symptoms of impaired cerebral circulation. These include sleeplessness, confusion, and poor performance in work. In addition, his patient suffered with chronic bone pain, a symptom that suggested to Monge M. that the bone marrow may be involved. A final footnote to this eloquent description is that the patient is now (1986) living and well in Lima, living proof of the reversibility of chronic mountain sickness by descent to sea level.

There is no clear pathologic definition of the disease and no grounds for predicting which individuals in a population may be susceptible. High-altitude natives have enlarged carotid bodies, the peripheral chemoreceptors for O_2. They also have impressive hypertrophy of the pulmonary vessel walls, a finding that is reminiscent of brisket disease in cattle. This discrepancy between pathologic and clinical findings in chronic mountain sickness has spawned a number of different points of view on its etiology.

One of the most intriguing aspects of chronic mountain sickness is its rarity among Himalayan peoples. The present consensus of opinion is that Sherpas are not susceptible to this illness as a result of a longer period for genetic adaptation to high altitude. However, the available studies are incomplete, and one of the authors once observed a Sherpa in Nepal whose hematocrit was 72 percent and who had typical symptoms of chronic mountain sickness. It would seem that careful comparisons between Sherpas and Indians are needed to settle the issue of genetic differences. These studies must be carried out by investigators who use comparable techniques in the two geographic areas. In addition, comparative studies should enlist the help of anthropologists and epidemiologists, because careful selection of subjects is of great importance, and physiologists generally are not accustomed to the required techniques of selection.

Comparative studies also must keep in mind the climatological differences between the various high-altitude areas of the world. For example, the altiplano of northern Chile is extremely desert-like in comparison to Peru. In this way it is more like the Tibetan plateau. The Peruvian highlands may be more comparable with the high valleys of Nepal in regard to rainfall and vegetation. Few studies have considered these differences, yet it is well known that adaptation to an arid environment is common in certain animals, such as the camelids.

11.3 Red Cells, Red Cell and Plasma Volumes, and Their Regulation

Although the symptoms of chronic mountain sickness are due to an increased blood volume, the syndrome is not usually thought to be a "hematologic" disease. This is due to the parallel that is often drawn between chronic mountain sickness and chronic obstructive pulmonary disease, and it has seemed natural to emphasize the respiratory etiology. Nevertheless, there is no clear quantitive relationship between PaO_2 and polycythemia in chronic mountain sickness. Hypoxemia undoubtedly stimulates the erythropoietic system; increases in the renal hormone erythropoietin have been documented. However, scant attention has been paid to the differences among individuals. It would be useful to know, for example, if the magnitude of the erythropoietin response to hypoxia or to bloodletting co-relates with the size of the red cell volume or the symptoms of chronic mountain sickness.

Having considered the possible mechanisms for a renal oxygen sensor, the authors favor the "vicious cycle" hypothesis. That is, increased viscosity that accompanies increased hematocrit could further reduce the supply of oxygen to the kidney tissues where erythropoietin is provided. This in turn may further stimulate a higher hematocrit, and so on. Unfortunately, the critical measurements of erythropoietin in subjects with various hematocrits at high altitudes have not been made.

There are no consistent differences between the red cells of high-altitude natives and those of sea-level residents. There is no evidence for nutritional deficiencies or for impaired hemoglobin synthesis, either in the high-hematocrit natives or in those with lower hematocrits. However, in chapter 3 important differences have been pointed out in different populations of high-altitude residents. That is, the hematocrits in Morococha (4,500 m) seem to be higher than the ones in Cerro de Pasco (4,300 m), and Santolaya has reported even more significant differences when comparing villages at a similar altitude in Chile. These findings emphasize the need for carefully planned epidemiologic studies. Systematic surveys of different communities and their environments need to be carried out to define what factors determine the hematocrit and its range of variation in a given location.

The classical measurements of red cell and plasma volume in chronic mountain sickness were carried out before double-label techniques were available. Now it is known that the hematocrit is not the same throughout the circulation, and estimation of the red cell mass from plasma volume determinations is very dangerous. Chapter 3 has reviewed available data and shown that the red cell mass in chronic mountain sickness is probably less than usually believed; contraction of the plasma volume could play a part in the very high hematocrits usually seen in this disorder. This concept is particularly provocative in that it points out the importance of understanding the control of red cell production. In addition, however, it suggests an entirely new area for investigation: regulation of the plasma volume.

These comments apply also to comparisons of South American, North American, and Asian populations. In fact, such interdisciplinary cooperation is even more important here, because additional social factors need to be controlled, such as seasonality and migration habits. The available data to suggest that hematocrits are lower in the Himalayas are not convincing when the variability in the Andean studies is considered. In addition, no comparative studies in the two areas have been performed by the same teams using the same techniques.

11.4   The Structure and Function of Hemoglobin at High Altitudes

The stimulus to red cell production is an inability to deliver O_2 to tissues, and hemoglobin is the protein responsible for its transport in the blood. Perhaps more is known about the molecular structure and function of hemoglobin than of any other human protein. Its affinity for oxygen is regulated by the interaction of its polypeptide subunits, under the influence of the allosteric effectors 2,3-diphosphoglycerate (2,3-DPG), H^+, and CO_2. These effectors regulate the position of the hemoglobin O_2 equilibrium curve so that its P50 (the PO_2 at half-saturation) seldom varies by more than a few torr.

Early studies by Barcroft in Cerro de Pasco suggested that the affinity of hemoglobin for O_2 increased at high altitudes, and this was taken as a favorable change in that O_2 in the lung could be taken up more efficiently. However, subsequent studies by Keys and co-workers and by Hurtado and others failed to support Barcroft's findings. In fact, these workers believed that O_2 affinity decreased in high-altitude natives and that this change was favorable for tissue O_2 delivery.

Lenfant and co-workers, who were the first to study the red cell metabolite 2,3-DPG in high-altitude natives, found it to be increased. Its concentration is regulated mainly by red cell pH, and it increases with alkalosis, as demonstrated by its increase in parallel with hyperventilation in newcomers to high altitudes.

In the authors' own work, new, automated techniques have been employed to study the in vivo position of the Oxygen Equilibrium Curve (OEC) in Morococha natives. These methods allow correlation of all effectors of hemoglobin oxygen affinity in individuals and show that, in general, the decreased O_2 affinity caused by 2,3-DPG is offset by the opposite effect of alkalosis itself to increase affinity. The net result is that the in vivo position of the OEC is not significantly different from that of sea-level residents. As altitude increases above about 4,000 meters, however, the affinity steadily increases, because at these altitudes alkalosis is more pronounced than is the increase in 2,3-DPG. Chapter 4 has shown that from a theoretical point of view Barcroft was correct in his opinion that increased O_2 affinity is beneficial in hypoxia, because of the improved rate of oxygenation of red cells in the pulmonary circulation.

Thus, in the author's own work or in the review of the literature, no convincing evidence has been found for blood oxygen affinity effects that cannot be explained on the basis of current understanding of hemoglobin structure and function. In studies of approximately 150 individuals in Morococha and Cerro de Pasco, no blood OEC's were found that could not be explained on the basis of known effects, including the Bohr effect.

A remaining area that is in need of further studies, however, is the definition of in vivo pH. This issue has been raised by the finding that polycythemia has an effect on the apparent measured pH. This may be an artifact induced by the interaction of red cells with the glass pH electrode, but proof is still lacking. The point is important in interpreting acid-base status and in determining the exact position of the OEC. Perhaps some of the newer methods to measure pH will clarify this matter.

11.5   Circulation

Polycythemia and hypoxia act together to increase the pulmonary circulatory pressure. This, in turn, increases the load on the right ventricle, and a progression of cardiac enlargement and ultimate failure mark the advanced cases of chronic mountain sickness. In modern times, cases seldom advance to this point, because the possibility of descent is readily available. Hemodynamic and electrocardiographic studies of high-altitude residents have pointed out the tremendous variability in expression of this pathophysiologic progression, and no guidelines are available to predict which individuals will develop heart failure.

The very low incidence of arteriosclerosis and systemic hypertension found in Andeans must protect them against the risks of high blood viscosity. Therefore, newcomers to high altitudes should be screened for these conditions if they are over age forty and they intend to remain at altitude for a long period of time. The authors have observed one case of myocardial infarction in a volunteer performing a simple Masters test; he later confessed he was a sea-level man who had suffered moderate hypertension while living at sea level. Thousands of more severe exercise tests have been conducted in true high-altitude natives of Morococha over the years without any untoward effects. This lack of systemic hypertension and arteriosclerosis seems to be an ideal model for the comparative study of the effects of Western habits on arterial disease.

Increased circulatory pressures and increased capillary density have the potential for increased blood flow in tissue beds, but this is probably offset by increased viscosity and resistance to flow. This is clearly demonstrated by dye dilution experiments in the pulmonary circulation. Thus, the polycythemic high-altitude resident develops a high-pressure, low-velocity type of circulation, which may preserve the amount of O_2 available that may also decrease the responsiveness of the hemodynamic system.

Circulatory adaptation to hypoxia is not complete; if it were, erythropoietin secretion would not be increased and polycythemia would not follow. Another indication that the circulatory system cannot fully compensate for hypoxia is that birth weight is reduced at high altitudes. Although much needs to be done to further define what factors regulate birth weight, the consensus is that diminished O_2 delivery to the fetus is responsive.

That cardiac output measurements in high-altitude natives have conflicted is probably due to differences in methods. A review of the literature
indicated, however, that Peruvian high-altitude natives (without excessive
polycythemia) seem to have cardiac outputs that are the same at a given O_2
uptake as at sea level, while natives of Leadville, Colorado, seem to have
somewhat reduced cardiac outputs. The authors' studies in bloodletting
suggest that the cardiac output is regulated at least in part by polycythemia,
in that output increases after removal of blood. This is an area in great need
of further work, because no data are available for large numbers of patients
that relate cardiac output, O_2 uptake, and hematocrit. Essential to such
studies will be the development of accurate noninvasive techniques.

Many observers of high-altitude natives have believed that some degree
of "tissue" adaptation must take place in native residents. It is true that such
natives are capable of impressive feats of exercise, but documentation of
such tissue adaptation is lacking. Capillary density studies carried out in the
myocardium indicate a proliferation. Similar studies in other organs have
not been done in humans and are badly needed. Myoglobin stores are
increased in muscles of natives, but the role of myoglobin, if indeed there is
one, still is not clear. The efficiency of oxidative phosphorylation in mitochondria is a new area of research, and preliminary studies suggest that in
hypoxic animals the efficiency is increased. With time, perhaps, these interesting studies will be extended to humans.

11.6   Ventilation

The chest dimensions of the high-altitude Quechua Indian are larger for his
height than are those of Sherpa or Tibetan natives. This appears to be related
to the length of time of exposure to hypoxia (in other words, to age) and may
reflect lifelong hyperventilation. The vital capacity of the Peruvian native,
however, while believed to be increased according to sea-level standards,
was not significantly different from sea-level predictions in a series of
almost 150 subjects in the authors' studies. Because the vital capacity normally decreases with age and the chest volume apparently increases, it
seems that the residual volume of the native chest also increases.

The diffusing capacity of the high-altitude native is increased, partly
owing to higher hemoglobin concentration. Bloodletting experiments suggest that other factors, such as a greater membrane surface area, contribute
as well. Very few studies have been done on this important question,
however.

Increased ventilation in response to hypoxia is a normal human reflex,
mediated by O_2 sensors in the carotid bodies. The reflex develops in the first
decade after birth, and its expression is influenced by the ambient PO_2
during this critical time. Chiodi was the first to show that high-altitude

residents responded less to hypoxia than do newcomers from sea level. This phenomenon has been confirmed in other South American natives, as well as in Asia.

A popular hypothesis to explain chronic mountain sickness has been that hypoventilation leads to greater erythropoietic stimulus in subjects who are already hypoxemic. One line of evidence to support this view is the impression that chronic mountain sickness is more common in older subjects. This is consistent with the hypoventilatory etiology, because the ventilatory reflex diminishes normally with age. Only a few longitudinal studies of hematocrit change with age have been carried out—too few to be conclusive—but this remains an attractive hypothesis. Another argument in favor is that chronic mountain sickness patients seem to undergo more blood desaturation during sleep than do controls, and administration of respiratory stimulants appears to reverse the polycythemia.

Against the hypoventilation hypothesis is the evidence that after bloodletting, PaO_2 increases and $PaCO_2$ decreases, both of which are signs of ventilatory stimulation. This would not be expected if depressed ventilatory drive were the etiology, and it raises the possibility that, in some subjects, polycythemia would exacerbate ventilatory depression—as seen in the Pickwick syndrome, for example. This area should be fruitful for future studies if careful measurements of the ventilatory reflexes can be carried out in high-altitude natives at different hematocrits.

Another argument against the hypoventilatory hypothesis is that in Tibet, more sojourners than natives seem to develop excessively elevated hematocrits. These newcomers would be expected to have intact hypoxia ventilatory drives and would be interesting to study; they could provide the opportunity to see whether depressed ventilatory drive in lowlanders would correlate with excessive polycythemia after migration to high altitudes.

11.7   Renal Function in High-Altitude Polycythemia

Human beings, unlike many lower-order organisms, are dependent on only one system, the kidney, for maintenance of electrolyte homeostasis. When hematocrits are very high, the kidney must make do with a very low plasma flow. Systematic exploration of the renal function in high-altitude natives in Morococha and Cerro de Pasco has been carried out in order to characterize the renal adaptations to this extreme condition.

Polycythemia reduces the filtration rate, increases the filtration fraction (the fraction of plasma that is filtered by the glomeruli), and markedly reduces the renal plasma flow. Surprisingly, the tubular functions remain intact. A slight increase in protein excretion is the only abnormality found in severe hypoxemia and polycythemia.

The physiologic response of the kidney in high-altitude natives is a useful model for general physiologic renal studies. A reduced plasma flow in the absence of ischemia is possible only in cases of polycythemia. The suggestion is made in chapter 7 that this model may be used in standard in vivo and in vitro studies of the kidney. The chapter also shows by a simple mathematical approach that, because the $(a - v)O_2$ difference across the kidney is small, this organ is sensitive to changes in the PaO_2, and the $P\bar{v}O_2$ drop found in high-altitude natives in the systemic circulation is even more severe in the kidney.

11.8 Exercise Capacity

Lowland sojourners to high altitudes have been impressed by the physical capabilities of high-altitude natives, be they residents of the Andes or the Himalayas. When the subjects have been carefully selected, however, objective attempts at measuring maximal $\dot{V}O_2$ have failed to show a superiority of natives over sea-level residents. One difference that *is* demonstrable is that high-altitude natives do not seem to have the endurance of sea-level athletes performing at the same altitude. The reason for this is not clear, but the possibility of polycythemia and a reduced cardiac output response to exercise needs to be investigated.

Lifelong residents of high altitudes demonstrate a reduced ventilatory response to exercise. This response is more complicated than hypoxic drive, although hypoxia must be a part of the reflex. The implications of this observation are that O_2 is taken up with less ventilatory effort in high-altitude natives than in sea-level natives, which can be considered either an efficient adaptation or a limitation, depending on the point of view. Taken to its extreme, this reduced reflex cannot be advantageous, as illustrated by an example in which a young man developed a bradyarrhythmia before he had any sensation of breathlessness.

In the authors' survey of subjects in Cerro de Pasco, no correlation has been found between exercise ventilation and hematocrit. In bloodletting experiments, however, polycythemia has been found to impose a "damping" effect on the cardiovascular system, slowing its response to an exercise challenge. In addition, lowering the hematocrit increases the "lactacid" energy production. Increased lactic acid during exercise also can be viewed positively (a higher capacity for exercise) or negatively (a lower anaerobic threshold), depending on the point of view.

11.9 The Comparative Physiology of Hypoxemic Polycythemia

There is no doubt that there is a genetic adaptation in animals that have been exposed to hypoxia for long periods of time. How long is a matter of speculation, but one of the adaptive changes seems to be an alteration of the hemoglobin molecule. Mammals and birds that are truly adapted have an increased hemoglobin O_2 affinity and limited polycythemia. This is true in amphibians, which are favored by the cold environment of the mountains (cold temperatures diminish the O_2 requirements of these animals).

The human animal does not seem to be naturally selected for high altitudes. The normal hemoglobin O_2 affinity and marked polycythemia of humans are shared with other animals who do not do well at high altitudes, such as the domestic creatures brought to the mountains by the Spanish. In this respect, comparative studies help to explain why humans show a limited capacity to acclimatize to the high mountains. Chronic mountain sickness, in the authors' view as well as that of others, is more an indication of this limited capacity than it is an isolated clinical entity. Further studies of animals selected on the basis of shorter generation times could serve as important models for understanding high-altitude adaptation.

11.10   Bloodletting

The hypothesis that any degree of polycythemia is a maladaptive response at high altitudes goes beyond the concept of chronic mountain sickness as a condition of "excessive" polycythemia. The reasoning behind it is based on clinical observations of both young and old people at high altitudes, in the interpretation of exercise and functional studies at both the ventilatory and the circulatory levels, and on lessons learned from comparative physiology. The authors' experimental approach has been to reduce the hematocrit to sea-level values by the use of controlled bloodletting. The clinical results have confirmed the known benefits of the procedure in chronic mountain sickness but also have added the fact that even a sea-level hematocrit is compatible with improvement of the clinical condition.

Physiologic studies of bloodletting subjects have indicated a change in the O_2 transport pattern. That is, in one subject studied with invasive techniques, while O_2 content decreased, cardiac output increased and was more responsive to exercise. Pulmonary ventilation improved in that alveolar O_2 increased, along with PaO_2 and a drop in $PaCO_2$. Pulmonary artery pressure dropped immediately after hemodilution in one subject and actually reached sea-level normal values in spite of continued hypoxia. The overall exercise capacity increased in some subjects and did not change in others, but it did not drop in any. This suggests that exercise was not limited by the decrease in hematocrit in these subjects.

The O_2 transport measurements after bloodletting suggest that polycythemia could be in part responsible for the hypoventilation in chronic mountain sickness patients; this concept deserves further study. It is of interest that several case reports have appeared in which polycythemia vera patients at sea level improved their arterial saturation after bloodletting, again suggesting a depressant effect of polycythemia on the control of respiration.

Still needed are long-term studies of bloodletting in high-altitude natives of differing hematocrits. It is the authors' subjective impression from informal follow-up of bloodletting subjects that the beneficial effects last much longer than would be expected if the red cells were replaced normally. This suggests that bloodletting may have interrupted a vicious cycle of desaturation, accelerated erythropoiesis, circulatory impairment, desaturation, and so on. Further studies incorporating the measurement of erythropoietin will be of interest.

11.11 The Integration of Physiologic Variables

When Joseph Barcroft (1934) wrote, "Every adaptation is an integration," he was not referring to the integration of a single physiologic parameter along a functional relationship, but rather to the integration of multiple physiologic parameters leading to the optimization of adaptive mechanisms. In hypoxia this complex process may begin with perturbation of one or a few variables, such as increased hematocrit and hyperventilation. These may lead to acid-base changes, increased viscosity, increased heart work, increased vascular pressure, anatomic changes in the vessel walls, and so on. At some point all these various reactions must come to a new equilibrium that defines the acclimatized state. The actual position of the equilibrium will depend on as many individual factors as there are differences among human beings. These modifying factors are the keys to understanding the tremendous variability at high altitude.

The authors' view of how the different variables may interact in chronic mountain sickness is summarized in figure 11.1. This diagram shows the broad physiologic units in the relationships among hypoxia and its physiological effects. Clearly, hypoxia is the central inciting cause of chronic mountain sickness; this is known because descent to sea level is always curative. Hypoxia has many known effects, including stimulation of erythropoietin and pulmonary hypertension. These result in a series of more-or-less predictable physiological changes. The question remains, however, as to why some individuals develop chronic mountain sickness and others do not, even when exposed to the same degree of ambient hypoxia.

There are at least five contributions to hypoxia in high-altitude natives (fig. 11.1): altitude itself, depressed ventilatory responsiveness, sleep desaturation, impaired lung function, and impaired circulation. Each of these is controlled by multiple factors. The exact pathway to chronic mountain sickness may differ from patient to patient, depending on the net balance of these contributing factors.

The likelihood that an individual will suffer from chronic mountain sick-

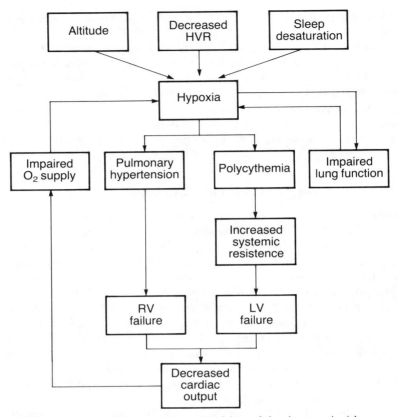

Figure 11.1.   Physiologic variables in the etiology of chronic mountain sickness.

ness depends on the balance of these factors that contribute to hypoxia. That is, a slight exaggeration in hypoxic ventilatory depression, sleep desaturation, and lung disease (even very mild chronic obstructive lung disease) could by themselves tip the balance toward chronic mountain sickness. This balance, which could be the subject of quantitation, would seem to lend itself to a mathematical model. The time has come for such a model to be developed. It should be possible to use relatively simple, noninvasive measurements on individuals to predict who will develop excessive polycythemia and who will not.

After a review of both the literature and our own experimental results and clinical observations, some of which extend over several decades, we think there is no reason to believe that chronic mountain sickness is a "disease" in the usual sense of the word. Rather, it can be viewed as an accumulation of physiologic responses, each one of which is slightly off the mean for the population. For example, there is a normal variation in hemoglobin concentration at sea level and a range of hypoxic ventilatory response, just as there is a range in athletic ability, body size, strength, and so on. If, under the added burden of hypoxia, an individual has a higher than normal hematocrit and a lower than normal ventilation rate, and is not in a highly conditioned, athletic state, perhaps the symptoms of chronic mountain sickness may appear.

The authors do not share Monge M.'s view, strictly, that chronic mountain sickness is a "loss of acclimatization," because we are not convinced that most humans are well suited to life at high altitudes. In this sense, humans do not adapt to hypoxia in the way that genetically adapted animals do. Instead, well-conditioned, stoic, strong humans live and reproduce at high altitudes, but we have yet to find one who would not prefer to live at sea level. Future efforts should be directed at identification of which individuals, by virtue of their genetic makeup, are unsuited to this hypoxic life.

11.12 A Public Health Note

This somewhat unorthodox view of chronic mountain sickness and of its apparent lack of clinical relevance leads to a more scientific approach to problems of public health of the Andean populations. Humans, especially if born at a high altitude, are subjected to a process of natural selection that allows them to lead normal lives and to employ remarkable capacities for physical exercise. However, any pulmonary disease will reduce this capacity, disturb the delicate new equilibrium of acclimatization, and reduce the chances for a normal life.

Although able to live a pastoral life, the acclimatized high-altitude resident will be at risk if his or her life becomes Westernized. Overweight, environmental pollution, high carbon monoxide levels, sedentarism, cigarette smoking—all factors that are important but tolerable at sea level—become catastrophic for the high-altitude native. Moreover, people in their fifties and sixties, who today are considered fully capable of normal life at sea level, can be incapacitated even in the absence of pulmonary disease by what is considered primary chronic mountain sickness.

The Andean countries of Peru, Chile, and Bolivia depend on mining as their main economic resource. The most important mines are located at high altitudes, and the Andean miner is not only susceptible to primary chronic mountain sickness but also is exposed to the unhealthy environment of this industry, which easily leads to pulmonary problems and secondary chronic mountain sickness. Visits to the mining tunnels have confirmed firsthand the assertion that miners do not use their protective masks. Apparently these devices were not designed for the hyperventilation of the high-altitude native, and the users feel the increased resistance to air flow.

The dryness of the atmosphere and the increased ventilatory rate in the absence of filtering devices must be factors that elevate the risk of pneumoconiosis in these high mining places. Add to this the disadvantages of excessive polycythemia, and the applied value of fundamental research at high altitudes becomes clear. Public health experts are now in a position to base recommendations on physiologic findings, rather than on the more empirical and dogmatic approaches that still pervade the high-altitude literature. In this regard it is satisfying to be able to help those miners who, along with their forebears, have cooperated as volunteers for so many in vivo studies conducted in an effort to better understand human physiology.

The authors hope that the information obtained from Andeans will stimulate interest in the public health problems of the Himalayan and Tibetan mountains, which have been less studied. Finally, there is no doubt that the pulmonary doctor practicing at sea level will find facts and concepts developed in high-altitude studies of direct relevance to physiologic and clinical problems in the hypoxic conditions of sea-level medicine.

The age of classical descriptive physiology seems to be coming to an end, and we are entering a era of molecular and cellular biology. Many of the studies summarized in this book have been central to the elucidation of fundamental physiological mechanisms and have, therefore, advanced our understanding of O_2 transport in general. However, for all this sophisticated physiologic information, few benefits have been returned to high-altitude natives or to the physician who must care for them. It is now possible to insist on better health care for high-altitude residents. This has been undertaken in North America by the University of Colorado group, who have studied the effects of respiratory stimulants on hematocrit and the practical matter of infant health. The problems in the Andes is greater, however, because of the large number of people who live at great altitudes and because public health care is, in general, less advanced.

It is time to recognize not only the great debt owed to research in high-altitude acclimatization, but also the obligation we owe to the hardy people who live in the high mountains. They do not have a large political voice, but they are as deserving of the fruits of modern medicine as are their sea-level counterparts. High-altitude research should continue along parallel lines of science, applied physiology, and public health. Understanding and solving the problems of high-altitude humans will tax our abilities to cross traditional lines of scientific disciplines and will require an "integrative" approach to understanding them as individuals.

Notes

Introduction

1. *The Singing Mountaineers: Songs and Tales of the Quechua People*, collected by Josí María Arguedas, ed. Ruth Stephan (Austin: University of Texas Press, 1957), 39.

Chapter One: The History of Chronic Mountain Sickness

1. A mercury pump is a manometric device to measure the gas content of blood.
2. Chemodectomas, tumors of the carotid bodies, are discussed in chapter 2.
3. Hemodilution is used throughout the book to indicate a procedure of removal of blood and replacement with an equal volume of plasma or a plasma substitute. It is to be distinguished from phlebotomy, where blood is simply removed. In hemodilution the blood volume remains constant, whereas in phletobomy it drops.

Chapter Two: High-Altitude Natives and Chronic Mountain Sickness

1. The altitude of Huarochirí is 3,000 meters.
2. Desamparados is the railway station at Lima, and is at sea level. Huacachina, a summer resort on the desertic coastal plain south of Lima (Ica), also is at sea level. It has a hotel near a sulfurous lagoon with swimming rats and a horrible smell. The waters are noted for their benefit to rheumatism.
3. *Hyperglobulia* is an outdated word used to mean an elevated red blood cell count.
4. Pertaining to osteocope, a severe pain in the bones, classically a symptom of syphilitic bone disease.

Chapter Three: Red Cells, Red Cell and Plasma Volumes, and Their Regulation

1. Unfortunately, some high-altitude studies report only hemoglobin concentrations; others report only hematocrits. Usually they are equally useful. However, the hematocrit, while simpler to measure in the field, has greater potential for error; the speed and radius of centrifugation are critical, and the required speed increases with hematocrit. A certain amount of plasma is always trapped within the column of packed red cells, and this may vary with the hematocrit and the condition.
2. In both methods, hemoglobin is converted to the cyanomet derivative with potassium ferricyanide. In the older method, this solution is compared to a set of reference standards through use of the naked eye. The accuracy is probably no better

than ± 1 g/dl, and it depends upon the experience of the observer. The newer method uses a spectrophotometer to quantitate the optical density, and its accuracy, about ± 0.1 g/dl, does not depend upon the accuracy of the observer.

3.   The method of obtaining blood is important in hematocrit determinations. For example, using a drop of blood from a fingertip puncture, the hematocrit can be significantly lower than that from a venepuncture if the finger must be "milked." In this case, extravascular fluid may be included in the blood sample. This error tends to introduce bias toward lower hematocrits in that blood is obtained with great difficulty from polycythemia subjects because of its high viscosity in this state.

4.   Ferritin, a storage compound for iron, is composed of a protein shell surrounding a ferric hydroxyphosphate core, which can contain up to five thousand iron atoms per molecule. The concentration of ferritin in the blood has been used as an index of total body iron stores.

5.   Normally the red cell synthesizes a slight excess of protoporphyrin, and the excess remains with the cell as free erythrocyte protoporphyrin (FEP). When hemoglobin synthesis is limited, this compound may increase dramatically. Although the normal concentration depends somewhat on the methods used to measure it, a composite normal range is $15-80$ µg/dl red cells. The FEP is one of the earliest and most sensitive indicators of iron deficiency: it may be increased up to fivefold in iron-deficient patients who have not yet developed anemia.

6.   Red cell volume is measured by injecting a known quantity of labeled red cells, sampling after waiting a suitable time for mixing in the circulation, resampling, and calculating a dilution factor. Plasma volume is measured in the same way, using a plasma label or a dye. The most popular red cell label is ^{51}Cr, a gamma-emitting isotope with a half-life of twenty-six days. A study at high altitude would require several weeks to ship equipment and supplies to the study site, and additional time to return, and as such it would result in such severe loss of radioactivity as to make systematic studies difficult.

7.   This method is based on the assumptions that all of the dye remains in the vascular system during the period of measurement, and that it is uniformly distributed in the circulation. These assumptions are only partially valid in most cases.

8.   The body hematocrit is the total red cell volume divided by the total blood volume. This value will deviate from the measured venous hematocrit if the capillary and large vessel hematocrits are different or if there is significant regional variation in hematocrit. Whether this is so in high-altitude natives is not known, but there is growing evidence for such regionalization in animals.

9.   The Farheaus effect refers to the tendency of the hematocrit to decrease as blood flows from a reservoir into tubes of smaller diameter. This property is not flow-rate dependent.

10.   *Relative, spurious,* or *Gaisbök's polycythemia* are terms used to indicate conditions in which the hematocrit is elevated by means of contracted plasma volume rather than by expanded red cell volume.

Chapter Four: The Structure and Function of Hemoglobin at High Altitudes

1. In this formula, α is the solubility coefficient for CO_2. Its value is temperature-dependent. The constant pK' is also temperature- and pH-dependent; therefore, the pH calculated from this formula is very sensitive to experimental error.

2. In the VanSlyke apparatus, gases are displaced from a known quantity of blood and measured using a mercury manometer.

3. The Adair equation used in these calculations relates oxygen pressure with hemoglobin saturation using four equilibrium constants for the successive reactions of oxygen with hemoglobin. This is only one of several useful methods of hemoglobin-oxygen binding.

4. The Bohr factor is a measure of the dependence of blood oxygen affinity on pH. It is expressed as the slope of the logP50-pH line.

Chapter Five: Circulation

1. The "indirect Fick" technique uses alveolar PCO_2 to estimate $PaCO_2$, and mixed venous PCO_2 is estimated by adjusting the inspired PCO_2 to a point at which CO_2 is neither taken up nor liberated in the lung. These values give $(a - \bar{v})CO_2$ from assumed blood CO_2 dissociation curves and, with $\dot{V}CO_2$, permit estimation of cardiac output.

2. According to this technique, the subject is forcibly ventilated with a mixture of O_2, air, and acetylene from an anesthesia bag. The bag contents are sampled at about 14 sec and 18 sec, and the rates of disappearance of O_2 and acetylene are calculated. The rate of O_2 uptake is estimated, and with the separately measured $\dot{V}O_2$, cardiac output is calculated. This method relies on the assumption that there is no recirculation during the time of the test. This is now known to be false, and this technique gives values lower than those obtained by the direct Fick technique.

Chapter Six: Ventilation

1. The residual volume is the volume of air in the lung that remains after the strongest possible expiration. It is, therefore, the total lung capacity minus the vital capacity. It cannot be measured directly but can be determined by indirect methods.

2. *Hypoxic ventilatory response* (HVR) is defined as the increase in ventilation that occurs in response to a given degree of hypoxia. As discussed later in the chapter, it is usually measured by rebreathing from an anesthesia bag and measuring the increase in ventilation as a function of decreasing PAO_2 while $PACO_2$ is held constant.

3. In order to measure directly the diffusing capacity for O_2, equation 6.1 requires measurement of $\dot{V}O_2$, PAO_2, and PcO_2. In practice, the PcO_2 must be the mean capillary PO_2, and measurement of this is not possible. This difficulty is circumvented by using CO as the test gas. When a small amount is given, it is taken up completely by hemoglobin because the affinity is two hundred times that for O_2, and the PcCO therefore can be assumed to be zero. Using the D_LCO derived in this

way, the D_LO_2 and D_LCO_2 can be calculated because they are 1.23 and 24.6 times more soluble than is CO.

4. Minute ventilation ($\dot{V}_E$) is defined as the amount of air at body temperature and pressure, saturated with water vapor (i.e., BTPS) exchanged by the lungs in one minute.

Chapter Ten: Bloodletting

1. Whether an alveolus exchanges gas depends on whether it is ventilated and perfused. The ventilation/perfusion ratio is the alveolar ventilation, $\dot{V}_A$, divided by the pulmonary capillary blood flow, $\dot{Q}_c$, the cardiac output. In normal, erect individuals, $\dot{V}_A/\dot{Q}_c = 4/5$ or $5/6$, with some variation from the bases of the lungs to the apices. Abnormalities, whether caused by ventilation or by perfusion, will impair gas exchange, particularly at high altitude, where alveolar PO_2 is reduced.

2. Normal mean pulmonary artery pressure at sea level is about 12 mm Hg, rising to about 18 mm Hg on severe exercise.

3. Hemodilution refers to the removal of red cells and replacement with a substitute such as a saline/albumin mixture. Phlebotomy, or simple bleeding, removes both red cells and plasma. The two techniques must be distinguished: the first should, in theory, leave the total blood volume unchanged, while in the second, blood volume initially contracts then is re-expanded by shifts of fluids between the various compartments of the body.

4. Note that this is not the same as maximal O_2 uptake, VO_{2max}, the usual measure of work capacity. These untrained subjects often stopped before VO_{2max} was reached.

5. Bulk viscosity refers to the viscosity measured in a standard glass viscometer. This is mainly a function of the hematocrit, and it should be appreciated that it is an in vitro property. In the intact animal, the actual, or effective, viscosity is a function of many other factors, such as local regulation of flow and pressure in individual capillary beds.

6. The minute ventilation usually increases linearly with $\dot{V}CO_2$ to a certain point, where the slope steepens. This point, the ventilatory threshold, is reproducible in an individual, and it may correspond to the anaerobic threshold, the point at which lactic acid begins to accumulate in the blood. Because there is some controversy in the literature about whether this point in fact corresponds to the anaerobic threshold, we use the more descriptive term, *ventilatory threshold.*

7. See chapter 6 for a discussion of the techniques for cardiac output measurement.

8. These studies report systolic and diastolic pressures. Because the pulmonary artery pressure does not follow a sine-wave pattern exactly, the true mean pressure is usually slightly less than the arithmetic mean. However, the difference is very small, and systolic/diastolic values of 23/15 mm Hg would give a mean pressure close to 19 mm Hg.

9. The VD/VT is the ratio of dead space to tidal volume. The dead space is the volume of gas that is inspired but does not reach alveoli. This volume includes the

mouth, throat, trachea, bronchi, and bronchiolar volumes, as well as the volume of the breathing value itself.

10. One form of the alveolar gas equation is

$$PaCO_2 = (\dot{V}CO_2 \times 0.863)/\dot{V}_A$$

11. The ejection fraction is the fraction of blood contained in the ventricles at the end of diastole that is ejected during systole.

Glossary

Acidosis   The result of any process which by itself adds excess CO_2 (respiratory acidosis) or nonvolatile acids (metabolic acidosis) to arterial blood. Acidemia does not necessarily result; compensating mechanisms (increase of HCO_3^- in respiratory acidosis, increase of ventilation and consequently decrease of arterial CO_2 in metabolic acidosis) may intervene to restore plasma pH to normal.

Alkalosis   The result of any process which, by itself, diminishes acids (respiratory alkalosis) or increases bases (metabolic alkalosis) in arterial blood.

$(a - \bar{v})O_2$ The difference between arterial and mixed venous blood-O_2 contents.

ATPS   Conditions of ambient temperature and pressure, saturated with water vapor.

AT   Anaerobic threshold, the exercise level at which lactic acid begins to accumulate in the arterial blood. This point roughly corresponds to the "ventilatory threshold," the point at which ventilation markedly increases with additional power output.

BE   Base excess, a measure of metabolic alkalosis or acidosis (negative values of base excess) expressed as the mEq of strong acid or strong alkali required to titrate a sample of 1 liter of oxygenated blood to a pH of 7.4 at $37°$ C, PCO_2 of 40 torr.

Blood viscosity   A measure of the "thickness" of the blood. Viscosity is usually measured in a rotating cone-and-plate viscometer or a glass viscometer at $37°$ C. The units of measure are centipoise, cp.

Body hematocrit   The "true" hematocrit: red cell volume (RCV) divided by total blood volume (TBV), the sum of red cell and plasma volumes.

Bohr effect   Dependence of O_2 saturation of hemoglobin on the H^+ concentration, or pH. Originally this term referred to the effect of CO_2, but modern usage refers only to the H^+ effect. An increase in the pH increases O_2 saturation of hemoglobin. The effect is usually expressed as $\Delta logPO_2/\Delta pH$ at a given saturation. For human blood at 10%–90% saturation, the Bohr effect at $37°$ C is about -0.48 for a ΔpH of 0.1 unit.

BTPS   Conditions of body temperature and barometric pressure, saturated with water vapor. These are the conditions existing in the gas phase of the lungs.

Cardiac output ($\dot{Q}$)   The volume of blood pumped by the heart, l/min.

Cardiac index (CI)   The cardiac output normalized for body size. The units are $l/min/m^2$.

CaO_2   Arterial O_2 content, ml/deciliter.

Chloride shift   (Hamburger effect.) The increase of red cell HCO_3^- concentration during CO_2 uptake results in a concentration gradient for HCO_3^- that favors diffusion of HCO_3^- from the red cells. In exchange, Cl^- diffuses from plasma into the red cells to maintain electroneutrality. Water also diffuses into the red cell, causing it to swell slightly.

Circulation time   Time between absorption of a substance in the venous blood and its appearance in the arterial circulation.

COPD   Chronic obstructive pulmonary disease, a term used to denote a loss of pulmonary function owing to long-term disease such as emphysema.

Cosm   Osmolav clearance.

Creatinine clearance   Rate of excretion of creatinine in the urine.

C$\bar{v}$O$_2$ Mixed venous O_2 content, usually obtained by sampling blood from the vena cava or the right atrium of the heart. Units are ml/deciliter.

D$_L$CO   Total lung diffusing capacity for CO. The diffusing capacities for O_2 and CO_2 are D$_L$CO$_2$ and D$_L$O$_2$. The amount of gas, commonly expressed as ml gas (STPD), diffusing between alveolar gas and pulmonary capillary blood per torr mean gas pressure difference per min, that is, ml O_2/(min × torr).

D$_M$CO   Membrane component of the diffusing capacity. Similar conventions for O_2 and CO_2 are used as for total lung diffusing capacities.

2,3-DPG   2,3-diphosphoglyceric acid, a glycolytic intermediate in the red cell that binds to hemoglobin to decrease its O_2 affinity.

ECG   Electrocardiogram.

ERBF   Effective renal blood flow.

ERPF   Effective renal plasma flow.

Erythropoietin   A hormone, produced in the human kidney, that stimulates erythropoiesis.

FEV$_1$ Forced expiratory volume in 1 sec, a measurement of pulmonary function. It is characteristically reduced in chronic obstructive pulmonary disease (see *COPD*).

FF   Filtration fraction of the kidney. The fractional amount of volume delivered to the kidney that is filtered.

Fick equation $Q = \dot{V}O_2/(a - \bar{v})O_2$, a fundamental relationship used in calculating the cardiac output in the steady state.

FIO$_2$ O_2 in inspired air, as a fraction.

FRC   Functional residual capacity (also functional residual air), the volume of gas remaining in the lungs at the resting expiratory level.

GFR   Glomerular filtration rate.

Hemodilution   Removal of blood and replacement with an equal volume of a plasma expander such as 5 percent albumin in saline. This is to be distinguished from simple phlebotomy because the blood volume is maintained.

HVR   Hypoxic ventilatory response, usually expressed as the increase in minute ventilation ($\dot{V}_E$) in response to decreasing inspired PO_2 (PIO_2).

Hematocrit   Fraction of blood that is red cells (%).

Hemoglobin   Concentration of hemoglobin in the blood, g/deciliter.

kpm   See *work*.

MCH   Mean corpuscular hemoglobin: hemoglobin/rbc.

MCHC   Mean corpuscular hemoglobin concentration: hemoglobin/hematocrit.

MCV   Mean corpuscular volume: hematocrit/rbc.

O$_2$ debt   Amount of oxygen consumed in excess of that taken up.

O$_2$ pulse O_2 taken up per heart beat. This is obtained by dividing the O_2 uptake ($\dot{V}O_2$) by the heart rate.

P50 PO_2 at which hemoglobin is half-saturated with O_2. For normal blood, P50 is about 28–29 torr at 37° C, pH 7.4, PCO_2 40 torr.

PA   Pulmonary artery.

PaCO$_2$ Arterial CO$_2$ partial pressure.
PACO$_2$ Alveolar CO$_2$ partial pressure.
PAH   Para-amino-hippurate, a compound used to measure the renal plasma flow (RPF).
PaO$_2$ Arterial O$_2$ partial pressure.
PAO$_2$ Alveolar O$_2$ partial pressure, often calculated from the alveolar air equation: PAO$_2$ = PIO − PaCO$_2$/R
PcCO$_2$ Capillary CO$_2$ partial pressure.
PcO$_2$ Capillary O$_2$ partial pressure.
PETCO$_2$ CO$_2$ partial pressure in end-tidal gas.
PECO$_2$ CO$_2$ partial pressure in the mixed expired gas.
PETO$_2$ O$_2$ partial pressure in end-tidal gas.
PEO$_2$ O$_2$ partial pressure in the mixed expired gas.
pHa   Arterial blood pH.
Phlebotomy   Removal of venous blood. This is to be distinguished from hemodilution, in that the blood volume is reduced and no replacement is provided.
PICO$_2$ CO$_2$ partial pressure in inspired gas.
P$_I$O$_2$ O$_2$ partial pressure in inspired gas.
Plethora   A clinical term used to describe an excess of blood. Subjects with plethora appear dull and red, with watery eyes and often with cyanotic (blue) lips.
Polycythemia vera   (Váquez's disease, polycythemia rubra vera.) A condition of overproduction of red blood cells in the bone marrow. Apparently production is autonomous because the rate is not related to hypoxia or the levels of erythropoietin, as it is in other states of increased red cell production.
PvO$_2$ Venous O$_2$ partial pressure.
P$\bar{v}$O$_2$ Mixed venous O$_2$ partial pressure.
PvCO$_2$ Venous CO$_2$ partial pressure.
P$\bar{v}$CO$_2$ Mixed venous CO$_2$ partial pressure.
$\dot{Q}$ Cardiac output.
$\dot{Q}$c   Capillary blood flow.
R   Respiratory quotient (non–steady state): $\dot{V}CO_2/\dot{V}O_2$.
rbc   Red blood cell count, usually expressed as millions of cells/mm^3.
RBF   Renal blood flow.
Red cell mass   Red cell volume, the volume of red cells in the body, ml/kg.
Residual air   Air remaining in the lungs after full expiration.
RPF   Renal plasma flow.
RQ   Respiratory quotient (steady state): $\dot{V}CO_2/\dot{V}O_2$.
SaO$_2$ Arterial saturation with O$_2$.
STPD   Conditions of standard temperature (0° C), pressure (760 torr), dry gas.
SV   Stroke volume, the volume of blood pumped from the heart in each ejection.
T^{c}H$_2$O   Maximal tubular free water clearance.
Thermodilution   A technique for the measurement of cardiac output in which a small quantity of iced saline is injected through a catheter in the pulmonary artery and detected at a distal site.
Tm   Tubular maximum capacity for reabsorption of a filtered substance. For example, the Tm for glucose (Tm$_G$) is 375 mg/min/1.73m^2.
Torr   Unit of measure for gas pressures, equal to 1 mm Hg.

Uosm   Urine solute concentration.

V   Volume.

V̇   Flow, volume/time.

V̇$_A$ Alveolar ventilation.

V̇$_A$/Q̇$_c$ Ventilation/perfusion ratio.

VC   Vital capacity, the maximal amount of air that can be inspired.

V̇CO$_2$ Rate of CO_2 production in the expired gas.

VD/VT   Ratio of dead space to tidal volume, often calculated by the equation
VD/VT = $(PaCO_2 - PECO_2)/(PaCO_2 - PICO_2)$.

V̇$_E$ Minute ventilation, usually expressed as 1/min (BTPS).

Vital capacity   See *VC*.

V̇O$_2$ Rate of O_2 uptake from the inspired gas, usually expressed as 1/min (STPD).

V̇O$_{2max}$ Maximal rate of O_2 uptake, defined as a rate that does not increase when the work rate is increased.

Work   The gravitational force acting on a stationary mass of 1 kg is 9.80 Newtons (N) and is equal to 1 kilopond (kp). A unit of work is done when a force of 1N acts through 1 meter and equals 1 Newton-meter, or 1 joule. When 1 kg is moved through a vertical distance of 1 meter against the force of gravity, the work performed is 9.80 joules, or 1 kilopond-meter (kpm). The external expression of work is power, expressed as work/time. This book uses the units kpm/min, but some authors also use watts. An approximate conversion is 600 kpm/min = 100 watts.

References

Abbrecht, P. H., and J. K. Littel (1972). Plasma erythropoietin in men and mice during acclimatization to different altitudes. *J. Appl Physiol* 32(1):54–58.

Acosta, J. de (1608). *Historia natural y moral de las Indias*. Madrid.

Adams, W. H., and S. M. Shresta (1974). Hemoglobin levels, vitamin B_{12}, and folate status in a Himalayan village. *Am J Cardiol* 27:217–19.

Adamson, J. W., A. Hayashi, G. Stamatoyannopoulos, and W. F. Burger (1972). Erythrocyte function and marrow regulation in hemoglobin bethesda (B145 histidine). *J Clin Invest* 51:2883–88.

Aggio, M. C., M. J. Montano, M. T. Bruzzo, and N. Giusto (1972). Possible inefficiency of polycythemia in tolerance to high altitude. *Acta Physiol Latinoam* 22:123–28.

Alexander, J. K., L. H. Hartley, M. Modelski, and R. F. Grover (1967). Reduction of stroke volume during exercise in man following ascent to 3,100 m altitude. *J Appl Physiol* 23(6):849–58.

Alippi, R. M., A. C. Giglio, A. C. Barcelo, C. E. Bozzini, R. Farina, and E. Rio (1979). Influence of dietary protein concentration and quality on response to erythropoietin in the polycythaemic rat. *Br J Haem* 43:451–56.

Altman, P. L., and D. S. Dittmer (1971). *Respiration and circulation*. Bethesda, Md.: Federation of American Societies of Experimental Biology.

Altschule, M. D., M. D. Volk, and H. Henstell (1940). Cardiac and respiratory function at rest in patients with uncomplicated polycythemia vera. *Amer J Med Sci* 200:478–483.

Anderson, T. W., J. R. Brown, J. W. Hall, and et al. (1968). The limitation of linear regression for the predictions of vital capacity and forced vital capacity. *Respiration* (Basel) 25:140–48.

Arias-Stella, J. (1969). Human carotid body at high altitudes. *Am J Cardiol* 55:82a.

Arias-Stella, J., and S. Recavarren (1973). On the pathology of chronic mountain sickness. *Path Microbiol* 39:283–86.

Arias-Stella, J., and M. Saldaña (1963). The terminal portion of the pulmonary arterial tree in people native to high altitudes. *Circulation* 28:915–28.

Arias-Stella, J., and M. Topilsky (1971). Anatomy of the coronary circulation at high altitude. *In* R. Porter and J. Knight (eds.): *High altitude physiology: Cardiac and respiratory aspects*. New York: Churchill Livingstone, pp. 149–57.

Arias-Stella, J., and J. Valcarcel (1973). The human carotid body at high altitudes. *Path Microbiol* 39:292–97.

Arias-Stella, J., H. Kruger, and S. Recavarren (1973). Pathology of chronic mountain sickness. *Thorax* 28:701–8.

Arnoud, J., J. C. Quilici, N. Guttierrez, J. Beard, and H. Vergnes (1979). Methaemoglobin and erythrocyte reducing systems in high-altitude natives. *Ann Hum Biol* 6:585–92.

Artigue, R. S., and W. A. Hyman (1976). The effect of myoglobin on the oxygen concentration in skeletal muscle subjected to ischemia. *Ann Biomed Eng* 4:128–37.

Aste-Salazar, H., and A. Hurtado (1944). The affinity of hemoglobin for oxygen at sea level and at high altitudes. *Am J Cardiol* 142:733–43.

Åstrand, I., P. O. Åstrand, I., Hallback, and A. Kilbom (1973). Reduction in maximal oxygen uptake with age. *J Appl Physiol* 35(5):649–54.

Åstrand, P., and I. Åstrand (1958). Heart rate during muscular work in man exposed to prolonged hypoxia. *J Appl Physiol* 13:75–79.

Auchincloss, J. H., R. Gilbert, and G. H. Baule (1966). Effect of ventilation on oxygen transfer during early exercise. *J Appl Physiol* 21:810–918.

Auckland, K. (1974). Renal blood flow. *In* K. Thurau and A. C. Guyton (eds.): *Kidney and urinary tract physiology II. International review of physiology.* Baltimore: University Park Press, pp. 23–80.

Balke, B. (1964). Work capacity and its limiting factors at high altitude. *In* W. H. Weihe (ed.): *The physiological effects of high altitude.* New York: Macmillan, pp. 233–47.

Banchero, N. (1983). Skeletal muscle capillarity in chronic hypoxia. *In* E. D. Chamberlayne and P. G. Condliffe (eds.): *Adjustment to high altitude.* Bethesda, Md.: U.S. Dept. of HHS, pp. 83–90.

Banchero, N., R. F. Grover, and J. A. Will (1971). Oxygen transport in the llama (*Lama glama*). *Resp Physiol* 13:102–15.

Banchero, N., S. R. Kayar, and A. J. Lechner (1985). Increased capillarity in skeletal muscle of growing guinea pigs acclimated to cold and hypoxia. *Resp Physiol* 62(2):245–56.

Banchero, N., F. Sime, D. Peñaloza, J. Cruz, R. Gamboa, and E. Marticorena (1966). Pulmonary pressure, cardiac output, and arterial oxygen saturation during exercise at high altitude and at sea level. *Circulation* 33:249–62.

Barbashova, Z. I. (1964). Cellular level of adaptation. *In* D. B. Dill, E. F. Adolph, and C. G. Wilber (eds.): *Handbook of physiology.* Baltimore: Williams and Wilkins, pp. 37–54.

Barclay-Piazza, P. A. (1982). *Perdida de la sensibilidad de los quimioreceptores de oxigeno en reatones de altura, comparacion con el humano.* B.Sc. thesis. Lima: Cayetano Heredia Univ.

Barclay-Piazza, P. A. (1983). *Control de la ventilación: Respuesta a la hiperoxia y a la hipercapnea en ratones de nivel del mar y sometidos a hipoxia hipobarica.* M.Sc. thesis. Lima: Cayetano Heredia Univ.

Barcroft, J. (1925). *The respiratory functions of the blood: Lessons from high altitude.* Cambridge: Cambridge Univ. Press, p. 176.

Barcroft, J. (1934). *Features in the architecture of physiological function.* London: Cambridge Univ. Press.

Barcroft, J., C. A. Binger, A. V. Bock, J. H. Doggart, H. S. Forbes, G. Harrop, J. C. Meakins, and A. C. Redfield (1923). Observations upon the effect of high altitude on the physiological processes of the human body carried out in the Peruvian Andes chiefly at Cerro de Pasco. *Philos Trans R Soc London Ser B* 211:351–480.

Baron, D. W., C. D. Ilsley, E. Sheiban, P. A. Poole-Wilson, and A. F. Rickards (1980). R wave amplitude during exercise: Relation to left ventricular function and coronary artery disease. *Br Heart J* 44:512–17.

Bartels, H., P. Hilpert, K. Barbey, K. Betke, K. Riegel, M. F. Lang, and J. Metcalfe (1963). Respiratory functions of blood of the yak, llama, camel, Dybowsky deer and African elephant. *Am J Physiol* 205:331–36.

Battaglia, P., G. Morpurgo, and S. Passi (1971). Variability of the Bohr effect in man. *Experientia* 27:321–22.

Battler, A., V. Froelicher, R. Slutsky, and W. Ashburn (1979). Relationship of QRS amplitude changes during exercise to left ventricular function and volumes and the diagnosis of coronary artery disease. *Circulation* 60:1004–13.

Bauer, J. H., L. R. Willis, R. W. Burt, and C. E. Grim (1975). Volume studies. II. Simultaneous determination of volume, red cell mass, extracellular fluid, and total water before and after volume expansion in dog and man. *J Lab Clin Med* 86(6):1009–17.

Beall, C. M. (1982). A comparison of chest morphology in high altitude Asian and Andean populations. *Hum Biol* 54(1):145–63.

Beall, C. M. (1983). Reappraisal of Andean high altitude erythrocytosis from a Himalayan perspective. *Sem Resp Med* 5(2):195–201.

Beall, C. M., and A. B. Reichsman (1984). Hemoglobin levels in a Himalayan high altitude population. *Am J Cardiol* 63:301–6.

Beaver, W. L., N. Lamarra, and K. Wasserman (1981). Breath-by-breath measurement of true alveolar gas exchange. *J Appl Physiol* 51(6):1662–75.

Becker, E. L., J. A. Schilling, and R. B. Harvey (1957). Renal function in man acclimatized to high altitude. *J Appl Physiol* 10:79–80.

Bencowitz, H. Z., P. D. Wagner, and J. B. West (1982). Effect of change in P_{50} on exercise tolerance at high altitude: A theoretical study. *J Appl Physiol* 53(6):1487–95.

Benesch, R., and R. E. Benesch (1969). Intracellular organic phosphates as regulators of oxygen release by haemoglobin. *Nature* 221:618–22.

Bergofsky, E. H.,and S. Holtzman (1967). A study of the mechanisms involved in the pulmonary arterial pressor response to hypoxia. *Circ Res* 20:506–19.

Berlin, N. I., J. H. Lawrence, and J. Gartland (1950). Blood volume in polycythemia as determined by P_{32} labeled red blood cells. *Am J Med* 9:747–51.

Bert, P. (1878). *La pressión barométrique*. Paris: Masson.

Bert, P. (1943). *Barometric pressure: Researches in experimental physiology.* Bethesda, Md.: Undersea Medical Society.

Bharadwaj, H. S., S. Verma, T. Zachariah, M. R. Bhatia, S. Kishnani, and M. S. Malhotra (1977). Estimation of body density and lean body weight from body measurements at high altitude. *Europ J Appl Physiol* 36:141–150.

Birgegard, G., O Miller, J. Caro, and A. Erslev (1982). Serum erythropoietin levels by radioimmunoassay in polycythemia. *Scand J Clin Invest* 29:161–67.

Biscoe, T. J. (1971). Carotid body: Structure and function. *Physiol Rev* 51:437–95.

Black, C. P., and S. M. Tenney (1980). Oxygen transport during progressive hypoxia in high altitude and sea level water fowl. *Resp Physiol* 39:217–39.

Blantz, R. C. (1977). Chap. 2, Glomerular filtration. *In* N. E. Kurtzman and M. Martinez-Maldonado (eds.): *Pathophysiology of the kidney.* Springfield, Ill.: Thomas, p. 65.

Bolton, W., and M. F. Perutz (1970). Three-dimensional fourier synthesis of horse deoxyhemoglobin at 2 Angstrom units resolution. *Nature* (London) 228:551–52.

Bonavía, D., F. León-Velarde, C. Monge C., M. Sánchez-Griñón, and J. Whittembury (1984). Tras las Huellas de Acosta 300 años después: Consideraciones sobre su descripción del "Mal de Altura." Universidad Católica, Lima. *Rev Hist Univ Catol.*

Bonavía, D., F. León-Velarde, C. Monge C., M. I. Sánchez-Griñón, and J. Whittembury (1985). Acute mountain sickness: Critical appraisal of the pariacaca story and on-site study. *Resp Physiol* 62:125–34.

Bradley, S. E., and G. P. Bradley (1945). Renal function during chronic anemia in man. *Blood* 2:192–202.

Brandfobrener, M., M. Landowne, and N. W. Shock (1955). Changes in cardiac output with age. *Circulation* 12:557–65.

Brody, D. A. (1956). A theoretical analysis of intracavitary blood mass influence on the heart-lead relationship. *Circ Res* 4:731–38.

Brooks, W. D. W. (1936). Circulatory adjustments in polycythemia rubra vera. *Proc Soc Roy Soc Med* 29:1379–83.

Brown, E. G., R. W. Krouskop, F. E. McDonnell, C. Monge C., F. Sarnquist, N. J. Winslow, and R. M. Winslow (1985). Simultaneous and continuous measurement of breath-by-breath oxygen uptake and arterial-venous oxygen content. *J Appl Physiol* 58:1138–39.

Buick, F. J., N. Gledhill, A. B. Froese, L. Spriet, and E. C. Meyers (1980). Effect of induced erythrocythemia on aerobic work capacity. *J. Appl Physiol* 48(4):636–42.

Bullard, R. W. (1972). Vertebrates at altitudes. *In* M. K. Yousef, S. M. Horvath, and R. W. Bullard (eds.): *Physiological adaptations: Deserts and mountains.* New York: Academic Press, pp. 209–25.

Bullard, R. W., C. Broumand, and F. R. Meyer (1966). Blood characteristics and volume in two rodents native to high altitude. *J Appl Physiol* 21:994–98.

Bulow, K. (1963). Respiration and wakefulness in man. *Acta Physiol Scand* sup 209:1–110.

Byrne-Quinn, E., I. E. Sodal, and J. V. Weil (1972). Hypoxic and Hypercapnic ventilatory drives in children native to high altitude. *J Appl Physiol* 32:44–46.

Cardich, A. (1960). Investigaciónes prehistóricas en los Andes Peruanos. *In* J. M. Baca (ed.): *Antigua Perú, espacio y teimpo.* Lima.

Cassin, S., R. D. Gilbert, C. F. Bunnell, and E. M. Johnson. (1971). Capillary development during exposure to chronic hypoxia. *Am J Physiol* 220:448–51.

Castle, W. B., and J. H. Jandl (1966). Blood viscosity and blood volume: Opposing influences upon oxygen transport in polycythemia. *Sem Hematol* 3(3):193–98.

Cerretelli, P. (1976). Limiting factors to oxygen transport on Mount Everest. *J Appl Physiol* 40(5):658–67.

Cerretelli, P. (1983). Energy metabolism during exercise at altitude. *In* E. D. Chamberlayne and P. G. Condliffe (eds.): *Adjustment to high altitude.* Bethesda, Md.: U.S. Dept. of HHS, pp. 61–64.

Cerretelli, P., and R. Debijadji (1964). Discussion. *In* W. H. Weihe (ed.): *The physiological effects of high altitude.* New York: MacMillan, pp. 242–47.

Chanutin, A., and R. R. Curnish (1967). Effect of organic and inorganic phosphates on the oxygen equilibrium curve of human erythrocyte. *Arch Biochem Biophys* 121:96–102.

Chapman, C. B., J. N. Fisher, and J. B. Sproule (1960). Behavior of stroke volume at rest and during exercise in human beings. *J Clin Invest* 39:1208–13.

Chedid, H., and W. Jao (1974). Hereditary tumors of the carotid bodies and chronic obstructive pulmonary disease. *Cancer* 33:1635–41.

Chiocchio, S. R., S. M. Hilton, H. J. Tramezzani, and P. Willshaw (1984). Loss of peripheral chemoreflexes to hypoxia after carotid body removal in the rat. *Resp Physiol* 57:235–46.

Chiodi, H. (1957). Respiratory adaptations to chronic high altitude hypoxia. *J Appl Physiol* 10(1):81–87.

Chiodi, H. (1970). Comparative study of the blood gas transport in high altitude and sea level camelidae and goats. *Resp Physiol* 11:84–93.

Chiodi, H. (1978). Aging and high altitude polycythemia. *J. Appl Physiol* 45: 1019–20.

Cohn, J. E., D. D. Carroll, B. W. Armstrong, R. H. Shephard, and R. L. Riley (1954). Maximal diffusing capacity of the lung in normal male subjects of different ages. *J Appl Physiol* 6:588–97.

Coindet, L. (1863). De l'acclimatement sur les altitudes du Mexique. *Gaz Hebd Med Chir* 10:817–21.

Cokelet, G. R. (1982). Speculation on a cause of low vessel hematocrits in the microcirculation. *Microcirculation* 2(1):1–18.

Collins, D. D., C. H. Scoggin, C. W. Zwillich, and J. V. Weil (1978). Hereditary aspects of decreased hypoxic response. *J Clin Invest* 62:105–110.

Correa, A. M. (1978). *Un modelo de hipoxia intermitente: Estudio en ratones de algunos prármetros sanguineos cerebrales.* B.Sc. thesis. Lima: Cayetano Heredia Univ.

Correa, A. M., C. Monge C., and J. Whittembury (1979). Hematología corporal y cerebral en ratones blancos aclimatados a la hipoxia hipobarica equivalente a 4500 m de altura. Abstracto no. 152. II *Journadas Cientivical*, Cayetano Heredia Univ.

Cosio, G. (1965). Trabajo minero a gran altura y los valores hemáticos. *Boletín, Instituto de Salud Occupacional*, Lima 10:5–12.

Cosio, G., and A. Yataco (1968). Valores de hemoglobins en relacion con la altura sobre el nivel del mar. *Rev Sal Occ* 13:5–17.

Crowell, J. W., and E. E. Smith (1966). Mathematical determination of the optimal hematocrit. *The Physiologist* 9:161.

Cruz, J. C., C. Diaz, E. Marticorena, and V. Hilario (1979). Phlebotomy improves pulmonary gas exchange in chronic mountain sickness. *Respiration* 38:305–13.

Cruz, J. C., and R. J. Zeballos (1975). Influencia racial sobre la respuesta ventilatoria a la hipoxia e hipercapnia. *Acta Physiol Latinoam* 25:23–32.

Cruz-Coke, R., A. P. Cristoffanini, M. Aspillaga, and F. Biancani (1966). Evolutionary forces in human population in an environmental gradient in Arica, Chile. *Hum Biol* 38:421–38.

Cuba-Caparó, A. (1950). *Policitemia y mal de montana en corderos.* M.D. thesis, Universidad Nacional Mayor de San Marcos. Lima: Editora Medica Peruana.

Cueva, S., H. Sillau, A. Valenzuela, H. Plog, and W. Cardenas (1970). Hipertensión pulmonar, hipertrofia cardiaca derecha y Mal de Altura en pollos parrilleros. *In* M. Moro and E. R. Zaldivar (eds.): *Cuarto boletín extraordinario.* Centro de Investigación IVITAUNM de San Marcos, Lima, pp. 142–46.

DeGraff, A. C., R. F. Grover, R. L. Johnson, J. W. Hammond, and J. M. Miller (1970). Increased diffusing capacity of the lung in persons native to 3,100 m in North America. *J Appl Physiol* 29(1):71–76.

Delgado, C. (1969). *Función de concentración renal en el habitante de la altura.* M.D. thesis, Lima, Peru: Cayetano Heredia Univ.

Dempsey, J. A., W. G. Reddan, M. L. Birnbaum, H. V. Forster, J. S. Thoden, R. F. Grover, and J. Rankin (1971). Effects of acute through life-long hypoxic exposure on exercise pulmonary gas exchange. *Resp Physiol* 13:62–89.

deWardener, H. E., R. P. McSwiney, and B. E. Miles (1951). Renal hemodynamics in primary polycythemia. *Lancet* 11:204–5.

Dhindsa, D. S., A. S. Hoversland, and J. Metcalfe (1971). Comparative studies of the respiratory functions of mammalian blood. VII. Armadillo (*Dasypus novemcinctus*). *Resp Physiol* 13:198–208.

Dill, D. B. (1973). Carlos Monge M. Dec 13, 1884–Feb. 15, 1970: Pioneer in Environmental Physiology. *The Physiologist* 16(1):103–9.

Dill, D. B. (1938). *Life, heat, and altitude: Physiological effects of hot climates and great heights.* Cambridge, Mass.: Harvard Univ. Press.

Dill, D. B., J. H. Talbott, and W. V. Consolazio (1937). Blood as a physiochemical system. XII. Man at high altitudes. *J Biol Chem* 118:649–66.

Dill, D. B., A. Graybill, A. Hurtado, and A. C. Taguini (1963). Gaseous exchange in the lungs in old age. *J Am Geriatr Soc* 11:1063–76.

diPrampero, P. E., P. Mognoni, and A. Veicsteinas (1981). The effect of hypoxia on maximal anaerobic alactic power in man. *In* W. Brendel and R. A. Zink (eds.): *High altitude physiology and medicine.* New York: Springer, pp. 88–93.

Doblar, D. D., V. Santiago, and N. H. Edleman (1977). Correlation between ventilatory and cerebrovascular responses to inhalation of CO. *J Appl Physiol* 43:455–62.

Douglas, G. S., and J. S. Haldane (1909). The cause of periodic or Cheyne-Stokes breathing. *J Physiol* 38:401.

Douglas, N. J., D. P. White, J. V. Weil, C. K. Pickett, R. J. Martin, D. W. Hudgel, and C. W. Zwillich (1982). Hypoxic ventilatory response decreases during sleep in normal men. *Am Rev Resp Dis* 125:286–89.

Durand, J., and J. P. Martineaud (1971). Resistance and capacitance of the skin in permanent and temporary residents at high altitude. In R. Porter and J. Knight (eds.): *High altitude physiology: Cardiac and respiratory aspects.* New York: Churchill Livingstone, pp. 159–70.

Eaton, J. W., T. D. Skelton, and E. Berger (1974). Survival at extreme altitude: Protective effect of increased hemoglobin-oxygen affinity. *Science* 185:743–44.

Edwards, C., D. Heath, and P. Harris (1971). The carotid body in emphysema and left ventricular hypertrophy. *J Path* 104:1–13.

Edwards, H. T. (1936). Lactic acid at rest and work at high altitude. *Am J Cardiol* 116:367–75.

Elsner, R. W., A. Bolstad, and C. Forno (1964). Maximum oxygen consumption of Peruvian Indians native to high altitude. *In* W. H. Weihe (ed.): *The physiological effects of high altitude.* New York: Macmillan, pp. 217–23.

Erslev, A. J. (1953). Humoral regulation of red cell production. *Blood* 8:349–57.

Erslev, A. J. (1981). Erythroid adaptation to altitude. *Blood Cells* 7:495–508.

Erslev, A. J., F. Caro, and A. Besarab (1985). Why the kidney: *Nephron* 41:213–16.

Erslev, A. J., J. Caro, R. Silver, and O. Miller (1981). The biogenesis of erythropoietin. *Exp Hemat* 8:1–13.

Erslev, A. J., P. J. McKenna, J. P. Copelli, R. J. Hamburger, H. E. Cohn, and J. E. Clark (1968). The rate of red cell production in two nephrectomized patients. *Arch Int Med* 122:230–35.

Espinos, D., J. L. Alvarez-Sala, and A. Villegas (1982). Relationship of red-cell 2,3-diphosphoglycerate with anemia, hypoxaemia and acid-base status in patients with cirrhosis of the liver. *Scand J Clin Invest* 42:613–16.

Fan, F. C., R. Y. Z. Chen, G. Schuessler, and S. Chien (1980). Effects of hematocrit variations on regional hemodynamics and oxygen transport in the dog. *Am J Physiol* 238:H545–52.

Farley, R. D., and J. F. Case (1968). Perception of external oxygen by the burrowing shrimp, *Callianassa californiensis Dana* and *C. affinis Dana*. *Biol Bull* 134:261–65.

Faura, J., J. Ramos, C. Reynarfarje, E. English, P. Finne, and C. Finch (1969). Effect of altitude on erythropoiesis. *Blood* 33(5):668–76.

Fernán-Zegarra, L., and F. Lazo-Toboada (1961). Mal de montana crónico. Consideraciones anatomopatologicas y referencias clinicos de un caso. *Revista Peruana de Cardiologia* 6:49.

Fishman, A. P., J. McClement, A. Himmelstein, and A. Cournand (1952). Effects of acute anoxia on the circulation and respiration in patients with chronic pulmonary disease studied during the "steady state." *J Clin Invest* 31:770–81.

Forster, R. E. (1964). Diffusion of gases. In W. O. Fern and H. Rahn (eds.): *Handbook of physiology, Respiration 1*. pp. 839–72. Washington, D.C.: American Physiological Society.

Frisancho, A. R. (1975). Functional adaptation to high altitude hypoxia. *Science* 187:313–19.

Frisancho, A. R., G. A. Borkan, and J. E. Klayman (1976). Pattern of growth of lowland and highland Peruvian Quechua of similar composition. *Hum Biol* 47:233–43.

Fulwood, R., C. L. Johnson, J. D. Bryner, E. W. Gunter, and C. R. McGrath (1982). *Hematological and nutritional biochemistry reference data for persons 6 months–74 years of age: United States, 1976–80*. DHHS Publication No. (PHS) 83–1682, National Center for Health Statistics.

Garruto, R. M., and J. S. Dutt (1983). Lack of prominent compensatory polycythemia in traditional native Andeans living at 4,200 meters. *Am J Cardiol* 61:355–66.

Garruto, R. M., and C. J. Hoff (1976). Genetic affinities and history. *In* P. T. Baker and M. A. Little (eds.): *Man in the Andes*. Stroudsburg, Pa.: Dowden, Hutchinson, and Ross, pp. 98–114.

Gayeski, E. J., and C. R. Honig (1978). Myoglobin saturation and calculated PO_2 in single cells of resting gracilis muscles. *In* I. A. Silver, M. Erecinska, and H. I. Bicher (eds.): *Advances in experimental medicine and biology. Oxygen transport to tissue—III*. New York: Plenum, pp. 77–84.

Giezendanner, P., P. Cerretelli, and P. E. DiPrampero (1983). Breath-by-breath alveolar gas exchange. *J Appl Physiol* 55(2):583–90.

Gilbert, D. L. (1983a). The first documented report of mountain sickness: The China or headache mountain story. *Resp Physiol* 52:315–26.

Gilbert, D. L. (1983b). The first documented description of mountain sickness: The Andean or Periacaca story. *Resp Physiol* 52:327–47.

Glaser, E. M., and J. McMichael (1940). Effect of venesection at the capacity of the lungs. *Lancet* 2:230–31.

Goldsmith, G. (1936). Cardiac output in polycythemia vera. *Arch Int Med* 58:1041–47.

Gonzales, E. (1971). *Hemodinámica renal en el nativo de altura estudiado a nivel del mar.* M.D. thesis. Lima: Peru: Cayetano Heredia Univ.

Grollman, A. (1932). *The cardiac output of man in health and disease.* Baltimore: Charles C. Thomas.

Grover, R. F., R. Lufchanowski, and J. K. Alexander (1971). *Hypoxia, high altitude, and the heart.* Basel: Karger.

Grover, R. F., J. T. Reeves, E. B. Grover, and J. E. Leathers (1967). Muscular exercise in young men native to 3,100 m altitude. *J Appl Physiol* 22(3):555–64.

Grover, R. F., J. T. Reeves, D. H. Will, and S. G. Blount (1963). Pulmonary vasoconstriction in steers at high altitude. *J Appl Physiol* 18:567–74.

Gupta, R., and A. Basu (1981). Variations in body dimensions in relation to altitude among the Sherpas of the eastern Himalayas. *Ann Hum Biol* 8(2):145–51.

Guyton, A. C., and T. Q. Richardson (1961). Effect of hematocrit on venous return. *Circ Res* 9:157–64.

Guyton, A. C., C. E. Jones, and T. G. Coleman (1973). *Cardiac output and its regulation.* 2nd ed. Philadelphia: Saunders.

Hackett, P., J. T. Reeves, C. D. Reeves, R. F. Grover, and D. Rennie (1980). Control of breathing in Sherpas at low and high altitude. *J Appl Physiol* 49:374–79.

Hackett, P. H., J. T. Reeves, R. F. Grover, and J. V. Weil (1984). Ventilation in human populations native to high altitude. *In* J. B. West and S. Lahiri (eds.): *Man at high altitude.* Bethesda, Md.: American Physiological Society, pp. 179–91.

Haldane, J. S., and J. G. Priestley (1905). The regulation of the lung—ventilation. *J Physiol* 32:225–66.

Hall, F. G. (1937). Adaptations of mammals to high altitudes. *J Mammol* 18:468–72.

Hall, F. G., D. B. Dill, and E. S. G. Barron (1936). Comparative physiology in high altitudes. *J Cell Comp Physiol* 8:301–13.

Halvorsen, S. (1966). The central nervous system in regulation of erythropoiesis. *Acta Haemat* 35:65–79.

Hamilton, W. F. (1964). Measurement of the cardiac output. *Handbook of physiology,* sec. 2, "Circulation," pp. 551–84.

Harris, P., and D. Heath (1977). *The human pulmonary circulation: Its form and function in health and disease.* Edinburgh: Churchill Livingstone.

Harrop, G. A., and E. H. Heath (1927). Pulmonary gas diffusion in polycythemia vera. *J Clin Invest* 4:53–70.

Hartley, L. H., J. K. Alexander, M. Modelski, and R. F. Grover (1967). Subnormal cardiac output at rest and during exercise at 3,100 m altitude. *J Appl Physiol* 23(6):839–48.

Haselton, P. S. (1972). The internal surface area in normal and emphysematous lungs. *J Path* 106:3.

Heath, D. (1971). Discussion. In R. Porter and J. Knight (eds.): *High altitude physiology: Cardiac and respiratory aspects*. Edinburgh: Churchill Livingstone, pp. 54–55.

Heath, D., and D. R. Williams (1981). *Man at high altitude*. Edinburgh: Churchill Livingstone.

Hebbel, R. P., J. W. Eaton, R. S. Kronenberg, E. D. Zanjani, L. G. Moore, and E. M. Berger (1978). Human llamas: Adaptation to altitude in subjects with high hemoglobin oxygen affinity. *J Clin Invest* 62:593–600.

Hebbel, R. P., R. S. Kronenberg, and J. W. Eaton (1977). Hypoxic ventilatory responses in subjects with normal and high oxygen affinity hemoglobins. *J Clin Invest* 60:1211–15.

Hecht, H. H., and J. H. McClement (1958). A case of "chronic mountain sickness" in the United States. *Am J Med* 25:470–77.

Hecht, H. H., H. Kuida, R. L. Lange, J. L. Thorne, and A. M. Brown (1962). Brisket disease II. Clinical features and hemodynamic observations in altitude-dependent right heart failure of cattle. *Am J Cardiol* 32:171–83.

Heistad, D. D., M. L. Marcus, J. C. Ehrhardt, and F. M. Abboud (1976). Effect of stimulation of carotid chemoreceptors on total and regional cerebral flow. *Circ Res* 38:20–25.

Hill, A. V. (1910). The possible effects of the aggregation of the molecules of hemoglobin on its oxygen dissociation curve. *J. Physiol* 40:4–7.

Holland, R. A. B., and R. E. Forster (1966). The effect of size of red cells on the kinetics of their oxygen uptake. *J Gen Physiol* 49:727–42.

Hoon, R. S., V. Balasubramanian, O. P. Mathew, S. C. Tiwari, S. C. Sharma, and K. S. Chadha (1977). Effect of high-altitude exposure for 10 days on stroke volume and cardiac output. *J Appl Physiol* 42(5):722–27.

Horvath, S. M., and J. F. Borgia (1984). Cardiopulmonary gas transport and aging. *Am Rev Resp Dis* sup 129:s68–s71.

Horvath, S. M., H. Chiodi, S. H. Ridgway, and S. Azar (1968). Respiratory and electrophoretic characteristics of hemoglobins of porpoises and sea lions. *Comp Biochem Physiol* 24:1027–33.

Horvath, S. M., A. Malenfant, F. Rossi, and L. Rossi-Bernardi (1977). The oxygen affinity of concentrated human hemoglobin solutions and human blood. *Am J Cardiol* 2:343–54.

Horwitz, L. D., J. M. Atkins, and S. J. Leshin (1972). Role of the Frank-Starling mechanism in exercise. *Circ Res* 31:868–75.

Huang, S. Y., X. H. Ning, Z. N. Zhou, Z. Z. Gu, and S. T. Hu (1984). Ventilatory function in adaptation to high altitude: Studies in Tibet. *In* J. B. West and S. Lahiri (eds.): *High altitude and man*. Bethesda, Md.: American Physiological Society, pp. 173–77.

Humphrey, P. R. D., J. Marshall, R. W. RossRussell, G. Wetherley-Mein, G. H. DuBoulay, T. C. Pearson, L. Symon, and E. Zulkha (1979). Cerebral blood-flow and viscosity in relative polycythaemia. *Lancet* (Oct):873–77.

Humphrey, P. R. D., J. Michael, and T. C. Pearson (1980). Red cell mass, plasma volume, and blood volume before and after venesection in relative polycythemia. *Brit J Haem* 46:435–38.

Hurtado, A. (1932a). Studies at high altitude: Blood observations on the Indian natives of the Peruvian Andes. *Am J Physiol* 100:487–505.

Hurtado, A. (1932b). Respiratory adaptations in the Indian natives of the Peruvian Andes. *Am J Cardiol* 17:137–65.

Hurtado, A. (1942). Chronic mountain sickness. *J Am Med Assoc* 120:1278–80.

Hurtado, A. (1960). Some clinical aspects of life at high altitudes. 53:247–58.

Hurtado, A. (1964). Animals in high altitudes: Resident man. *In* Dill, D. B. (ed.): *Handbook of physiology,* 843–60. Adaptation to the environment. Washington, D.C.: Am Physiol. Soc.

Hurtado, A. (1971a). Discussion of paper by S. Lahiri. *In* R. Porter and J. Knight (eds.): *High altitude physiology: Cardiac and respiratory aspects.* Edinburgh: Churchill Livingstone, p. 112.

Hurtado, A. (1971b). The influence of high altitude on physiology. *In* R. Porter and J. Knight (eds.): *High altitude physiology: Cardiac and respiratory aspects.* Edinburgh: Churchill Livingstone, pp. 3–13.

Hurtado, A., C. F. Merino, and D. Delgado (1945). Influence of anoxemia on erythropoietic activity. *Arch Int Med* 75:284–323.

Hurtado, A., T. Velásquez, C. Reynafarje, R. Lozano, R. Chavez, H. Aste-Salazar, B. Reynarfarje, S. Sánchez, and J. Munoz (1956). Mechanisms of natural acclimatization: Studies on the native resident of Morococha, Peru, at an altitude of 14,900 feet. Report 56-1 to the Air University, School of Aviation Medicine, USAF, Randolph AFB, Texas. P. 57.

Isaacs, R. (1923). Pathologic physiology of polycythemia vera. *Arch Int Med* 31:289.

Isaaks, R. E., and D. R. Harkness (1980). Erythrocyte organic phosphates and hemoglobin function in birds, reptiles and fishes. *Am Zool* 20:115–29.

Isaaks, R. E., and D. R. Harkness (1983). Erythrocyte organic phosphates and hemoglobin function in domestic mammals. *In* N. S. Agar and P. G. Board (eds.): *Red blood cells of domestic mammals.* Amsterdam: Elsevier Science Pubs., pp. 315–37.

Jacobson, L. O., E. Goldwasser, W. Freed, and L. Plzak (1957). Role of the kidney in erythropoiesis. *Nature* (London) 179:633–34.

Johnson, R. L., S. S. Cassidy, R. F. Grover, J. E. Schutte, and R. H. Epstein (1985). Functional capacities of lungs and thorax in beagles after prolonged residence at 3,100 m. *J Appl Physiol* 59(6):1773–82.

Jones, N. L. (1976). Use of exercise in testing respiratory control mechanisms. *Chest* 70:169–73.

Jorfeldt, L., and J. Wahren (1971). Leg blood flow during exercise in man. *Clinical Science* 41:459–73.

Jourdanet, D. (1863). *De l'anemie des altitudes et de l'anemie en general dans ses rapports avec la pressión de l'atmosphere.* Paris: Balliere, p. 44.

Kannel, W. B., T. Gordon, P. A. Wolf, and P. McNamara (1972). Hemoglobin and the risk of cerebral infarction: The Framingham study. *Stroke* 3(4):409–20.

Katz, A. M. (1977). *Physiology of the heart.* New York: Raven Press.

Kentala, E., J. Heikkila, and K. Pyorala (1973). Variation of QRS amplitude in exercise ECG as an index predicting result of physical training in patients with coronary heart disease. *Acta Med Scand* 194:81–86.

Keys, A. (1936). The physiology of life at high altitudes: The international high altitude expedition to Chile, 1935. *Sci Month* (Oct): 289–311.

King, A. B., and S. M. Robinson (1972). Ventilation response to hypoxia and acute mountain sickness. *Aerosp Med* 43:419–21.

Klein, H. (1983). Isovolemic hemodilution in high-altitude polycythemia. *In* E. D. Chamberlayne and P. G. Condliffe (eds.): *Adjustment to high altitude*. NIH Pub. no. 83-2496, U.S. Dept. of HHS. Bethesda, Md.: USPHS, pp. 47–52.

Koller, L. D., J. H. Exon, and J. E. Nixon (1979). Polycythemia produced in rats by environmental contaminants. *Arch Environ Health* 34:252–55.

Kollias, J., E. R. Buskirk, R. F. Akers, E. K. Prokop, P. T. Baker, and E. Picon-Reátegui (1968). Work capacity of long-time residents and newcomers to altitude. *J Appl Physiol* 24(6):792–99.

Kreuzer, F., M. Tenney, J. C. Mithoefer, and J. Remmers (1964). Alveolar arterial oxygen gradient in Andean natives at high altitude. *J Appl Physiol* 19:13–16.

Kryger, M. H., and R. F. Grover (1983). Chronic mountain sickness. *In* T. L. Petty and R. M. Cherniack (eds.): *Seminars in respiratory medicine*. Vol. 5, Man at Altitude. New York: Thieme-Stratton, pp. 164–68.

Kryger, M. H., R. D. Glas, R. E. Jackson, D. McCullough, C. H. Scoggin, R. F. Grover, and J. V. Weil (1978a). Impaired oxygenation during sleep in excessive polycythemia of high altitude: Improvement with respiratory stimulation. *Sleep* 1:3–17.

Kryger, M. H., R. E. McCullough, D. Collins, C. H. Scoggin, J. V. Weil, and R. F. Grover (1978b). Treatment of excessive polycythemia of high altitude with respiratory stimulant drugs. *Am Rev Resp Dis* 1217:455–64.

Kryger, M. H., R. E. McCullough, R. Doekel, D. Collins, J. V. Weil, and R. F. Grover (1978c). Excessive polycythemia of high altitude: Role of ventilatory drive and lung disease. *Am Rev Resp Dis* 118:659–66.

Lahiri, S. (1971). Genetic aspects of the blunted chemoreflex ventilatory response to hypoxia in high altitude adaptation. *In* R. Porter and J. Knight (eds.): *High altitude physiology: Cardiac and respiratory aspects*. Edinburgh: Churchill Livingstone, pp. 103–24.

Lahiri, S., and J. S. Milledge (1965). Sherpa physiology. *Nature* (London) 207: 610–12.

Lahiri, S., K. Maret, and M. G. Sherpa (1983). Dependence of high altitude apnea on ventilatory sensitivity to hypoxia. *Resp Physiol* 52:281–301.

Lahiri, S., J. S. Milledge, G. P. Chattopadhyay, A. K. Bhattacharyya, and A. K. Sinha (1967). Respiration and heart rate of Sherpa highlanders during exercise. *J Appl Physiol* 23(4):545–54.

Lahiri, S., R. G. Delaney, J. S. Brody, M. Simpser, T. Velásquez, E. K. Motoyama, and C. Polgar (1976). Relative role of environmental and genetic factors in respiratory adaptation to high altitude. *Nature* (London) 261:133–35.

Lahiri, S., J. S. Brody, E. K. Motoyama, and T. M. Velásquez (1978). Regulation of breathing in newborns at high altitude. *J Appl Physiol* 4(5):673–78.

Lahiri, S., K. Maret, M. G. Sherpa, and R. M. Peters (1984). Sleep and periodic breathing at high altitude: Sherpa natives vs sojourners. *In* J. B. West and S. Lahiri (eds.): *Man at high altitude,* Bethesda, Md.: American Physiological Society, pp. 73–90.

Lanning, E. P. (1965). Early man in Peru. *Sci Am* 223:68–76.

Larsen, O. A., and N. A. Lassen (1964). Cerebral hematocrit in normal man. *J Appl Physiol* 19:571–74.

Lasker, G. W. (1962). Differences in anthropometric measurements within and between three communities in Peru. *Hum Biol* 34:63–70.

Lawson, H. C. (1964). The volume of blood—A critical examination of methods for its measurement. *Handbook on physiology Circulation 1,* 23–49. Washington, D.C.: American Physiological Society.

Lenfant, C., J. D. Torrance, and C. Reynafarje (1971). Shift of the O_2-dissociation curve at altitude: mechanism and effect. *J Appl Physiol* 30(5):625–31.

Lenfant, C., P. Ways, C. Aucutt, and J. Cruz (1969). Effect of chronic hypoxic hypoxia on the O_2-Hb dissociation curve and respiratory gas transport in man. *Resp Physiol* 7:7–29.

Lertzman, M., B. M. Frome, L. G. Israels, and R. M. Cherniak (1964). Hypoxia in polycythemia vera. *Ann Int Med* 60: 409–17.

Levine, B. A., and K. R. Sirinek (1981). Cardiac output determination by thermodilution technique: The method of choice in low flow states. *Proc Soc Exp Biol Med* 167:279–83.

Lichty, J. A., R. Y. Ting, P. D. Bruns, and E. Dyar (1957). Studies of babies born at high altitude. I. Relation of altitude to birth weight. *Am J Dis Child* 93:666–69.

Loew, P. G., and G. Thews (1962). Die altersabhangigkeit des arteriellen saurstoffdruckes bei der berufsatigen bevolkerung (The dependency of age for arterial oxygen pressure in working population). *Klin Woch* 40 (21):1093–98.

Lozano, R., and C. Monge C. (1965). Renal function in high-altitude natives and in natives with chronic mountain sickness. *J Appl Physiol* 20(5):1026–27.

Lozano, R., C. Torres, C. Marchena, J. Whittembury, and C. Monge C. (1969). Response to metabolic (ammonium chloride) acidosis at sea level and at high altitude. *Nephron* 6:102–9.

Lutz, P. L., I. S. Longmuir, and K. Schmidt-Nielsen (1974). Oxygen affinity of bird blood. *Resp Physiol* 20:325–30.

MacNeish, R. S. (1971). Early man in the Andes. *Sci Am* 224:36–46.

Manoach, M., S. Gitter, E. Grossman, D. Varon, and S. Gassner (1971). Influence of hemorrhage on the QRS complex of the electrocardiogram. *Am Heart J* 82(1):55–61.

McCullough, R. E., J. T. Reeves, and R. L. Liljegren (1977). Fetal growth retardation and increased infant mortality at high altitude. *Arch Environ Health* 32: 36–39.

McGrath, J. J. (1971). Acclimation response of pigeons to simulated high altitude. *J Appl Physiol* 9:191–97.

McVergnes, J. P., M. D. Blayo, J. Coudert, G. Autezani, P. Dediu, and J. Duvand (1973). Cerebral blood flow and metabolism in high altitude residents. *Stroke* 4:345–50.

Mela, L., and M. Wagner (1983). Adaptation of mitrochondrial metabolism to hypoxia. *In* E. D. Chamberlayne and P. G. Condliffe (eds.): *Adjustment to high al-*

titude. NIH Pub. no. 83-2493, U.S. Dept. of HHS. Bethesda, Md.: USPHS, pp. 91–94.

Merino, C. F. (1950). Studies on blood formation and destruction in the polycythemia of high altitude. *Blood* 5(1):1–31.

Merino, C. F. (1956). *The plasma erythropoietic factor in the polycythemia of high altitudes.* Report 56-103 to the Air University, School of Aviation Medicine, USAF, Randolph AFB, Texas. p. 103.

Merino, C. F., and C. Reynafarje (1952). Bone marrow studies in the polycythemia of high altitudes. *J Lab Clin Med* 142:637–47.

Messmer, K. (1975). Hemodilution. *Surg Clin N Am* 55(3):659–78.

Milledge, J. S., and P. M. Cotes (1985). Serum erythropoietin in humans at high altitude and its relation to plasma renin. *J Appl Physiol* 59:360–64.

Milledge, J. S., and S. C. Sørensen (1972). Cerebral arteriovenous oxygen difference in man native to high altitude. *J Appl Physiol* 32:687–89.

Mirand, E. A., and G. P. Murphy (1971). Erythropoietin alterations in human liver disease. *NY St J Med* 71:860–64.

Monge M., C. (1937). High altitude disease. *Arch Int Med* 59: 32–40.

Monge, M., C. (1929). *Les erythremias de l'altitude: Les rapports avec la maladie de Váquez. Etude physiologique et pathologique.* Paris: Masson et Cie.

Monge M., C. (1925). Sobre un caso de enfermedad de Váquez. Communicacion presentada a la Academia Nacional de Medicina, Lima. pp. 1–6.

Monge M., C. (1928). La enfermedad de los Andes. *Anales de la Facultad de Mecicina,* Universidad de Lima. pp. 1–309.

Monge M., C., and C. Monge C. (1966). *High altitude diseases: Mechanism and management.* Springfield, Ill.: Charles C. Thomas.

Monge M., C. (1942). Life in the Andes and chronic mountain sickness. *Science* 95(2456):79–84.

Monge M., C. (1948). *Acclimatization in the Andes: Historical confirmation of "Climatic Aggression" in the development of Andean man.* Baltimore: Johns Hopkins Press.

Monge C., C. (1983). Hemoglobin regulation in hypoxemic polycythemia. *In* E. D. Chamberlayne and P. G. Condliffe (eds.): *Adjustment to high altitude.* U.S. Dept. of HHS. Bethesda, Md.: USPHS pp. 53–56.

Monge C., C., and C. Monge M. (1968). Adaptation of domestic animals. *In* E. S. E. Hafez (ed.): *Adaptation of domestic animals.* Philadelphia: Lea and Febiger, pp. 194–201.

Monge C., C., and J. Whittembury (1974). Increased hemoglobin oxygen affinity at extremely high altitudes. *Science* 186:843.

Monge C., C., and J. Whittembury (1976a). High altitude adaptations: Whole animal. *In* J. Bligh, J. L. Cloudsley-Thompson, and A. G. Macdonald (eds.): *The environmental physiology of animals.* London: Blackwell Scientific Pub., pp. 289–308.

Monge C., C., and J. Whittembury (1976b). Chronic mountain sickness. *Johns Hopkins Med J* 139:87–89.

Monge C., C., and J. Whittembury (1982). Chronic mountain sickness and the physiopathology of hypoxemic polycythemia. *In* J. R. Sutton, N. L. Jones, and

C. S. Houston (eds.); *Hypoxia: Man at altitude*. New York: Thieme-Stratton, Inc., pp. 51–56.

Monge, C., C., R. Lozano, and A. Carcelén (1964). Renal excretion of bicarbonate in high altitude natives and in natives with chronic mountain sickness. *J Clin Invest* 43(12):2303–9.

Monge C., C., R. Lozano, and J. Whittembury (1965). Effect of blood-letting on chronic mountain sickness. *Nature* (London) 207:770.

Monge C., C., A. Cazorla, G. Whittembury, Y. Sakata, and C. Rizo-Patron (1955). A description of the circulatory dynamics in the heart and lungs of people at sea level and at high altitude by means of the dye dilution technique. *Acta Physiol Latinoam* 5:189–210.

Monge C., C., R. Lozano, C. Marchena, J. Whittembury, and C. Torres (1969). Kidney function in the high-altitude native. *Fed Proc* 28:1199–1203.

Moore, L. G., and G. J. Brewer (1981). Beneficial effect of rightward hemoglobin-oxygen dissociation curve shift for short-term high altitude adaptation. *J Lab Clin Med* 98(1):145–54.

Moore, L. G., P. Brodeur, O. Chumbe, J. D'Brot, S. Hofmeister, and C. Monge (1986). Maternal ventilation, hypoxic ventilatory response in infant birth weight during high altitude pregnancy. *J Appl Physiol* 60:1401–60.

Moore, L. G., S. S. Rounds, D. Jahnigen, R. F. Grover, and J. T. Reeves (1986). Infant birth weight is related to maternal arterial oxygenation at high altitude. *J Appl Physiol* 52:695–99.

Moret, P. R. (1971). Coronary blood flow and myocardial metabolism in man at high altitude. *In* R. Porter and J. Knight (eds.): *High altitude physiology: Cardiac and respiratory aspects*. Edinburgh: Churchill Livingstone, pp. 131–48.

Moret, P. R., E. Cobarrubias, J. Coudert, and F. Duchosal (1972). Cardiocirculatory adaptation to chronic hypoxia. III. Comparative study of CO, pulmonary and systemic circulation between sea level and high altitude residents. *Acta Cardiol* 27:596–619.

Morpurgo, G., P. Arese, A. Bosia, G. P. Pescarmona, M. Luzzana, J. G. Modiano, and S. R. Ranjit (1976). Sherpas living permanently at high altitude: A new pattern of adaptation. *Proc Nat Acad Sci* (Washington, D.C.) 73:747–51.

Morpurgo, G., P. Battaglia, L. Bernini, A. M. Paolucci, and G. Modiano (1970). Higher Bohr effect in Indian natives of Peruvian highlands as compared with Europeans. *Nature* (London) 227:387–89.

Morpurgo, G., P. Battaglia, N. D. Carter, G. Modiano, and S. Passi (1972). The Bohr effect and the red cell 2,3-DPG and Hb content in Sherpas and Europeans at low and high altitude. *Experientia* 28:1280–84.

Morrison, P., and R. Elsner (1962). Influence of altitude on heart and breathing rates in some Peruvian rodents. *J Appl Physiol* 17:467–70.

Morrison, P. R., K. Kerst, C. Reynafarje, and J. Ramos (1963). Hematocrit and hemoglobin levels in some Peruvian rodents from high and low altitudes. *Int J Biometeor* 7:51–58.

Muños, M. S. (1983). *Equilibriu ácido-básico en ratones sometidos a hipoxia inter-mitente*. M.Sc. thesis. Lima: Cayetano Heredia Univ.

Naeraa, N., E. S. Peterson, E. Boye, and J. W. Severinghaus (1966). pH and

Reynafarje, C., J. Faura, A. Paredes, and D. Villavicencio (1968). Erythrokinetics in high-altitude adapted animals (Llama, alpaca, vicuña). *J Appl Physiol* 24:93–97.

Reynafarje, C., J. Ramos, J. Faura, and D. Villavicencio (1964). Humoral control of erythropoietic activity in man during and after altitude exposure. *Proc Soc Exp Biol Med* 116:649–50.

Rich, I. N., and B. Kubanek (1980). Release of erythropoietin from macrophages mediated by phagocytosis of crystalline silica. *J Reticuloendothel Soc* 31(1): 17–30.

Richardson, T. Q., and A. C. Guyton (1959). Effect of polycythemia and anemia on cardiac output and other circulatory factors. *Am J Cardiol* 197:1167–70.

Richter, T., J. R. West, and A. J. Fishman (1957). The syndrome of alveolar hypoventilation and diminished sensitivity of the respiratory center. *N Engl J Med* 256:1165–70.

Riegel, K. P. (1980). Blood volume and hematocrit in various organs in newborn piglets. *Ped Res* 14:1324–27.

Robinson, S. (1938). Experimental studies of physical fitness in relation to age. *Arbeitsphysiol* 10:251.

Rodman, T., and H. P. Chase (1959). The primary hyperventilation syndrome. *Am J Cardiol* 26:808–17.

Root, W. S., F. J. W. Roughton, and M. I. Gregersen (1946). Simultaneous determinations of blood volume by CO and dye (T1824) under various conditions. *Am J Physiol* 146:739–55.

Rossi-Fanelli, A., and E. Antonini (1958). Studies on the oxygen and carbon monoxide equilibrium of human myoglobin. *Arch Biochem Biophys* 77:478–79.

Rothammer, I., and W. J. Schull (1982). Adaptación genética a la altura en una población de habla Aymara de las provincias de Parinacota y Arica. *In* Las poblaciones humanas del altiplane Chileno: Aspectos geneticos, reproductivos y socioculturales. Santiago: UNESCO.

Rotta, A., A. Cánepa, A. Hurtado, T. Velásquez, and R. Chavez (1956). Pulmonary circulation at sea level and high altitudes. *J Clin Invest* 9:328–36.

Roughton, F. J. W., and R. E. Forster (1957). Relative importance of diffusion and chemical reaction rates in determining rate of exchange of gases in the human lung with special reference to true diffusing capacity of pulmonary membrane and volume of blood in the lung capillaries. *J Appl Physiol* 11(2):290–302.

Ruiz, L., and D. Peñaloza (1970). Altitude and cardiovascular diseases. Progress report to the World Health Organization.

Ruiz, L., M. Figueroa, C. Horna, and D. Peñaloza (1968). Systemic blood pressure in high altitude residents. Progress report to the World Health Organization.

Ruiz, L., M. Figueroa, C. Horna, and D. Peñaloza (1969). Prevalencia de la hipertensión arterial y cardiopatía isquémica en las grandes alturas. *Arch Inst Cardiol Méx* 39:474–89.

Rushmer, R. F. (1959). Constancy of stroke volume in ventricular responses to exertion. *Am J Cardiol* 196:745.

Saldaña, M. J., L. E. Salem, and R. Travezan (1973). High altitude hypoxia and chemodectomas. *Human pathol* 4:251.

Saltin, B., and P. Åstrand (1967). Maximal oxygen uptake in athletes. *J Appl Physiol* 23:353–58.

Samaja, M., A. Veicsteinas, and P. Cerretelli (1979). Oxygen affinity of blood in altitude Sherpas. *J Appl Physiol* 47(2):337–41.

Samaja, M., and R. M. Winslow (1979). The separate effects of H⁺ and 2,3-DPG on the oxygen equilibrium curve of human blood. *Br J Haem* 41:373–81.

Sánchez, C., C. Merino, and M. Figallo (1970). Simultaneous measurement of plasma volume and red cell mass in polycythemia of high altitude. *J Appl Physiol* 28(6):775–78.

Santolaya, B. R. (1983). *El norte grande de Chile: Asenatmientos humanos y desarrollo de ecosistemas d'ridos.* Santiago: Facultdad de Arquitectura y Urba.

Santolaya B. R., J. Araya C., A. Vecchiola C., R. Prieto P., R. M. Ramirez, and R. Alcayaga A. (1981). Hematocrito, hemoglobina y presión de oxígeno arterial en 270 hombres y 266 mujeres sanas y residentes de altura (2,800 m). *Rev Med Hosp Roy H. Glover* 1:17–29.

Scherf, D., and C. Bornemann (1968). The electrocardiogram after acute hemorrhage. *Dis Chest* 53:99–100.

Schmidt-Nielsen, K., and J. L. Larimer (1958). Oxygen dissociation curves of mammalian blood in relation to body size. *Am J Cardiol* 195:424–28.

Schoene, R. B., S. Lahiri, P. H. Hackett, R. M. Peters, J. S. Milledge, C. J. Pizzo, F. H. Sarnquist, S. J. Boyer, D. J. Graber, K. H. Maret, and J. B. West. (1984). Relationship of hypoxic ventilatory response to exercise performance on Mount Everest. *J Appl Physiol* 56(6):1478–88.

Scott, H. W., and S. R. Elliott (1950). Renal hemodynamics in congenital heart disease. *Bull Johns Hopkins Hosp* 86:58–71.

Severinghaus, J. W., and A. B. Carcelén (1964). Cerebrospinal fluid in man native to high altitude. *J Appl Physiol* 19(2):319–21.

Severinghaus, J. W., C. R. Bainton, and A. Carcelén (1966). Respiratory insensitivity to hypoxia in chronically hypoxic man. *Resp Physiol* 1:308–34.

Severinghaus, J. W., H. Chiodi, E. I. Eger, B. Brandstater, and T. F. Hornbein (1966). Cerebral blood flow in man at high altitude. *Circ Res* 19:274–82.

Severinghaus, J. W., M. Stupfel, and A. F. Bradley (1956). Variations of serum carbonic acid pK′ with pH and temperature. *J Appl Physiol* 9:197–200.

Sherwood, J. B., and E. Goldwasser (1979). A radioimmunoassay for erythropoietin. *Blood* 54(4):885–93.

Sime, F. (1973). *Ventilación humana en hipoxia crónica etiopatogenia de la enfermadad de Monge o desadaptación crónica a la altura.* Ph.D. thesis. Instituto de Investigaciónes de la Altura. Lima: Cayetano Heredia Univ.

Sime, F., C. Monge C., and J. Whittembury (1975). Age as a cause of chronic mountain sickness (Monge's disease). *Int J Biometr* 19(2):93–98.

Singer, R. B., and A. B. Hastings (1948). An improved clinical method for the estimation of disturbances of the acid-base balance of human blood. *Medicine* 27:223–42.

Sirotzky, L. (1974). *Eliminaciqurinaria de proteinas en el nativo de altura.* M.D. thesis. Lima: Cayetano Heredia Univ.

Sjöstrand, T. (1953). Volume and distribution of blood and their significance in regulating the circulation. Part I. Variations in blood volume. *Physiol Rev* 33:202–28.

Smith, H. W. (1951). *The kidney: Structure and function in health and disease*. New York: Oxford Univ. Press.

Snyder, G. K., E. E. Wilcox, and E. W. Burnham (1985). Effects of hypoxia on muscle capillarity in rats. *Resp Physiol* 62(1):135–40.

Sørensen, S. C., and J. W. Severinghaus (1968a). Respiratory sensitivity to acute hypoxia in man born at sea level living at high altitude. *J Appl Physiol* 25(1): 211–16.

Sørensen, S. C., and J. W. Severinghaus (1968b). Irreversible respiratory insensitivity to acute hypoxia in man born at high altitude. *J Appl Physiol* 25(3): 217–20.

Sørensen, S. C., N. A. Lassen, J. W. Severinghaus, J. Coudert, and M. P. Zamora (1974). Cerebral glucose metabolism and cerebral blood flow in high-altitude residents. *J Appl Physiol* 37:305–10.

Starling, E. H. (1918). *The Linacre lecture on the law of the heart*. London: Longmans, Green.

Stenberg, J., B. Ekblom, and R. Messin (1966). Hemodynamic response to work at simulated altitude, 4,000 m. *J Appl Physiol* 21(5):1589–94.

Stewart, H. J., C. H. Wheeler, and N. F. Crane (1941). Circulatory adjustments in polycythemia vera. *Am Heart J* 21:511.

Stradling, J. R., and D. J. Lane (1980). Polycythemia vera and central sleep apnea. (Letter). *Br Med J* 280:404.

Strohl, K. P., and J. M. Fouke (1983). Periodic breathing at altitude. *Sem Resp Med* 5(2):169–74.

Swanson, G. D. (1980). Breath-to-breath considerations for gas exchange kinetics. *In* P. Cerretelli and B. Whipp (eds.): *Exercise Bioenergetics and Gas Exchange*. Amsterdam: Elsevier/North Holland, pp. 211–22.

Talbott, J. H., and D. B. Dill (1936). Clinical observations at high altitude: Observations on six healthy persons living at 17,500 feet and a report of one case of chronic mountain sickness. *Am J Med Sci* 192:626–29.

Tenney, S. M. (1974). A theoretical analysis of the relationships between venous blood mean tissue oxygen pressures. *Resp Physiol* 20:238–96.

Tenney, S. M., and L. C. Ou (1970). Physiological evidence for increased tissue capillarity in rats acclimatized to high altitude. *Resp Physiol* 8:137–50.

Theilen, E. O., M. H. Paul, and D. E. Gregg (1954). A comparison of effects of intra-arterial and intravenous transfusion in hemorrhagic hypotensions on coronary blood flow, systemic blood pressure, and ventricular end diastolic pressure. *J Appl Physiol* 7(5):248–52.

Thomas, D. J., J. Marshall, R. W. Ross-Russell, G. Wetherley-Mein, G. H. Du-Boulay, T. C. Pearson, L. Symon, and E. Zilkha (1977a). Cerebral blood flow in polycythemia. *Lancet* (July 23):161–63.

Thomas, D. J., J. Marshall, R. W. Ross-Russell, G. Wetherley-Mein, G. H. Du-Boulay, T. C. Pearson, L. Symon, and E. Zilkha (1977b). Effect of haimatocrit on cerebral blood flow in man. *Lancet* (Nov. 5):941–43.

Thomas, L. J. (1972). Algorithms for selected blood acid-base and blood calculations. *J Appl Physiol* 33(1):154–58.

Thorling, E. B., and A. J. Erslev (1968). The tension of oxygen and its relation to hematocrit and erythropoiesis. *Blood* 31(3):332–43.

Tohgi, H., H. Yamanouchi, M. Murakami, and M. Kameyama (1978). Importance of the hematocrit as a risk factor in cerebral infarction. *Stroke* 9(4):369–74.

Torrance, J. D., C. Lenfant, J. Cruz, and E. Martecorena (1970–71). Oxygen transport mechanisms at high altitude. *Resp Physiol* 11:1–15.

Torres, C., R. Lozano, J. Whittembury, and C. Monge (1970). Effect of angiotensin on the kidney of the high altitude native. *Nephron* 7:489–98.

Townes, B. D., T. F. Hornbein, R. B. Schoene, F. H. Sarnquist, and I. Grant (1984). Human cerebral function at extreme altitude. *In High Altitude and Man*, ed. J. B. West, and S. Lahiri. Washington, D.C.: American Physiological Society.

Tramezzani, J. H., E. Monita, and S. R. Chiocchio (1971). The carotid body as a neuroendocrine organ involved in control of erythropoiesis. *Proc Nat Acad Sci* 68(1):52–55.

Traystman, R. J., R. S. Fitzgerald, and S. Loscutoff (1978). Cerebral circulatory responses to arterial hypoxia in normal and chemodenervated dogs. *Circ Res* 42:649–57.

Treger, A., D. B. Shaw, and R. F. Grover (1965). Secondary polycythemia in adolescents at high altitude. *J Lab Clin Med* 66:304–14.

Turek, A., and F. Kreuzer (1981). Effect of shifts of the O_2 dissociation curve upon alveolar-arterial O_2 gradients in computer models of the lung with ventilation-perfusion mismatching. *Resp Physiol* 45(2):133–40.

Turek, Z., and F. Kreuzer (1976). Effect of a shift of the oxygen dissociation curve on myocardial oxygenation at hypoxia. *In* J. Grote, D. Reneau, and G. Thews (eds.): *Oxygen transport to tissue*. Vol. 2. New York: Plenum Pub.

Turek, Z., N. Grandtner, and F. Kreuzer (1972). Cardiac hypertrophy, capillary and muscle fiber density, muscle fiber diameter, capillary radius and diffusion distance in the myocardium of growing rats adapted to a simulated altitude of 3,500 m. *Pflugers Arch* 335:19–28.

Turek, Z., F. Kreuzer, and L. J. C. Hoofd (1973). Advantage or disadvantage of a decrease of blood oxygen affinity for tissue oxygen supply at hypoxia: A theoretical study comparing man and rat. *Pflugers Arch* 342:185–97.

Turek, Z., F. Kreuzer, and M. B. E. Ringnalda (1978). Blood gases at several levels of oxygenation in rats with a left-shifted blood oxygen dissociation curve. *Pflugers Arch* 376:7–13.

Turek, Z., B. E. M. Ringnalda, M. Grandtner, and F. Kreuzer (1973). Myoglobin distribution in the heart of growing rats exposed to a simulated altitude of 3,500 m in their youth or born in the low barometric chamber. *Pflugers Arch* 340:1–10.

Turek, Z., B. E. M. Ringnalda, L. J. C. Hoofd, A. Frans, and F. Kreuzer (1972). Cardiac output, arterial and mixed venous blood saturation, and blood O_2 dissociation curve in growing rats adapted to a simulated altitude of 3,500 m. *Pflugers Arch* 335:10–18.

Turek, Z., B. E. M. Ringnalda, O. Moran, and F. Kreuzer (1980). Oxygen transport in guinea pigs native to high altitude (Junin, Peru, 4,105 m). *Pflugers Arch* 384:109–15.

Valdivia, E. (1956). *Mechanisms of natural acclimatization: Capillary studies at high altitudes*. Report 55-101 to the Air University, School of Aviation Medicine, USAF, Randolph AFB, Texas. P. 101.

Valdivia, E. (1959). Total capillary bed in striated muscle of guinea pigs native to the Peruvian Mountains. *Am J Physiol* 194:585–89.

Valentine, W. N., T. G. Hennessy, E. Lang, R. Longmire, R. McMillan, W. Odell, J. F. Ross, and J. L. Scott (1968). Polycythemia: Erythrocytosis and erythremia. *Ann Int Med* 69(3):587–606.

van Assendelft, O. (1984). Anemia and Polycythemia: Interpretation of laboratory tests and differential diagnosis. *In* J. A. Koepke (ed.): *Laboratory hematology.* New York: Churchill Livingstone, pp. 865–902.

Vanier, T., M. J. Dulfano, C. Wu, and J. F. Desforges (1963). Emphysema, hypoxia, and the polycythemic response. *N Eng J Med* 269:169–78.

VanSlyke, D. D., A. B. Hastings, A. Hiller, and J. Sendroy (1928). Studies of gas and electrolyte equilibria in blood, XIV: The amounts of alkali bound by serum albumin and globulin. *J Biol Chem* 79:769–80.

Váquez, H. (1892). Sur une forme speciale de cyanose s'accompagnant d'hyperglobulie excessive et persistante. *Compt Rend Soc Biol* (Paris) 44:384.

Vatner, S. F., and Braunwald, E. (1975). Cardiovascular control mechanisms in the conscious state. *N Engl J Med* 293(19):970–76.

Velásquez, T. (1956). *Maximal diffusing capacity of the lungs at high altitudes.* Report 56-108 to the Air University, School of Aviation Medicine, USAF, Randolph AFB, Texas.

Velásquez, T. (1972). Análisis de la Función Respiratoria en la Adaptación a la Altitud. Doctoral Thesis, Universidad Nacional Mayor de San Marcos, Lima.

Velásquez, T., C. Martinez, W. Pezzia, and N. Gallardo (1968). Ventilatory effects of oxygen in high altitude natives. *Resp Physiol* 5:211–20.

Viault, F. (1890). Sur l'augmentation considerable du nombre des globules rouges dans le sang chez les habitants des hautes plateaux de l'amerique du sud. *Compt Rend Soc Biol* (Paris) 30:917–18.

Wade, J. P. H., G. H. DuBoulay, J. Marshall, T. C. Pearson, R. W. Ross-Russell, T. A. Shirley, L. Symon, and G. Weatherly-Mein (1980). Cerebral blood flow, haematocrit, and viscosity in subjects with a high oxygen affinity variant. *Acta Neurol Scand* 61:210–15.

Wasserman, K. (1984). The anaerobic threshold measurement to evaluate exercise performance. *Am Rev Resp Dis* sup 129:s35–s40.

Wasserman, K., and J. B. Whipp (1975). State of the art: Exercise physiology in health and disease. *Am Rev Resp Dis* 112:219–49.

Wasserman, L. R., Dobson, R. L., and J. H. Lawrence (1949). Blood oxygen studies in patients with polycythemia and normal subjects. *J Clin Invest* 28:60–65.

Weil, J. V., E. Bryne-Quinn, I. E. Sodal, G. F. Filley, and R. F. Grover (1971). Acquired attenuation of chemoreceptor function in chronically hypoxic man at high altitude. *J Clin Invest* 50:186–95.

Weil, J. V., G. Jamieson, D. W. Brown, and R. F. Grover (1968). The red cell mass–arterial oxygen relationship in normal man. *J Clin Invest* 47:1627–39.

West, J. B. (1981). *High Altitude Physiology: Benchmark Papers in Human Physiology.* Stroudsburg, Pa.: Hutchinson Ross Pub.

West, J. B., and P. D. Wagner (1981). Predicted gas exchange on the summit of Mt. Everest. *Resp Physiol* 42:1–16.

West, J. B., P. H. Hackett, K. H. Maret, J. S. Milledge, R. M. Peters, C. J. Pizzo, and R. M. Winslow (1983). Pulmonary gas exchange on the summit of Mt. Everest. *J Appl Physiol* 55(3):678–87.

Whipp, B. J., and K. Wasserman (1972). Oxygen uptake kinetics for various intensities of constant-load work. *J Appl Physiol* 33(3):351–56.

Whittembury, J. (1983). Chronic intermittent hypoxia in mice: a high-altitude model. *In* Chamberlayne, E. D., and P. G. Condliffe (ed.): *Adjustment to high altitude.* U.S. Dept. of HHS. Bethesda, Md.: USPS, pp. 79–82.

Whittembury, J., and C. Monge C. (1972). High altitude, hematocrit, and age. *Nature* (London) 238:278–79.

Whittembury, J. R. Lozano, C. Torres, and C. Monge C. (1968). Blood viscosity in high altitude polycythemia. *Acta Physiol Latinoam* 18:355–59.

Willison, J. R., G. H. DuBoulay, E. A. Paul, R. W. Ross-Russell, D. G. Thomas, J. Marshall, T. C. Pearson, and L. Symon (1980). Effect of high haematocrit on alertness. *Lancet* 1:846–48.

Winslow, R. M. (1983). Bloodletting at high altitude. *Sem Resp Med* 5(2):188–94.

Winslow, R. M., and S. S. McKneally (1986). Analysis of breath-by-breath exercise data from field studies. *Int J Clin Monit and Comput* 2:167–90.

Winslow, R. M., C. Monge C., E. G. Brown, H. G. Klein, F. Sarnquist, and N. J. Winslow (1985). The effect of hemodilution on O_2 transport in high-altitude polycythemia. *J Appl Physiol* 59(5):1495–1502.

Winslow, R. M., C. Monge C., N. J. Winslow, C. G. Gibson, and J. Whittembury (1985). Normal whole blood Bohr effect in Peruvian natives of high altitude. *Resp Physiol* 61(2):197–208.

Winslow, R. M., C. Monge C., and H. G. Klein (1986). Red cell mass and plasma volume in Andean natives with excessive polycythemia. *Acta Physiol Latinoam:* in press.

Winslow, R. M., M. Samaja, and J. B. West (1984). Red cell function at extreme altitude on Mount Everest. *J Appl Physiol* 56(1):109–16.

Winslow, R. M., M. L. Swenberg, R. L. Berger, R. I. Shrager, M. Luzzana, M. Samaja, and L. Rossi-Bernardi (1977). Oxygen equilibrium curve of normal human blood and its evaluation by Adair's equation. *J Biol Chem* 252(7): 2331–37.

Winslow, R. M., J. M. Morrissey, R. L. Berger, P. D. Smith, and C. G. Gibson (1978). Variability of oxygen affinity or normal blood: An automated method of measurement. *J Appl Physiol* 45:289–97.

Winslow, R. M., N. Statham, C. Gibson, E. Dixon, O. Moran, and J. DeBrot (1979). Improved oxygen delivery after plebotomy in polycythemic natives of high altitude. *Blood* 54:61A.

Winslow, R. M., C. Monge C., N. J. Statham, C. G. Gibson, S. Charache, J. Whittembury, O. Moran, and R. L. Berger (1981). Variability of oxygen affinity of blood: Human subjects native to high altitude. *J Appl Physiol* 51:1411–16.

Winslow, R. M., M. Samaja, N. J. Winslow, L. Rossi-Bernardi, and R. I. Shrager (1983). Simulation of the continuous O_2 equilibrium curve over the physiologic range of pH, 2,3-diphosphoglycerate, and pCO_2. *J Appl Physiol* 54(2):524–29.

Wintrobe, M. M. (1981). *Clinical hematology.* Philadelphia: Lea and Febiger.

Woodson, R. D. (1984). Hemoglobin concentration and exercise capacity. *Am Rev Resp Dis* sup 129:s72–s75.

Wranne, B., R. D. Woodson, and J. C. Detter (1972). Bohr effect: interaction between H^+, CO_2, and 2,3-DPG in fresh and stored blood. *J Appl Physiol* 32(6):749–54.

Xu-Chu, H., G. Zheng-zhong, N. Xue-han, Z. Chang-fu, L. Hua-ying, F. Zhong-ming, C. Zheng-zheng, and P. Tie-chen (1981). The role of respiratory function in the pathogenesis of severe hypoxemia in chronic mountain sickness. *In* Proceedings of *Symposium on Quinghai-Xizang (Tibet) Plateau* (Beijing, China), vol. 2: *Environment and ecology.* Beijing: Science Press.

Yagil, R., U. A. Sod-Moriah, and N. Meyerstein (1974). Dehydration and camel blood. II. Shape, size, and concentration of red blood cells. *Am J Physiol* 226:301–4.

Zucali, J. R., M. Lee, and E. A. Mirand (1978). Carbon Dioxide effects on erythropoietin and erythropoiesis. *J Lab Clin Med* 92(4):648–55.

Index

Acclimatization
  definition, 1–2
  loss of, 10
Acid, renal excretion, 133
Acosta, Father, 5
Adair equation, 67
Adaptation
  genetic, 1–2, 20
  Himalayas vs. Andes, 167
Adaptive disease, 10–12
Age
  chronic mountain sickness, 111
  PaO$_2$, 109
Aldosterone, 123
Alpaca, 162
  blood viscosity, 170
Alveolar-arterial O$_2$ gradient, 103
American Medical Expedition to Everest
    (1981), 17, 93, 113
Ammonia, renal excretion of, 133
Anaerobic threshold, Andean natives, 148
Angiotensin, 123, 135
Animal models, 173
Arias-Stella, J., 14, 28
Artemia salina, erythropoiesis, 175
Aste-Salazar, H., 62
Atrial peptides, 124

Balke, B., 145
Banchero, N., 86, 169
Barbashova, Z., 170
Barcroft, J.
  acclimatization, 8
  blood oxygen affinity, 55
  Cerro de Pasco expedition, 8, 59
  description of miners, 142
  integrative physiology, 213
Bar-headed goose, 162
Barrel chest, 21, 23
Barron, E. S. G., 12, 62
Beall, C., 17
Berger, R., 67
Bernard, C., 6
Bert, P., 59
  high-altitude polycythemia, 6, 177
Bicarbonate, renal excretion, 133

Birds, O$_2$ affinity, 164–65
Blood-brain barrier, 105
Blood doping, 31
Bloodletting, 177–202
Blood volume, lung, 90, 103
Body composition, 20–21
Bohr effect, 58
  high-altitude natives, 70–71
Brain hematocrit, 173–74
Breath-holding time, 109
Brisket disease, 28, 79, 172

Camelids, 162, 170, 171
Capillaries, skeletal muscle, 95
Capillary proliferation, 52–53, 79
Cardiac output
  acute hypoxia, 78
  control of, 76, 84
  and exercise, 151–52
  and hemodilution, 196
  and high-altitude natives, 85
  measurement of, 84
Carotid bodies, 30
Castle, W., 76
Cerebrospinal fluid, 105
Cerretelli, P., 153
Chemodectoma, 30, 105
Chemoreceptors, 104, 105
Chest. *See* Morphometry
Chickens, chronic mountain sickness, 172
Chile, 12, 16
Chinchilla, 162
Chiodi, H., 17, 171
Chloride shift, 74
Chronic lung disease, red cell volume, 53–54
Chronic mountain sickness
  acid-base balance, 133
  age, 111
  animals, 168
  blood oxygen affinity, 74
  bone pain, 27
  carotid bodies, 30
  chext X ray, 23
  circulation time, 90
  classification, 28–29

Chronic mountain sickness (*contd.*)
  cor pulmonale, 79, 83
  definition, 1, 5, 203, 204
  ECG, 23
  electrocardiogram, 81
  etiology, 213–14
  exercise, 87
  first case, 9, 23–27
  gross pathology, 27
  Himalayas, 17, 205
  history, 203–4
  lung function, 104
  pathologic definition, 205
  physical examination, 21–23
  plasma volume, 53–54
  polycythemia vera, 27
  public health and, 215–16
  pulmonary histology, 29
  red cell volume, 49
  respiratory stimulants, 114–15
  Sherpas, 17, 205
  sleep, 114
  symptoms, 21
  ventilation, 114
Chuquicamata, Chile, 16
Circulation
  cerebral, 91
  coronary, 79
  and polycythemia, 75
  pulmonary, 89
  renal, 119, 124
  skeletal muscle, 94
Circulation time, 89
Cobo, B., 20
Coindet, L., 6
Concentrating capacity, urinary, 136
Coronary artery disease, 78
Cor pulmonale
  animals, 172–73
  humans, 79–81
Cosio, G., 37
Cow, O_2 affinity, 164
Creatinine clearance, 139
Critical altitude, 40

Desert, adaptation to, 171
Diffusion, facilitated, 95–96
Dill, D. B., 12, 74, 110, 144
Diving mammals, O_2 affinity, 164

Ectotherms, O_2 affinity, 165
Electrocardiogram, 23, 81
Erythropoiesis
  at high altitudes, 44
  inhibitor of, 45
  nutrition, 41
Erythropoietin
  assay, 43
  extrarenal, 42
  normal production, 42–43
Exercise
  acid-base balance, 153
  athletes at altitude, 146
  blood gases, 186
  cardiac output, 87, 151–52, 156
  economy, 159–60
  hemodilution, 182
  high-altitude natives, 142–43
  lactic acid, 153, 186
  Leadville, Colorado, 156
  oxygen affinity, 153
  oxygen pulse, 151
  polycythemia, 158
  protocols, 143
  Sherpa, 157
  ventilation, 147–51

Farheaus effect, 52
Faura, J., 44, 45
Fernan-Zegarra, 28
Ferritin, 41–42
Fick equation
  cardiac output, 85
  diffusion, 102
Fick principle, 84
Filtration fraction, 124
Framingham study, 92–93
FRC (functional residual capacity), 189–90

Garruto, R., 19
GFR (glomerular filtration rate), 122, 128–29
Gilbert, D., 17–18
Goat, red blood cells, 170
Golden mantle ground squirrel, 167
Gonzales, E., 129
Gray squirrel, O_2 affinity, 164
Grover, R., 15–16
Guinea pig, O_2 affinity, 164
Guyton, A., 75

Haldane effect, 58
Hall, F., 62, 162
Heart rate
  exercise, 88
  hemodilution, 184
  maximal, 151
  phlebotomy, 184
Heath, D., 13, 29
Hematocrit
  age effects, 33–34
  body vs. capillary, 50–54
  brain, 173–74
  geographic effects, 34
  high-altitude natives, 33
  normal variation, 33
  optimal, 31, 90, 170
Hemodilution, 49, 177
  blood viscosity, 180
  cardiac output, 196
  electrocardiogram, 82–83, 189
  exercise, 182
  gas exchange, 189
  hemodynamics, 189
  stroke volume, 197
  2,3-DPG, 181
  ventilation-perfusion ratio, 195–96, 198
Hemoglobin
  Bohr effect, 58
  CO_2 effect, 58
  cooperativity, 57
  function, 35, 58
  Haldane effect, 58
  Hill plot, 64
  measurement, 34–35
  mutant, 43, 66–67
  normal values, 31–32
  oxygen affinity, 43, 55
  structure, 57
  See also Hematocrit
Henderson-Hasselbalch formula, 61
Hill, A. V., 55
Hill equation, 62
Himalayas, 17
Hurtado, A., 13–14, 144
Hypertension
  pulmonary, 172
  systemic, 78
Hypoventilation, primary, 29
Hypoxia, psychomotor function, 93
Hypoxic ventilatory drive, measurement,
  106

Inca Empire, 19–20
Infant mortality, 118
Infertility, 20
Institute of Andean Biology, 12
Integrative physiology, 213
Iron, 41–42, 44–45

Jandl, J., 76
Jauja, Peru, 20
Jourdanet, D., 6

Keys, A., 12, 62
Kidney, erythropoietin production, 42
Kollias, J., 146
Kryger, M., 16, 114–15

Lactic acid, exercise, 153, 186
Leadville, Colorado, 15–16, 156
Llama, 162
Lung capacities, 99–101

Mayorga, J., 7
Merino, C., 14, 44–45
Microcytosis, 170
Mitochondria, 96
Monge C., C., 12
Monge M., C.
  controversy with Barcroft, 10
  early contributions, 9
  loss of acclimatization, 1–2
Monge's disease
  classification, 29
  eponym, 11, 12–13
Monge's syndrome, classification, 28
Morphometry, body, 20
Morpurgo, G., 71
Muscle, myoglobin, 95–96
Myoglobin, 95–96, 200

National Institutes of Health, 67
Nepal, 34–36

Optimal hematocrit, 90
Osmotic clearance, renal, 136
Osmotic fragility, red cells, 39, 170
Oxygen
  debt, 200
  delivery, renal, 47–48
  equilibrium curve, blood, 55
  pulse, exercise, 151
  reservoir, 200

Oxygen (*contd.*)
  tissue, 170
  uptake, maximal, 143

P50
  exercise, 153
  in vivo, 63
  PAH clearance, 122
Pekin duck, 162
Peñaloza, D., 15, 78
Periodic breathing, 111–12
pH
  effect of polycythemia, 69
  red cell, 60–62
Phlebotomy, 177, 179
Phosphofructokinase, 64
Pigeons, pulmonary hypertension, 173
Plasma volume, 48–54
Pollution, air, 36
Polycythemia, 23
  animals, 168
  blood pressure, 77
  circulation, 75
  coagulation, 177
  compensatory mechanism, 8
  cor pulmonale, 179
  exercise, 158
  gas exchange, 178
  kidney model, 141
  pulmonary function, 178
  red cell volume, 53–54, 188
  renal circulation, 125–26
  renal function, 129–32
  sojourners, 116
  ventilation, 113–14
  vital capacity, 188
Polycythemia vera, O_2 transport, 178
Porpoise, O_2 affinity, 164
Preadaptation, 171
Pregnancy, high-altitude natives, 118
Proteinuria, 138
Protoporphyrin, free erythrocyte, 41–42
Pugh, L., 142
$P\bar{v}O_2$, animals, 168

Quechua, gene pool, 19

Rahn, H., 168
Red cell
  animals, 170
  camel, 171

  morphology, 39
  osmotic fragility, 170
  oxygenation rate, 170
  pH, 60–62
  volume, 48–54
Renal blood flow, 121
  anemia, 47
  congenital heart disease, 46–47
  polycythemia, 46
  viscosity effects, 46
Renal circulation, 119
Renal excretion
  acid, 133
  ammonia, 133–34
  bicarbonate, 133
Renal oxygenation, 138
Renal plasma flow, 122
Renal tubular transport, 122
Renin, 123
Reynafarje, C., 14, 45
Roger, G. H., 11
Rossi-Bernardi, L., 67
Roughton, F., 59
Ruiz, L., 78

Saldaña, M. J., 14
Samaja, M., 64, 71
Sánchez, C., 14, 51, 53
Santolaya, R., 16
Schmidt-Nielsen, K., 163
Schoene, R., 159–60
Severinghaus, J., 14, 69, 109
Sheep, red cells, 170
Sherpa
  blood oxygen affinity, 71
  chronic mountain sickness, 17
  exercise, 157
  hematocrit, 162
  vital capacity, 101
Silicosis, 36
Sime, F., 14
Sleep, ventilation, 94–95, 111–12
Sodium reabsorption, 135
Soroche, 5
Starling, E., 84
Subacute mountain sickness, 117

Talbott, S. H., 12
Tibetans, ventilation, 116–17
Toads, high-altitude, 165
Tolentino, Saint Nicholas, 20

Transfusion, autologous, 31
2,3-DPG
  animals, 164
  discovery, 64
  hemodilution, 181
  physiological effects, 64
  regulation, 202

Váquez's disease, 9, 23
Velásquez, T., 13–14
Venous PO_2, renal, 138
Venous return, cardiac, 76
Ventilation
  age, 33–34, 109
  blunted, 97
  control, 104
  CO_2 drive, 106
  development, 107
  exercise, 107, 147, 184–85
  genetic control, 104
  high-altitude natives, 108
  hypoxic drive, 106
  pregnancy, 118

sleep, 94–95, 111–12
threshold, 184–85
Ventilation-perfusion ratio, 103, 195–96, 198
Ventilatory drive, 30
Ventricular hypertrophy, 30
Viault, F., 6
Vicuña, 162
Viscosity
  blood, animal, 170
  hemodilution, 180
Vital capacity
  Andean, 101
  comparative studies, 101–2
  Sherpa, 101

Water reabsorption, tubular, 136
Weil, J., 16
Whittembury, J., 15, 69
Winslow, R., 5, 15

Yellow-bellied marmot, 167

**Hypoxia, Polycythemia, and Chronic
Mountain Sickness**

Designed by Chris L. Smith.
Composed by the Composing Room of
Michigan, Inc., in Times Roman text and
display. Printed by the Maple Press
Company on 50-lb. Glatfelter Smooth
Antique and bound in Joanna's Arrestox A
(navy) and stamped in gold.